D0538357

MASTERING Documentation

SECOND EDITION

MASTERING Documentation

SECOND EDITION

Springhouse Corporation
Springhouse, Pennsylvania

Staff

Vice President
Matthew Cahill

Art Director
John Hubbard

Managing Editor
H. Nancy Holmes

Clinical Director
Judith A. Schilling McCann, RN, MSN

Clinical Editors
Carla M. Roy, RN, BSN, CCRN (project manager); Joanne Bartelmo, RN, MSN, CCRN; Jill Curry, RN, BSN, CCRN; Beverly Tscheschlog, RN; Tracy L. Yeomans, RN, BSN, CCRN

Editors
Doris Weinstock (project manager), Peter H. Johnson

Copy Editors
Brenna H. Mayer (manager), Priscilla DeWitt, Barbara Long, Pamela Wingrod

Designers
Arlene Putterman (associate art director), Debra Moloshok (book designer), Linda Franklin (project manager), Donna S. Morris

Typographers
Diane Paluba (manager), Joyce Rossi Biletz, Valerie Molettiere

Manufacturing
Deborah Meiris (director), Patricia K. Dorshaw (manager), Otto Mezei (book production manager)

Editorial Assistants
Beverly Lane, Marcia Mills, Liz Schaeffer

Indexer
Barbara Hodgson

The clinical procedures described and recommended in this publication are based on research and consultation with nursing, medical, and legal authorities. To the best of our knowledge, these procedures reflect currently accepted practice; nevertheless, they cannot be considered absolute and universal recommendations. For individual application, all recommendations must be considered in light of the patient's clinical condition and, before administration of new or infrequently used drugs, in light of the latest package-insert information. The authors and the publisher disclaim responsibility for any adverse effects resulting directly or indirectly from the suggested procedures, from any undetected errors, or from the reader's misunderstanding of the text.

Printed in the United States of America.

MD2-010199

A member of the Reed Elsevier plc group

Library of Congress Cataloging-in-Publication Data

Mastering documentation. — 2nd ed.
p. cm.
Includes bibliographical references and index.
1. Nursing records.
RT50.M38 1999
610.73—dc21
DNLM/DLC
for Library of Congress 98-42247
ISBN 0-87434-952-4 (alk. paper) CIP

Contents

Contributors

Marguerite S. Ambrose, RN, MSN, CCRN, CS
Assistant Professor
Allegheny University of the Health Sciences
Philadelphia

Karen T. Bruchak, RN, MSN, MBA
Assistant Administrator, Cancer Clinical Programs
University of Pennsylvania Cancer Center
Philadelphia

Gina Chapman, RN, MSN
Clinical Development Specialist
Allegheny University Hospitals, Bucks County
Warminster, Pa.

Nancy Cirone, RN,C, MSN, CDE
Director of Education, Bucks/Parkview
Allegheny University Hospitals, Bucks County
Warminster, Pa.

Denise Del Serra Detato, RN, MBA, MSN, CNA
Director of Patient Services
North Penn Visiting Nurse Association
Lansdale, Pa.

Ann Boyle Grant, RN, PhD
Dean of Instruction, Health and Sciences
Cuesta College
San Luis Obispo, Calif.

Ann Helm, RN, BSN, MS, JD
Nurse-Attorney
Associate Professor
Department of Preventive Medicine
Oregon Health Sciences University
Portland

Ellen J. Mangin, RN, MSN, CRNP, CS
Director of Resident Services
Rydal Park of Philadelphia Presbyterian Homes
Rydal, Pa.

Krystyna Matlack, RN, CPHQ, MMGT
Quality Analyst
Hospital of the University of Pennsylvania
Philadelphia

Carol M. Weir, RN, RGN
Product Manager
Thornberry Ltd.
Wyomissing, Pa.

Acknowledgments

The publisher and editors thank the following institutions for their help in preparing this book.

Doylestown Hospital
Doylestown, Pa.

Heritage Home Health
Meredith, N.H.

Our Lady of Lourdes Medical Center
Camden, N.J.

St. Mary's Manor
Lansdale, Pa.

Chestnut Hill Rehabilitation Hospital
Philadelphia

Allegheny University Hospitals
Philadelphia and Bucks County

Care Computer Systems, Inc.
Bellevue, Wash.

Foreword

Nurses often view documentation as a necessary chore, but one that is not as important as providing expert hands-on care. Many of us postpone documenting procedures, physical assessment findings, and patient outcomes until after everything else is completed. Think back to when you last charted. You'll probably recall that your documentation took place during the patient's afternoon nap, after morning care had been completed and just before visiting hours, or while the patient was having a respiratory therapy treatment.

Yet documentation is one of the most critical skills that nurses perform. Although we tend to approach documentation casually, our entire nursing career could depend upon the accuracy and completeness of our charting. How much should be charted? Where should the information be charted? These questions are crucial when documenting the patient's continuity of care as well as our expert nursing care. And they take on added urgency when the adequacy of patient care becomes the focus of a lawsuit.

One of the most difficult situations to document is patient care that a court of law might view as substandard or negligent. Imagine, for example, the following situation: A patient is admitted to your unit with acute respiratory failure and pneumonia. You arrive for your shift just as the admitting doctor is reviewing the patient's laboratory findings and latest chest X-rays. It is apparent to all that the patient's respiratory distress is not compatible with life and that he needs immediate endotracheal intubation and mechanical ventilation.

But the intubation is difficult and the doctor, after giving medications that paralyze the patient's respiratory muscles, has now twice intubated the esophagus. The patient is ashen, with blue mucous membranes, and the electrocardiogram is revealing a bradycardia of 24 beats per minute. The patient has no palpable blood pressure, and his pupils are fixed and dilated.

How do you begin to document in this type of situation? Do you resort to narrative charting, starting with the time that the medications were given, and fail to note any further times until the patient is pronounced dead by the doctor? Do you note when the Code Blue was called or merely that a Code Blue was initiated? Do you write down approximate times when various medical personnel arrived or when other procedures, such as the insertion of a central venous line, were initiated?

The second edition of *Mastering Documentation* is designed to assist you with these difficult questions. The book begins with a thorough discussion of the importance of nursing documentation in the context of the medical record. Chapter 2 reviews the legal and ethical implications of documentation, including the very types of issues that are implied in the patient scenario just mentioned. Chapter 3 explores the link between documentation and quality management and reimbursement, and chapter 4 reviews the different documentation systems (such as focus charting, the PIE format, and charting by exception) that are currently used in various health care settings.

To help you write your own notes, *Mastering Documentation,* Second Edition, devotes three chapters to documentation in specific nursing settings: acute care, long-term care, and home care. This is followed by a chapter on documenting the nursing process, which covers how standards of data collection are met and what to include in nursing notes about patient education. Chapter 9 gives practical examples of how to chart everyday events, such as patient falls, disruptive visitors, and family members who are unwilling or unable to adequately care for an elderly relative in the home setting.

The last two chapters of the book address the legal implications of documentation. Chapter 10 highlights charting practices that increase your potential legal liability. Chapter 11 discusses malpractice lawsuits, including your role during the pretrial collection of evidence, how to preserve the medical record, what to do if you need representation by an attorney, how to protect your assets, and how to defend yourself on the witness stand.

The final section of the book contains an extensive glossary of important terms as well as seven useful appendices. These appendices present the most current North American Nursing Diagnosis Association (NANDA) taxonomy, the American Nurses Association Standards of Nursing Practice, the 1998 Nursing Care and Documentation Standards of the Joint Commission on Accreditation of Healthcare Organizations, and commonly accepted abbreviations and symbols. They also include a current listing of nursing organizations and documentation guidelines for common nursing diagnoses.

New in the second edition are completed samples of the widely used MDS 2.0 and Oasis-B forms as well as examples of official Medicare forms 485 and 486. Special logos throughout the text reinforce vital information that will assist you in your documentation. "Charting Guidelines" suggests ways to improve your documentation skills; "Better Charting" signals a completed form with handwritten notations; "Charting Timesaver" shows you how to save time documenting; "Using Computers" outlines effective use of computers in documentation; and "On Trial" provides information, including actual court cases, that will help you avoid lawsuits and perilous charting.

As I reviewed and read the second edition of *Mastering Documentation,* I was amazed at the thoroughness of the text and the helpful reminders that will assist me the next time I document my nursing care. Even though I teach this topic, I learned many finer points that will make my documentation more accurate and legally defensible in the future. I thoroughly recommend this text to nurses new in the discipline as well as those more seasoned in a variety of nursing settings. I am sure that we all can learn many new and valuable skills from this second edition of *Mastering Documentation.*

Ginny W. Guido, RN, MSN, JD
Professor and Chair
Department of Nursing
Eastern New Mexico University
Portales

1

Nursing Documentation and the Medical Record

Broadly speaking, documentation refers to the preparation and maintenance of records that describe a patient's care. If you document with attention to detail, you'll clearly show the quality of care your patient received, the outcome of that care, and the treatment he still needs.

The detailed information you assemble will be scrutinized by many reviewers, including other health care team members; accrediting, certifying, and licensing organizations; quality improvement monitors; peer reviewers; and Medicare and insurance company reviewers. Your documentation may also be examined by attorneys and judges. And researchers and educators may use it to improve patient care and to provide continuing education.

This chapter spells out what you need to document satisfactorily for these reviewers and to enhance the quality of patient care. After summarizing the history of documentation, it describes the development of the medical record and covers the two basic types: source-oriented and problem-oriented. Next, the chapter reviews the principles of sound documentation, including using computers to promote efficiency. It then discusses current nursing documentation requirements, policies, and trends.

Overview of documentation

Traditionally, nurses recorded their *observations* of patients, creating documents only under the direction of doctors. The chief purposes of these documents was to demonstrate that doctors' orders had been followed, that the facility's policies had been observed, and that all requisite care had been provided. Charting began as a checklist of cursory observations, such as whether the patient "ate well" or "slept well." Beyond such simple notations, nurses were reluctant to record their own ideas.

Florence Nightingale, the 19th-century British nurse, is customarily regarded as the founder of nursing documentation. In *Notes on Nursing,* she stressed the importance of gathering patient information in a clear, concise, organized manner. As her theories gained acceptance, nurses began to be trained in her concept of lucid, formal nursing documentation. Gradually, nurses' perceptions and observations about patient care gained credence and respect.

Much later, in the 1970s, nurses began creating their own vocabulary for documentation based on *nursing diagnoses.* This was the first attempt to answer the increasingly urgent call for standards based on nursing data and nursing interventions. However, nursing diagnoses have thus far failed to gain acceptance as the basis for independent reimbursement. Insurance companies and Medicare do not reimburse for nursing services rendered under a nursing diagnosis.

The current reimbursement trend is to compensate nurses, especially nurse practitioners and home health care nurses, for skilled care that meets eligibility requirements. This care includes assessing a patient's condition, creating a plan of care, and following a strict treatment regimen.

More than ever before, nursing documentation plays a vital role in ensuring reimbursement by verifying — and justifying — a nurse's actions.

Understanding the medical record

Typically, a patient's medical record contains many forms, including the initial assessment and demographic forms, daily assessment flow sheets, problem or nursing diagnosis lists, plan of care or clinical pathways, and other flow sheets. Forms vary according to the individual facility's policies and procedures and in response to a welter of organizational, regulatory, and patient-related requirements. (See *What makes up the medical record?* pages 4 and 5.)

Because of the medical record's complexity, many nurses organize the data by category, placing undue focus on format over content. However, a medical record is more than a dry summary of a patient's illness and recovery. It's an incremental record of a patient's daily care and a road map of actual and potential patient care problems and appropriate interventions. In addition to being well organized, the record should also be easy to read and accessible to all members of the health care team and, ultimately, the reviewers.

Many nurses approach the medical record with trepidation — needlessly. Think of the medical record as an ally, not an enemy. It serves as a focus for organizing your thoughts about patient care and recording your actions. Used properly, it can help you identify problem areas, plan better patient care, and evaluate the care given.

Nursing documentation makes up one critical part of the complete medical record, which contains contributions from all health care team members. Your contribution has many purposes. It communicates your assessments and the care you gave, and it allows you, the nurse, to take credit for what you have observed and done. It also assists all caregivers in coordinating treatment, ensures reimbursement, and provides legal protection for you and your employer. (See *Guarding against liability,* page 6.)

Purpose of the medical record

The medical record provides evidence of the quality of patient care. It is used by various groups to help evaluate and enhance patient care.

Evidence of the quality of care

To verify the quality of your care, you must describe what you've done for your patient and provide evidence that it was necessary. You also should describe your patient's response to the care and any changes made in his plan of care. And you must be sure to document this information in accordance with professional practice standards — those published by the American Nurses Association (ANA) and the Joint Commission on Accreditation of Healthcare Organizations (JCAHO), for instance.

Another organization, the National Committee for Quality Assurance (NCQA), is the newest credentialing body. The NCQA performs several functions, including accreditation of managed care plans and certification of quality assurance specialists, either through the national office or through state affiliates. Although the NCQA does not mandate a specific method of quality evaluation, it does reinforce the importance of using JCAHO, Medicare, and other standards to evaluate and improve patient care in all health care settings.

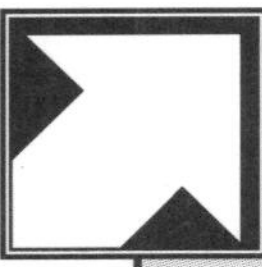

CHARTING GUIDELINES

What makes up the medical record?

Each health care facility has its own medical record-keeping system, typically composed of the documents listed below. Depending on the patient's needs, the medical record may include some or all of these items.

Face sheet

The first page of the medical record, this form includes information identifying the patient by name, birth date, social security number, address, and marital status. It also lists his closest relative or guardian, food or drug allergies, admitting diagnosis, assigned diagnosis-related group, and the attending doctor.

Medical history and physical examination

Completed by the doctor, this form contains the patient's initial medical examination and evaluation data.

Initial nursing assessment form

This document contains nursing data, including the patient's health history, physical and psychosocial assessments, baseline functional status, demographics, and pertinent social environment information.

Doctor's order sheet

This is the record of the doctor's medical orders.

Problem or nursing diagnosis list

Known as a problem list or a nursing diagnosis list in health care facilities that follow the problem-oriented medical record system, this record lists the patient's problems. Some health care facilities list nursing diagnoses on a separate form.

Nursing plan of care

This is a statement of the nurse's plan of patient care. Usually included with the basic medical record forms, it's sometimes kept in a separate folder at the nurses' station until the patient's discharge.

Graphic sheet

Known by various titles assigned by the health care facility, this form is a type of flow sheet that tracks the patient's temperature, pulse rate, respiratory rate, blood pressure and, possibly, daily weight. Additional graphic sheets may be designed for recording such information as skin care, blood glucose levels, urinalysis results, neurologic assessment data, and patient intake and output. These forms allow the nurse to show that a certain task or assessment was completed by simply dating, initialing, or checking off the appropriate column.

Medication administration record

This document contains a record of each medication a patient receives, including the dosage, administration route, site, date, and time.

Accreditation, certification, and licensure

Organizations, most notably the JCAHO, accredit health care facilities that meet their standards. (Some states also require all health care facilities — including home health care facilities — to become licensed.) Health care facilities need JCAHO accreditation not only to demonstrate that they provide quality care, but also to ensure their eligibility for government funds. The federal government also contracts with state organizations that certify health care facilities as being eligible to receive Medicare reimbursement.

Nurses' progress notes
This record details patient care information, nursing interventions, and the patient's responses.

Doctors' progress notes
Like the nurses' progress notes, this record contains the doctor's observations and notes on the patient's progress. It includes treatment data as well.

Diagnostic findings
These forms contain diagnostic and laboratory data — for example, hematology, pathology, and radiology test results.

Health care team records
This part of the medical record includes information from other professional personnel, such as physical therapists, respiratory therapists, and social workers.

Consultation sheets
These forms include evaluations made by doctors, clinical specialists, and others consulted for diagnostic and treatment recommendations.

Discharge plan and summary
This document presents a brief account of the patient's time in the health care facility and plans for care after discharge. Pertinent data may include dietary and medication instructions and follow-up medical appointments or referrals.

In deciding whether a facility should receive accreditation, an accrediting organization looks at the structure and function of the facility and reviews medical records to ensure that the facility meets the required standards. Then, at regular intervals, the organization checks the facility for compliance. The accrediting organization conducts surveys to assess the standard and quality of care and audits the facility to ensure that it's complying with those standards.

Most accrediting organizations have some common standards for documentation. For example, most require that each patient's medical record contain an assessment, a plan of care, medical orders, progress notes, and a discharge summary. Several organizations even spell out what these components must contain. Then, the nurse-manager must establish and implement documentation guidelines that meet the accrediting organization's requirements. These guidelines should specify the format that must be used as well as the topics that must be covered in the documentation.

Quality management

Mandated by state and JCAHO regulations, quality management activities are designed, conducted, and analyzed by designated employees of the health care facility. The quality management committee traditionally included doctors, nurses, and administrative personnel but has since expanded to include pharmacists, physical therapists and, often, consumers (such as a patient, family member, or community representative).

This committee seeks, develops, monitors, and evaluates new ways to improve the quality of patient care. Committee members must choose well-defined, objective, readily measurable indicators and collect data systematically over time to measure how often a performance standard is being followed and how well it's working. They may need to develop new indicators or even new standards, or they may need to redesign old ones. They then use

Guarding against liability

Good documentation should offer legal protection to you, the patient's other caregivers, and the health care facility.

Admissible in court as a legal document, the medical record provides proof of the care received by the patient and the standards by which the care was provided. Medical records typically serve as evidence in disability, personal injury, and mental competence cases. They're also used in malpractice cases, and how and what you document — or don't document — can mean the difference between winning and losing a case, not only for you but also for your employer.

For the best legal protection, make sure that your documentation shows that you not only adhere to professional standards of nursing care but also follow your employer's policies and procedures — especially in high-risk situations.

statistical techniques to translate the data into useful information for assessment. Improvement actions are based on results of the measurement and evaluation process, and successful quality improvement depends on effective teamwork.

Quality management has been steadily changing since the mid-1980s because of a perception that improvement efforts were ineffective and not far-reaching enough, targeting only individuals and regulators. The trend has now shifted toward emphasizing clinical outcomes as a way to create meaningful improvement both clinically and financially. Regulatory agencies now mandate that facilities submit certain quality management indicators to them on a regular basis for review and to establish a continuous accreditation process. The need to manage costs has become everybody's responsibility. Through proper documentation, each member of the health care team is held accountable for the care given to the patient.

Peer review

Peer review organizations are mandated by federal law to evaluate the quality of care provided in health care facilities. These organizations consist of employees who are paid by the federal government. They evaluate a sample of a health care facility's medical records and compare their findings with established generic standards or *screens* — a list of basic conditions that a group of similar health care facilities should meet. The reviewers use these screens to determine whether the health care facility or particular caregivers provided appropriate care. (See *How PROs evaluate performance.*)

Reimbursement requirements

Documentation helps determine the amount of reimbursement a health care facility receives. The federal government, for instance, uses a prospective payment system based on diagnosis-related groups (DRGs) to determine its Medicare reimbursements, paying a fixed amount for a particular diagnosis.

For the health care facility to receive payment, the patient's medical record at discharge must contain the correct DRG codes and show that the patient received the proper care for his DRGs. Your documentation should support your nursing diagnoses and

How PROs evaluate performance

Your nursing documentation is vitally important to peer review organizations (PROs), which can fine or sanction a health care facility that fails to provide quality care. Using established screens, PROs scrutinize medical records to determine whether a health care facility or particular caregivers have provided appropriate patient care. The screens identify the following problem areas.

Necessary admission
Reviewers look at the medical record to determine whether a health care facility justifiably admitted a particular patient and whether the patient received appropriate treatment.

Nosocomial infection
If the reviewers find that a health care facility has an excessive rate of nosocomial infection, the reviewers must examine the medical records to determine the causes.

Medical stability
If the record shows that a patient has a pattern of elevated temperature after insertion of an indwelling catheter, reviewers may question whether health care personnel have maintained the patient's medical stability.

Unscheduled returns to surgery
Reviewers are alert for unscheduled surgery, such as repeat surgery for infection.

Discharge planning
Reviewers check whether the health care facility provides a formal discharge planning process, as evidenced by the forms that the facility uses.

Avoidable trauma and death
When a patient dies unexpectedly during or after surgery or after a return to the critical care unit within 24 hours of being transferred out of the unit, PROs must determine whether the health care facility could have prevented the death.
If they find that the facility or specific caregivers were negligent, they can discipline those at fault and suggest steps to minimize the recurrence of such incidents.

Medicare complaints
PROs review complaints made by Medicare patients about care received at health care facilities. If they find problems with the quality of care a patient received, they can impose fines or sanctions or deny reimbursement for care provided.

indicate that appropriate patient teaching and discharge planning were provided.

Faulty documentation can have a direct impact on the amount of reimbursement a facility receives. For example, a home health care agency can be denied payment retroactively for home care visits deemed unreasonable and unnecessary — a determination strongly influenced by documentation.

Numerous patients have been discharged from home health care plans because the payer would no longer agree to pay for improperly documented care. This has the added negative effect of denying patients the care they need. (For more information, see chapter 3, Quality Management and Reimbursement.)

Organization of the medical record

There are many methods of organizing the medical record. Each health care facility selects the method — or a variation of it — that best suits its needs and the current legal and regulatory requirements.

Source-oriented narrative record

The source-oriented method requires members of each discipline — the sources — to record information in a separate section of the medical record. This system has several disadvantages. The first is that segregating entries according to discipline discourages communication among personnel; the reader must consult various parts of the record to gain a complete picture of the patient's care. Another problem with this type of documentation is its lack of coordination. Information is disjointed, topics are seldom clearly identified, and data are difficult to retrieve.

Although the source-oriented narrative record met charting needs in the past, the demand for detailed documentation of every aspect of patient care has made this method cumbersome because of its lack of boundaries. In addition, the narrative method does not consistently indicate that prudent patient care was given according to facility and regulatory standards.

These drawbacks created the need for a better way to organize the medical record. Some of the alternative charting formats that have been developed are:

- SOAP (Subjective-Objective-Assessment Plan)
- PIE (Problem-Intervention-Evaluation)
- Focus. (For more information on these formats, see chapter 4, Documentation Systems.)

ADL (activities of daily living) flow sheets are often used along with the above charting methods.

There will always be a place for narrative documentation, especially in subjective evaluation charting. However, narrative entries should be concise and relevant to the topic; they should not duplicate material already written on a flow sheet or plan of care.

Problem-oriented medical record

The problem-oriented medical record consists of baseline data, a problem list, a plan of care for each problem, and progress notes. Baseline data, which are obtained from all departments involved in patient care, focus on the patient's present complaints and illness. They include the patient's social and emotional status, medical status, health history, initial assessment findings, and diagnostic test results.

A problem list is then distilled from this baseline data to construct a plan of care. The plan of care addresses each of the patient's problems; these problems are routinely updated both in the plan of care and in the part of the medical record known as progress notes.

Charting by exception

This type of record consists of baseline data, a problem-oriented plan of care, flow sheets, and progress notes. Baseline data include significant demographics, health history, and functional status. Initial and ongoing health and psychosocial assessments are documented only as exceptions to preprinted guidelines prepared for each body system.

The plan of care depends heavily on clearly written standards of routine nursing care throughout the facility and within a particular unit. Only deviations from these standards need to be documented in a narrative fashion. Evaluations of patient status and response to care can be easily documented on a well-designed flow sheet with a few concise narrative notes to clarify any deviations from the expected outcome.

Charting by exception (CBE) is being used successfully at many facilities. Its main drawback is that sometimes the standards are inaccessible to staff who are responsible for the charting and to those who review the information.

Other formats

Many health care facilities have adapted the source-oriented or problem-oriented method to better meet their documentation needs. In the home health care setting, for example, nurses have created many documentation forms — including the initial assessment form, problem list, day-visit sheet, and discharge summary — to better reflect the services and essential quality of care they provide. These forms were designed to meet the nurse's documentation needs while at the same time complying with state and federal laws and other regulations.

Elements of sound documentation

Sound documentation demonstrates a logical approach to problem solving. Nursing documentation typically begins with assessment data, which provide a baseline definition of the patient's health care needs or problems currently and throughout hospitalization. Next, nursing documentation provides evidence that patient care has been planned, and it continues by reflecting nursing interventions and the patient's response and progress.

Essentially, effective documentation is a systematic, accurate, well-written account of nursing practice. To produce sound documentation, you'll need to set aside time for completing charts and other forms. Try to schedule a regular time for charting so that your records are current and updated. You'll need to use proper forms to ensure accuracy and consistency.

Legible, accurate, and clearly written charts that demonstrate professionalism and diligence will withstand litigation, ensure reimbursement, and satisfy reviewer requirements of the medical record.

Besides learning and applying documentation fundamentals, mastering documentation skills may involve improving existing documentation habits, using more efficient methods, adopting new systems, and applying new technology to documentation.

Of course, your documentation requirements will differ depending on where you work — in a hospital, nursing home, home health care agency, or other community facility. For instance, perioperative, critical, and emergency care areas have specialized criteria and forms for documenting nursing care. And requirements may change depending on the patient population — for example, requirements in obstetric settings differ from those in geriatric settings.

Three Cs

Documentation is both demanding and complex, a professional challenge for novice and expert alike. When documenting, remember the three Cs of good charting — Clarity, Conciseness, and Consistency. Make sure that you use correct spelling and approved abbreviations and symbols, avoid altering notations, and write legibly and neatly. Include your signature along with the date and time of posting.

Documentation should demonstrate the nursing process — from assessment, nursing diagnosis, and planning care to nursing interventions and evaluation. It should also demonstrate attention to precharting plans (such as the plan of care, Kardex, or activity sheets). What's more, it must comply with standards established by accrediting and licensing organizations, state and federal agencies, insurance companies, and your health care facility.

Efficient methods

To ensure thoroughness and accuracy, you must adopt efficient documentation methods. Such methods may include tape-recorded dictation and transcription services; computerized documentation; and special charting forms, such as standardized flow sheets, checklists, admission forms, initial care plans, and progress notes.

These methods provide data about the intensity of nursing care provided and the patient's condition. They help you make precise entries and supply information that can be retrieved easily.

New systems and formats

Several effective documentation systems currently in use were developed to respond to the expanded purposes and functions of the medical record — a result of the changes within the health care delivery system and the technological advances in health care.

Because narrative charting takes considerable time but rarely provides a quantifiable measure of a patient's condition, most health care facilities have implemented more efficient documentation systems. Among them are SOAP charting, Focus charting, the CBE method, computerized charting, and others.

SOAP charting, a vital component of the problem-oriented medical record, organizes record keeping by Subjective, Objective, Assessment, and Planning data. A variation, SOAPIE charting, adds two more categories: Intervention and Evaluation. Focus charting provides a specific structure for progress notes.

The CBE method uses standards carefully set by the facility, which provide a "normal" assessment baseline for nurses and therapists to chart from. If a patient is assessed as being within normal limits according to the standard, "WNL" (within normal limits) is entered in the chart. Otherwise, whatever is charted reflects what's deemed as *not* normal, the exception.

Clinical pathways can successfully combine the recording of data, the Kardex, and the traditional plan of care. Careful development of the pathway and the forms reflecting its implementation is crucial to the success of this format.

Each of these documentation systems has advantages, disadvantages, and distinguishing features that may make it more or less suitable for a given situation. CBE, for example, is most appropriate for summarizing patient care, whereas Focus charting is better suited for reporting a patient's rapidly changing condition. (For detailed information on these systems, see chapter 4, Documentation Systems.)

Charting by computer

Today, computers play an increasing role in completing the medical record from admission through discharge. Nursing plans of care, progress notes, medication records, vital signs records, intake and output sheets, and patient acuity may be recorded on computers. Some hospitals have installed bedside workstations to allow quick entry of information and access to it. Other facilities even have individualized forms for each area of nursing practice and provide a computer form that allows the nurse to select the assessment finding for a given patient and add information as needed.

An effective computerized documentation system must have the capacity to:

- record and send data to the appropriate departments
- adapt easily to the health care facility's needs
- display highly selective information on command
- provide easy storage access and retrieval for all trained personnel while maintaining the highest standards of patient confidentiality.

Benefits

The benefits of computerized charting include improved legibility, fewer errors, decreased recording time and costs, improved communication among health care team members, and greater access to medical data for patient care, education, research, and quality improvement. In addition, quick access to laboratory test findings and procedure results decreases the fragmentation of patient care.

Charting by computer also establishes a database about each patient that can be referred to during any subsequent admissions. This computer-based patient record provides information to the health care team when a patient isn't able to answer questions and the family is unavailable for interview.

In addition, an ongoing computer record provides:

- complete and accurate patient data that are available at all times
- a history of previous admissions that would alert current caregivers to adverse patient conditions that they might not be aware of, such as allergies or adverse reactions to medications
- a lifelong record of a patient's health events, including the interventions and outcomes
- the ability to transmit records reliably across long distances while maintaining confidentiality, thus ensuring access to the records whenever and wherever the patient may be.

Computerized charting is an especially efficient communication tool in home health care because patient charts can be sent over a telephone line between a laptop computer and the agency. The nurse or therapist no longer needs to take the time to travel back to an office to get information, thus reducing both professional time and travel expenses. (See *Charting home care in the electronic era,* page 12.)

Nurses are also being consulted by software companies, who wish to design products that will fit their needs. In all likelihood, more hospitals and home care agencies will adopt computerized charting as computer hardware and software become less expensive and more accessible.

Technological advances

With the increasing use of computerized documentation in home health care, internet-

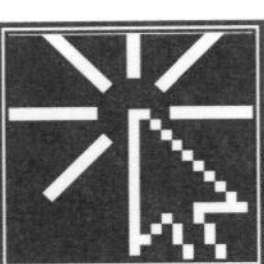

USING COMPUTERS

Charting home care in the electronic era

More and more home health care agencies are embracing computerized charting. Growing in popularity are computer notebooks and palmtops — portable devices combining hardware and software — that allow for documentation at the press of a finger.

Speeding reimbursement

In addition to handling the more routine aspects of documentation, computerized charting offers uniformity and thoroughness and ensures timely updates and speedy reimbursement.

Cutting paperwork

This technology also speeds and streamlines paperwork for the home care agency. In the past, completing certain charts and other paperwork was the sole responsibility of the office nurse-manager. She would review the field nurse's written information, apply it to accepted reimbursement tables and the health care agency's internal forms, and send the data to the appropriate office for processing.

Today, the properly equipped field nurse can obtain the appropriate data and complete the necessary forms during her health care visit by using a portable computer.

compatible computer products are not far off. Nurses will soon be able to chart in "real time" while out in the field.

Currently, information is downloaded from remote computers to the agency server at predetermined times, usually early in the morning, and throughout the day as needed. Internet and digital technology development will allow this exchange to be instantaneous. Because the data is recorded on computerized flow sheets, information is more accessible, with much of the vital data displayed on graphs for easy interpretation.

The fax machine is already in widespread use. Home health care agencies communicate with their nurses mainly by fax, and this efficient mode of communicating information will likely carry over into more areas of nursing.

Nursing informatics

In acknowledging the importance of computers in nursing, the ANA has recognized a field known as nursing informatics as an area of specialization. Nursing informatics aims to standardize documentation, improve communication, support decision making, develop and share new knowledge, and enhance the quality, effectiveness, and efficiency of health care, while advancing the science of nursing through the use of data, information, and knowledge.

Requirements of nursing documentation

State and professional organizations mandate certain documentation requirements. Some requirements are incorporated into laws, such as nurse practice acts, which vary from state to state. Other requirements — for example, evidence of accountability or a health care facility's documentation policies — are not mandated by law but are accepted under the general scope of nursing as practiced today.

Adherence to nurse practice acts

Nurse practice acts are state laws designating the specific activities that nurses can perform in that state. Cumulative changes in the regulations that govern nursing have led to substantial redefinitions or revisions of the acts in many states. Today, state regulations consider nurses to be managers of care as well as practitioners.

These and other revisions in state laws and regulations require that complete descriptions of nursing judgment and provision of care be documented in nurses' records as evidence that nurses have complied with standards.

Accountability

Proper nursing documentation provides evidence that the nurse has acted as required or ordered. She must demonstrate her accountability by complying with the documentation requirements established by the health care facility, professional organizations, and state law.

Policies affecting documentation

Health care facilities usually establish documentation policies that meet the requirements of insurance agencies and accrediting bodies. A facility's board of trustees typically appoints a committee to investigate various documentation systems and to make recommendations on adopting a particular format and style of documentation.

The health care facility may then decide to adopt a new system or modify an existing system to support its goals and preserve its accreditation and licenses.

Meeting requirements in special settings

In acute or critical care, long-term care, intermediate care, or home care environments, documentation requirements may be considerably more demanding. In such environments, be especially careful to review your facility's documentation policies and follow them accurately.

Acute or critical care

Documentation policies in acute or critical care settings generally require you to record assessment findings, nursing interventions, patient responses, and patient outcomes. Much of critical care unit documentation is entered on flow sheets accompanied by commentary and critical data, such as an electrocardiogram strip.

Long-term and intermediate care

These settings offer more time to document but documentation is highly regulated. State laws and Medicare's conditions of participation determine to a large extent what must be recorded. Some institutions choose the CBE documentation system for these settings.

Home care

Again, Medicare's conditions of participation strongly influence the documentation required. To increase efficiency and avoid licensing, accreditation, and reimbursement difficulties, most home health care agencies have abandoned narrative notes in favor of individualized visit sheets and physical discomfort forms.

Understanding length of stay and patient awareness

As the average patient's length of hospitalization continues to decline, documentation must include all exceptional problems and interventions. This becomes particularly important when reimbursing agents and insurance companies insist on evidence to justify a patient's extended stay in the health care facility.

Patient awareness also influences documentation. Patients today are increasingly aware of the nurse's role in documentation and of their own right to view the medical record. More and more patients may ask you for a copy of the medical record. Though the patient is entitled to this information, you should always consult your legal department for advice. The doctor should also be notified and should be present when the patient reviews the chart to answer any questions and explain terms. Keep in mind that the request to see the medical record may be preliminary to a lawsuit.

Understanding utilization review

Reimbursing agents maintain control over health care providers through utilization review programs that focus on length of hospital stay, treatment regimen, validation of diagnostic tests and procedures, and verification that medical supplies and equipment were used. To determine if utilization is proper, they commonly rely on nursing documentation.

Among specific data you may need to document (to comply with utilization review policy) are the types and quantity of I.V. access devices, infusion pumps, drains, tubes, and other equipment that you've used. Unfortunately, doctors don't usually record their use of supplies. Utilization review policies can also affect where treatment occurs — in the hospital, doctor's office, or patient's home, for example.

Current trends in documentation

Since the early 1990s, handwritten plans of care have been regarded as a thing of the past. The JCAHO no longer requires a formal plan of care, concluding that it doesn't necessarily affect patient outcomes. As a result, new documentation tools have arisen, including standardized plans of care, clinical pathways, and patient-outcome time lines.

Standardized plans of care

Today, standardized plans of care that correspond with a diagnosis-related group (DRG) or other guidelines are growing in use. The emphasis is on concise plans of care that reflect the patient's needs. Here, home health care nurses are on the cutting edge because Medicare's conditions of participation require that plans of care be tailored to specific patient needs.

Clinical pathways

The clinical pathway (also known as critical pathway, care map, or care track) is a blend of medical and nursing plans of care. It is a sequence of processes and events that move a patient toward an expected outcome. As a roadmap to care, it outlines such key elements as expected patient outcomes, essential medical and nursing interventions, and other patient variables for each DRG.

Doctors and nurses are responsible for establishing a clinical pathway for each DRG. The clinical pathway defines a patient's daily care requirements and desired outcomes that are consistent with the average length of stay for the specified DRG.

Clinical pathways are the patient care plan of the future. They ensure that patient care is consistent and carried out in an appropriate sequence. They also demonstrate quality and consistency of care to third-party payers, and enable the health care industry to prepare for the effects of prospective payment and managed care on reimbursement for services. They are especially useful when moving toward an automated system because they provide a structured approach in manageable categories.

Patient-outcome time lines

Another valuable documentation tool, the patient-outcome time line allows all practitioners to note essential diagnostic tests, interventions, patient outcomes, and other parameters to attain the average length of stay for each DRG.

For example, the patient-outcome time line for a patient who has had abdominal surgery might recommend that he be out of bed and into a chair the day after surgery and walking in the hallway 4 days after surgery. This plan will also list key interventions needed to achieve the expected outcomes and will be used to monitor the patient's progress during each shift.

Conclusion

Documentation will continue to change rapidly, which makes it all the more essential for you to understand and explore new approaches as documentation systems become more efficient and improve communication among health care personnel. New technology —and new ways of organizing your observations—should help you save time, eliminate confusion and, most important, improve patient care.

Selected references

American Nurses Association. *Nursing Quality Indicators: Definitions and Implications.* Washington, D.C.: American Nurses Publishing, 1996.

Barnette, J.E., and Clendenen, F. "Making the Transition to Critical Pathways—A Community Behavioral Health Center's Approach," *Best Practices and Benchmarking in Healthcare* 1(3):147-56, May-June 1996.

Boldreghini, S., et al. "Difference in Nursing Documentation Before and After Computerization: A Pilot Study," *Online Journal of Nursing Informatics* 2(1), Winter 1998.

Charting Made Incredibly Easy. Springhouse, Pa.: Springhouse Corp., 1998.

Chase, S.K. "Charting Critical Thinking: Nursing Judgments and Patient Outcomes," *Dimensions of Critical Care Nursing* 16(2):102-11, March-April 1997.

Joint Commission on Accreditation of Healthcare Organizations (JCAHO). *Comprehensive Accreditation Manual for Hospitals: The Official Handbook.* Oakbrook Terrace, Ill.: JCAHO, 1998.

Marrelli, T.M. *Nursing Documentation Handbook,* 2nd ed. St. Louis: Mosby–Year Book, Inc., 1996.

Moulton, P.J., et al. "Implementing Clinical Pathways: One Agency's Experience," *Home Healthcare Nurse* 15(5):343-54, May 1997.

Porrier, G. P., and Oberleitner, M.G. *Clinical Pathways in Nursing: A Guide to Managing Care from Hospital to Home.* Springhouse, Pa.: Springhouse Corp., 1999.

Windle, P.E., et al. "Documentation to Achieve Patient Outcomes Through Critical Pathways," in *Handbook of Nursing Case Management: Health Care Delivery in a World of Managed Care.* Edited by Flarey, D.L., et al. Gaithersburg, Md.: Aspen Pubs., Inc., 1996.

2

Legal and Ethical Implications of Documentation

Nurses are ethically and legally accountable to all of their patients. The scope of your professional responsibility is set out by your state's Nurse Practice Act and by other state and federal regulations. Documenting the nursing care provided in the patient's medical record is one way of accepting that responsibility and of being accountable to the patient and your profession. Your documentation demonstrates that the patient care you provide meets the needs of the patient at a specific point in time and meets the accepted standards of nursing practice mandated by law, your profession, and the health care facility in which you practice. It also assures the patient that every effort has been made to guarantee his well-being.

The purpose of the medical record is to communicate important clinical information to your patient's other caregivers. Documentation is a form of communication that is more important today than ever because of the increasing number and variety of providers who see the patient. If you deliver the appropriate standard of nursing care and chart that information in an acceptable and timely manner, you'll protect your patient's interests as well as your own. Failure to document appropriately has been a pivotal issue in many malpractice cases. The adage "If it isn't documented, it wasn't done" holds true in court.

Although the actual medical record, X-rays, laboratory reports, and other records belong to the institution, the *information* contained in them belongs to the patient, who has a right to obtain a copy of the materials. If a health care facility refuses to release a patient's records, the perceived reluctance may not bode well for the facility if the case comes to trial. In *Deford and Thompson v. Westwood Hills Health Care Center, Inc.*, Doctors Regional Medical Center and Barnes Hospital, St. Louis City, Missouri Circuit Court, Case No. 922-9564 (1992), a patient died after a nurse attempted to insert a feeding tube. Seven months later, when the family requested the patient's records, Westwood Hills staff mistakenly believed they were not authorized to release them and so refused. Copies of the records were finally released more than a year later. The case resulted in an $80,000 verdict against Westwood Hills on a wrongful death claim.

Knowing what your legal and ethical obligations are and scrupulously documenting to show that the care you provide meets these standards are keys to conveying information, meeting your patient's health care needs, and protecting yourself legally.

This chapter discusses the important legal and ethical issues involved when documenting your patient's condition and your nursing care. These include the legal relevance of the medical record, malpractice litigation, how policies and procedures affect legal decisions, risk management programs, quality assurance programs, and ethical considerations in patient care.

Legal relevance of medical records

Accurately and completely documenting the nature and quality of your nursing care helps the other members of the health care team confirm their impressions of the patient's condition and progress — or may signal the need for adjustments in the therapeutic regimen. This clinical account of a patient's condition, treatment, and responses is also used as evidence in the courtroom — for example, in malpractice suits, workers' compensation litigation, personal injury cases, and, possibly, criminal cases.

If you think of the medical record first and foremost as a clinical communication that you documented carefully, you needn't panic if the court subpoenas it. However, if you think only of legal implications or document to protect yourself, your part of the medical record will sound self-serving and defensive. Such documentation tends to have a negative impact on a judge and jury.

Standards of documentation

The type of nursing information that appears in a medical record isn't dictated by standards set by the courts. It's governed by standards developed over the years by the nursing profession and by state laws.

Documentation that meets these standards communicates the patient's status, medical treatment, and nursing care. Professional organizations such as the American Nurses Association (ANA) and regulatory agencies, such as the Joint Commission on Accreditation of Healthcare Organizations (JCAHO) and the Health Care Financing Administration, have established that documentation must include ongoing assessment, variations from the assessment, patient teaching, responses to therapy, and relevant statements made by the patient.

Although documentation goals have changed little since their inception, documentation methods have changed dramatically. For example, nurses no longer need to spend valuable time writing long narrative notes. Instead, many facilities today use such methods as flow sheets, graphic records, checklists, and charting by exception (in which only exceptions from articulated standards of care are charted). While flow sheets save valuable nursing time, they've been criticized as being too abbreviated and lacking important narrative information about the patient's condition. If used prudently, however, flow sheets can trigger or remind a nurse what actions are indicated.

Timely communication

The purpose of charting is communication, with an emphasis on timeliness. When the patient's condition deteriorates or changes in therapy are clearly indicated, you must not only chart this information, but also contact the doctor as soon as possible, and chart the fact that you contacted the doctor, the time the contact was made, and the doctor's response. If the doctor is not responding appropriately in your opinion, you must contact the next individual in the chain of command. Failure to do so is a breach of duty to the patient and leaves you vulnerable to a malpractice lawsuit.

There are numerous legal cases involving failure of the nurse to notify the doctor of changes in the patient's condition. When such notification is not documented, it is nearly impossible to prove that the doctor was called in a timely manner and that all critical information was communicated. These cases are often extremely serious, resulting in death or permanent disability.

In a California case, *Malovec v. Santa Monica Hospital,* Los Angeles County, California Superior Court, Case No. SC 019-167 (1994), a woman in labor repeatedly asked the charge nurse to call the Chief of Obstetrics because her obstetrician refused to perform a cesarean section despite guarded fetal heart tracings. The charge nurse refused and the baby was born with cerebral palsy and spastic quadriplegia. A confidential settlement was reached.

Errors or omissions

Errors or omissions can severely undermine your credibility in court. A jury could reasonably conclude that you didn't perform a function if it wasn't charted. If you failed to chart something and need to enter a late entry, date it the day you entered it.

In the case of *Anonymous v. Anonymous,* Suffolk Superior Court, Boston (1993), failure to chart led to a $1 million settlement. A 2-year-old was admitted to Children's Hospital for correction of a congenital urinary defect. Postoperative orders required blood pressure, pulse, and temperature to be taken every 4 hours, and respiratory rate and reaction to analgesia every hour. However, the child's care was not charted for 5 hours. The child was found in cardiorespiratory arrest and died from an overdose of a narcotic infusion. The responsible nurse admitted failing to assess the child strictly according to the orders; she also claimed that she had assessed the child adequately but had been "too busy" to chart her observations.

Failure to comply with a facility's policy can also constitute an omission. In *Wallace v. Sacred Heart Hospital,* Escambia County, Florida (1997), a nurse failed to apply Posey restraints to a patient who had a history of stroke and seizure disorder and was at high risk for falls. Early one morning, the patient was discovered trying to walk to the bathroom. A nurse found her and assisted her back to bed but neglected to apply restraints. An hour later the patient was found on the floor with a fractured left hip. The nurses involved failed to follow the hospital's policy for patients at high risk for falls and the doctor's order for restraints. A confidential settlement was reached during mediation.

Corrections and alterations

Any necessary corrections to the medical record should be made *only* by drawing a line through the initial charting, signing it, and dating it. Then you can proceed to supply the proper entry. *Never erase, obliterate, or otherwise alter a record.* Completely defensible malpractice cases have been lost because of chart alterations. The jury simply concluded the nurse was covering up something. Also, *never try to make the record "better" once you learn a malpractice case has been filed.* Attorneys have methods for analyzing papers and inks and can easily detect discrepancies.

Malpractice and documentation

Although you document first to serve your patient and to convey information, never lose sight of documentation's legal import. Depending on how well you administer care and record your activities and observations, the records may or may not support a plaintiff's accusation of nursing malpractice. Legally, malpractice focuses on these four elements: duty, breach of duty, causation, and damages.

Duty and breach of duty

The term *duty* refers to your obligation to provide patient care and to follow appropriate standards. The courts have ruled that a nurse has a duty to provide care once a nurse-patient relationship is established. The relationship may be established in person — at admission, for example — or at a distance — say, during a telephone conversation. (Even telephone calls must be carefully documented, especially with outpatient care and telephone triage on the rise.)

Breach of duty, a failure to fulfill your nursing obligations, can be difficult to prove because nursing responsibilities typically overlap those of doctors and other health care providers. A key question that is asked when a possible breach of duty is being investigated is "How would a reasonable, prudent nurse with comparable training and experience have acted in the same or similar circumstances?" In judging a nurse to have breached her duty, the courts must prove that the nurse failed to provide the appropriate care — as they did in the following case.

In *Collins v. Westlake Community Hospital,* 312 N.E. 2d 614 (Ill. 1974), a 6-year-old boy was hospitalized for a fractured leg, which was put in a cast and placed in traction. Although the doctor ordered the nurse on duty to monitor the condition of the boy's toes, the medical record lacked documentation that she did so. In fact, 7 hours elapsed between documented nursing entries in the medical record. The boy's leg was later amputated, and the parents sued on behalf of their son. Because a nurse is responsible for continually assessing patients and because documentation of these assessments didn't appear in the record, the nurse was found to have breached her duty to this child.

In another case, *Wickliffe v. Sunrise Hospital,* Clark County, Nevada District Court, Case No. 185939 (1988), a 13-year-old girl underwent Harrington rod surgery for scoliosis without complications. In the recovery room, she was found without pulse or respiration. Although she was resuscitated, she remained comatose and eventually died. The family accused the nurses of failing to check the girl's vital signs every 15 minutes as required by hospital policy. The authenticity of two pages of nursing notes was in dispute, with one page having entries of 11:20, 11:30, and 12:40 and another page covering from 11:50 to 12:40. The notes had different tab forms, were irregular in context, and were unlike other pages in the medical record. The jury concluded that the second page of notes was a later addition to the record and that a breach of duty had occurred when vital signs weren't recorded between 11:30 and 12:40. The jury awarded the family $1.75 million.

Causation

Once the plaintiff establishes a breach of duty, he must then prove that this breach caused the injury. Of the four malpractice elements, causation is the most difficult to prove. For the nurse to be liable, she must have *proximately caused* the injury by an act or an oversight. The principle of *proximity* is important because, in a typical health care facility, so many caregivers are involved in a patient's care. Even if a nurse did commit malpractice, it's conceivable that the patient's injury was caused by something other than the nursing intervention. For instance, even if a nurse gave a patient an overdose of a medication and the patient later vomited blood, the cause of the vomiting might actually be a surgical error and have nothing to do with the medication.

It's important to distinguish between bad outcomes and malpractice. A bad outcome is not malpractice *per se.* There are many inherent risks in health care, such as an adverse reaction to a blood transfusion received during surgery. If the medical record indicates that the blood was the correct type, that all policies and procedures were properly followed, and that the hospital policy set a reasonable standard, the patient has no cause for a claim — he simply had an unexpected reaction to the blood transfusion.

Some patients assume that a bad outcome is due to malpractice because they had unrealistic expectations or received an inadequate explanation of a condition or procedure. That's why careful communication before and during treatment is crucial. Many patients sue because the health care provider did not communicate with them enough and they are unhappy with the results of their care. Again, they won't be successful in suing for malpractice unless they can prove that the standard of care was not met. Nurses and other providers can help prevent some lawsuits simply by communicating well with their patients to establish realistic expectations of care.

Damages

To show malpractice, the patient's attorney must prove that injury occurred because of breach of duty and causation. It is not sufficient that the patient be disgruntled or dissatisfied; usually the injury must be physical, not just emotional or mental. If the patient has sustained a true physical injury, the attorney can then sue for damages. These damages represent the amount of money the court orders the defendant to pay to the plaintiff when a case is decided in the plaintiff's favor.

Policies and documentation

Although most discussions about documentation center on writing in the patient's chart, other types of documentation also affect nurses. One example is the documentation of policies and procedures contained in health care facility employee and nursing manuals. Deviation from these rules suggests that an employee failed to meet the facility's standards of care.

Whether such policies establish a standard of care has been debated in some malpractice cases. But in *every* nursing malpractice case, the actions of the nurse are compared with the appropriate nursing standard of care. The jury measures the nurse's actions or omissions against the performance of a reasonable, prudent nurse with comparable training and experience, using accepted, regularly updated national standards as guidelines. Keep in mind, however, that the defense can always challenge the presumption of the standard — by introducing expert testimony or by other methods.

In a case related to a health care facility's policies, the court was pressed to distinguish between a hospital's policies and "goals." In *H.C.A. Health Services v. National Bank,* 1745 S.W. 2d 120 (Ark. 1988), three nurses were working in a nursery composed of three connecting rooms. One nurse cared for a baby in the first (admissions) room. The other two nurses went into the second room, which housed 11 babies (two of whom were premature and one of whom was jaundiced). There was no documentation that for 1½ hours any of the nurses went into the third room, which had six babies. Documentation did show that when the first nurse finally entered the third room, she found that one of the infants had stopped breathing and had no heartbeat.

Both the hospital's executive director and the nurse who found the baby testified that, according to the hospital's manual, no infant is ever to be left alone without a member of the nursery staff present. However, they also testified that this was a goal — not a policy. Another doctor testified that the baby's problem would have been avoided if a nurse had been present. The court disagreed with the distinction between policies and goals and ruled against the hospital and nurses and in favor of the plaintiff.

Risk management and documentation

Sometimes, documentation reveals potential problems within a health care facility — for example, a particular procedure that repeatedly leads to patient injury or another type of accident. To reduce injuries and accidents, minimize financial loss, and meet the guidelines of the JCAHO and other regulatory agencies, health care facilities have instituted risk management programs. Based on similar programs first used in industry, risk management programs initially focused on maintaining and improving facilities and equipment and ensuring the safety of employees, visitors, and patients. Today, however, risk management (and quality management) efforts focus on identifying, evaluating, and reducing the risk of patient injury throughout the health care system.

The primary objectives of a risk management program are:

- to ensure optimal patient care
- to reduce the frequency of preventable injuries and accidents leading to liability claims by maintaining or improving quality of care
- to decrease the chance of a claim being filed by promptly identifying and following up on adverse events (incidents)
- to help control costs related to claims by identifying trouble spots early and intervening with the patient and his family.

Coordinating risk management and quality management

Rather than support two separate programs, many health care facilities now coordinate their risk management and quality management programs to ensure that they fulfill their legal duty to provide reasonable care. In doing so, the facility may also coordinate the programs' educational efforts — for example, in reaching out to a specific employee, such as a nurse or doctor, who's been identified as having a particular problem, or to a larger population, such as new residents and nurses.

The health care facility should place a high priority on teaching new residents and nurses about risk management and quality management. Required teaching topics for new employees include malpractice claims, staff members' particular reporting obligations, proper informational and reporting channels, and principles of risk management and quality management.

Keep in mind, however, that a coordinated system usually continues its dual focus on different aspects of health care delivery. Risk management focuses more on the patients' and families' perception of the care provided, whereas quality management (also known as quality improvement) focuses on the role and functions of the health care provider. (For more information on quality management programs, see chapter 3, Quality Management and Reimbursement.)

A reputation for safe, reliable, effective service is a health care facility's primary defense against liability claims. Systematic, well-coordinated risk management and quality management programs demonstrate to the public that the facility is managed in a legally responsible way. When complaints do arise, risk managers handle them promptly to contain the damage and minimize liability claims.

Identifying adverse events

A key part of a risk management program involves developing a system for identifying *adverse events*—events, such as patient falls, that would be considered an abnormal consequence of a patient's condition or treatment. These events may or may not be caused by a health care provider's breach of duty or the standard of care.

The most common "early-warning systems" for detecting adverse events are incident reporting and occurrence screening. These systems are crucial because they permit early investigation and intervention, thus helping to minimize additional adverse consequences and legal action. They also provide valuable databases for building strategies to prevent repeated incidents.

Incident reporting

In *incident reporting,* certain criteria are used to define events that must be reported by doctors, nurses, or other health care staff, either when they're observed or shortly after. Examples of such events include the unplanned return of a patient to the operating room and a medication error requiring intervention. *All errors must be reported* because it's impossible to predict which ones will require intervention.

Occurrence screening

In contrast, *occurrence screening* flags adverse events through a review of all or some of the medical charts. These reviews use generic criteria (such as a nosocomial infection, a fall, or an unexpected death). More specific reviews may focus on specialty- or service-specific criteria, such as an incorrect sponge count during surgery. Over the years, generic and focused criteria have been developed for reporting and screening systems, and a growing body of literature exists to compare the effectiveness of various approaches.

Although these early-warning systems pinpoint much useful information, they aren't effective without a strong organizational structure, the commitment of key staff (such as doctors, nurses, administrators, and chiefs of high-risk services, such as perinatal care) to analyze the information, and cooperation between risk management and quality management departments.

Other sources of information

In addition to incident reports and occurrence screening, nurses and patient representatives are a primary source of information for identifying adverse events as well as health care dangers or trends.

Nurses

Nurses are typically the first to recognize potential problems because they spend so much time with patients and their families. They can identify patients who are dissatisfied with their care, particularly those with complications that might result in injuries.

Patient representatives

Another information source is the patient representative's office, which keeps a file of patient concerns and complaints. By evaluating these concerns and complaints for trends, patient representatives can provide an early-warning signal of health care problems that need to be addressed, ranging from staffing to faulty equipment. They are also trained to recognize litigious patients, and they maintain communication with the patient and family after an incident has occurred.

Other departments

Other departments can also provide information about adverse events. For example, the billing department may become aware of a patient who threatens to sue after receiving his bill. Or the first clue of an impending lawsuit may come from the medical records office, when a patient or attorney requests a copy of the medical record.

Reports from the engineering department about the safety of the hospital environment and from purchasing, biomedical engineering, and the pharmacy on the safety and adequacy of products and equipment are also informative.

Trending reports of adverse events from various departments can identify areas that need attention more quickly than a focused departmental review. For instance, medication errors may correlate with new nurses or decreased staffing. Patient falls may correlate with staffing problems, problems with history taking in fall-prone patients, safety hazards, or a combination of these factors.

Of course, reports from all sources should be documented thoroughly. For nurses, this means charting on the patient's medical record and filling out incident reports and related nursing documents.

Managing adverse events

Once the risk manager learns of a potential or actual lawsuit, he or she notifies the medical records department and the hospital's insurance carrier or attorney (or both). The medical records department makes copies of the patient's chart and files the original in a secure place to prevent tampering.

A claim notice should also trigger a quality-management peer review of the medical record. This review may be conducted by the chairperson of the department involved, the risk management or quality management department, or an external reviewer to measure the health care provider's conduct against the professional standards of conduct for the particular situation. This review helps the risk manager determine the claim's merit and also helps to define the hospital's responsibility for care in particular situations. It also identifies areas where changes are needed, such as policy, training, staffing, or equipment.

Completing incident reports

An incident report is a formal report, written by doctors, nurses, or other staff members,

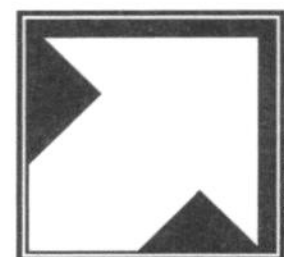

CHARTING GUIDELINES

Tips for writing an incident report

When a malpractice lawsuit reached the courtroom in years past, the plaintiff's attorney wasn't allowed to see incident reports. Today, however, the plaintiff in many states is legally entitled to a record of the incident if he requests it through proper channels.

When writing an incident report, keep in mind the people who may read it and follow these guidelines.

Write objectively
Record the details of the incident in objective terms, describing exactly what you saw and heard. For example, unless you actually saw a patient fall, write: "Found patient lying on the floor." Then describe only the actions you took to provide care at the scene, such as helping the patient get back into bed or assessing him for injuries.

Include only essential information
Document the time and place of the incident and the name of the doctor who was notified.

Avoid opinions
Don't commit your opinions to writing in the incident report. Rather, verbally share your suggestions or opinions on how an incident may be avoided with your supervisor and risk manager.

Assign no blame
Don't admit to liability and don't blame or point your finger at colleagues or administrators. Steer clear of such statements as "Better staffing would have prevented this incident." State only what happened.

Avoid hearsay and assumptions
Each staff member who knows about the incident should write a separate incident report. If one of your patients is injured in another department, the staff members in that department are responsible for documenting the details of the incident.

File the report properly
Don't file the incident report with the medical record. Send the report to the person designated to review it according to your facility's policy.

that informs hospital administrators about an adverse event suffered by a patient. Incident reports are continually being revised, and some may be computerized. (Computer processing permits classifying and counting of incidents to indicate trends.) If you're filing an incident report and need more room than the form allows, check your facility's policy; additional blank pages may not be protected from disclosure to a patient's attorney. (See *Tips for writing an incident report* and *Completing an incident report.*)

State, federal, and military statutes protect quality management and peer review documents from disclosure to a patient's attorney on the grounds that health care providers should be allowed to freely and thoroughly investigate claims of adverse events without having to worry about being sued for what they discover; however, incident reports may not be thus protected. Because the patient's attorney may be able to obtain a copy of an incident report, the document should be factual and succinct. Keep in mind that while names

BETTER CHARTING

Completing an incident report

When you discover a reportable event, you must fill out an incident report. Forms vary, but most include the following information.

INCIDENT REPORT

Name Greta Manning
Address 7 Worth Way, Boston, MA
Phone (617) 555-1122
Addressograph if patient

DATE OF INCIDENT	TIME OF INCIDENT
1-30-99	1442

EXACT LOCATION OF INCIDENT (Bldg, Floor, Room No, Area)
4-Main, Rm. 447

TYPE OF INCIDENT
(CHECK ONE ONLY) ☐ PATIENT ☐ EMPLOYEE ☑ VISITOR ☐ VOLUNTEER ☐ OTHER (specify)

DESCRIPTION OF THE INCIDENT (WHO, WHAT, WHEN, WHERE, HOW, WHY)
(Use back of form if necessary)
Patient's wife found on floor next to bed. States she was trying to put siderail of bed down to sit on pt's bed and fell.

Patient fall incidents

FLOOR CONDITIONS ☑ CLEAN & SMOOTH ☐ OTHER ____ ☐ SLIPPERY (WET) | FRAME OF BED ☑ LOW ☐ HIGH | NIGHT LIGHT ☐ YES ☑ NO

WERE BED RAILS PRESENT? ☐ NO ☐ 1 UP ☐ 2 UP ☐ 3 UP ☑ 4 UP | OTHER RESTRAINTS (TYPE AND EXTENT) N/A

AMBULATION PRIVILEGE ☐ UNLIMITED ☐ LIMITED WITH ASSISTANCE ☐ COMPLETE BEDREST ☐ OTHER

WERE NARCOTICS, ANALGESICS, HYPNOTICS, SEDATIVES, DIURETICS, ANTIHYPERTENSIVES, OR ANTICONVULSANTS GIVEN DURING LAST 4 HOURS?
☐ YES ☑ NO DRUG AMOUNT TIME

Patient incidents

PHYSICIAN NOTIFIED — Name of Physician J. Reynolds, MD — DATE 1-30-99 — TIME 1445 — COMPLETE IF APPLICABLE

Employee incidents

DEPARTMENT | JOB TITLE | SOCIAL SECURITY #
MARITAL STATUS

All incidents

NOTIFIED C. Jones, RN — DATE 1-30-99 — TIME 1500 | LOCATION WHERE TREATMENT WAS RENDERED

NAME, ADDRESS AND TELEPHONE NUMBERS OF WITNESS(ES) OR PERSONS FAMILIAR WITH INCIDENT - WITNESS OR NOT
Janet Adams (617) 555-0912 1 Main St., Boston, MA

SIGNATURE OF PERSON PREPARING REPORT	TITLE	DATE OF REPORT
Connie Smith, RN	RN	1-30-99

PHYSICIAN'S REPORT — To be completed for all cases involving injury or illness (DO NOT USE ABBREVIATIONS) (Use back if necessary)

DIAGNOSIS AND TREATMENT
Received patient in Emergency Department after reported fall in husband's room. 12 cm x 12 cm ecchymotic area noted on right hip. X-rays negative for fracture. Good range of motion. Ice pack applied. ——— J. Reynolds, MD

DISPOSITION sent home

PERSON NOTIFIED OTHER THAN HOSPITAL PERSONNEL NAME AND ADDRESS	DATE	TIME
R. Manning (daughter), address same as pt	1-30-99	1500

PHYSICIAN'S SIGNATURE	DATE
J. Reynolds, MD	1-30-99

of individuals who know about the incident are important, placing those names on the report may result in their being called to testify or give a deposition regarding the incident. Still, the goal of completing the incident report is to be truthful, timely, and objective.

Historically, nurses have been reluctant to complete incident reports for such events as medication errors because they feared retribution. The problem with this is that failure to complete a report may create the appearance that you're intentionally hiding information.

Documenting an incident in the medical record

When documenting an incident in the patient's medical record, keep the following in mind:

- Write a factual account of the incident, including the treatment and follow-up care provided and the patient's response. If you don't document the incident, the plaintiff's lawyer might think you're hiding something. This documentation shows that the patient was closely monitored after the incident. If the case goes to court, the jury may be asked to determine if the patient received appropriate care after the incident.
- Include in the progress notes and in the incident report anything the patient or his family says about their role in the incident, for example, "Patient stated, 'The nurse told me to ask for help before I went to the bathroom, but I decided to go on my own.'" This kind of statement helps the defense attorney prove that the patient was guilty of contributory or comparative negligence. Contributory negligence is conduct that contributed to the patient's injuries. Comparative negligence involves determining the percentage of each party's fault. For example, the nurse might be found 25% negligent and the patient 75% negligent.

Overview of malpractice lawsuits

National claims data show that the number of lawsuits naming the nurse as a specific defendant continues to increase. The expanding role of nurses, changes in managed care, shorter hospitalizations, and more acute home care have challenged the nurse-patient relationship. Nurses have less time to establish relationships with patients than they once did because patients now move out of the acute care system very quickly or are transferred to other units. All of this can lead to unfamiliarity, which may lead to errors. Try to establish rapport with your patients, but remember that nothing replaces good nursing care.

Although your chances of actually being sued are still small, the fear of a malpractice suit can be stress-producing. It's important to remember, however, that the majority of malpractice cases are settled out of court well before a trial date; of those that do go to trial, a vast majority are decided in favor of the health care provider.

Preliminary steps in a lawsuit

When a patient (the plaintiff) believes harm was caused by the action or negligence of a health care provider, he may file a lawsuit. Most of these claims are settled out of court. A plaintiff who was injured because the health care provider was negligent deserves compensation without going through the stress and expense of litigation. All parties named as defendants (usually doctor, hospital, and nurse) as well as the insurance companies and attorneys try to work toward a fair settlement.

A patient's refusal to pay his bill is sometimes the first sign a facility has that the patient was dissatisfied with his care. Depending on how the billing office is integrated with the quality management and risk management departments, steps may be taken at this time to investigate the patient's concerns. If they appear to be valid, a settlement offer may be made before litigation is even considered.

Sometimes a patient will try to obtain a copy of his medical record in an effort to learn about the care he received and then base a complaint on what he perceives as "mistakes." Although the patient has a right to a copy of the record, X-rays, and other reports, the facility can charge the patient for copying costs.

The first step for some patients may be to contact a malpractice attorney through family or friends. The attorney will interview the patient. If the case appears to have merit, the attorney will probably order a copy of the medical record or a specific section dealing with the event in question.

The plaintiff's attorneys usually work on a contingency basis, meaning that they're not paid for their work unless they win the case. This procedure is intended to prevent attorneys from taking meritless cases. However, the patient must pay for filing the case with the court, retaining expert witnesses, and other costs. Some cases with actual merit are not filed because the expense of trying the case outweighs any dollar amount that could be awarded for damages.

Preparations for adjudication

If the parties can't agree on a settlement or the plaintiff is dissatisfied with the settlement offer, he may take his claim to court for adjudication (a judicial decision). If the case appears to have merit and records have been obtained, the plaintiff's attorney will send the records to an expert for a preliminary review. If the attorney fails to do this, he runs the risk that the case will be dismissed as a frivolous claim. Some attorneys have nurses working full time or on a contract basis to do preliminary reviews.

Activity on the defendant's side may begin when the medical records department receives an attorney's request for a copy of the medical record and notifies the risk management department. This department begins an immediate review of the situation, and the health care facility's insurance carrier is notified. The doctor involved in the lawsuit will also be notified and given an opportunity to review the record.

Remember: No one should make changes in the medical record after a lawsuit has been initiated. If the record is incomplete or inaccurate, this should be clarified in a dated addendum. The jury will think that you were covering up something if you try to explain changes made to the medical record after it was requested by a lawyer.

Complaint

If the expert review indicates that the standard of practice was breached and injury that can be proximately related to that breach occurred, the attorney will file a *complaint*—a summary of what the injured party aims to prove. Most states allow patients to file a complaint up to 2 years from the time the alleged act of malpractice occurred or was discovered. In some jurisdictions, several years may elapse before the case goes to trial.

The complaint is filed in the courthouse, and copies are presented to each defendant or agent. This legal document notifies the defendant of the plaintiff's charges and gives the latest date on which an answer to the complaint can be filed.

In most jurisdictions, the complaint goes to a lower court judge. In jurisdictions with an arbitration system, an arbitration panel receives the complaint and initially hears the case. The case may then be appealed to the designated court. In cases involving the military or the Department of Veterans' Affairs, the case will be filed in federal court.

Discovery

Once the attorney files the complaint, the *discovery* period begins. Discovery has two purposes: to give each party time to gather evidence and learn all the facts and allegations involved in the case, and to encourage an out-of-court settlement when appropriate. In complex malpractice suits, the discovery period can last 1 or 2 years or even longer. When this period is over, both sides are ready to testify in court.

Deposition

The most important type of discovery for a nurse-defendant is the *deposition,* or testimony under oath. During a deposition, attorneys question the defendants, plaintiffs, and witnesses one by one while a court stenographer records the questions and answers. The nurse will be asked questions by the plaintiff's lawyer and sometimes by other lawyers representing additional parties.

If the nurse has her own malpractice insurance, she'll be represented by the insurer's attorney to protect her interests. At a minimum, her employer's attorney will be present to protect the interests of the health care facility. Many nurses believe they're adequately protected by their employer's attorney. This is not true; the interests of the employer and the nurse may diverge. For instance, if you fail to fulfill a policy or a procedure 100%, the facility could say you were outside the scope of employment; or you may no longer be employed by the facility when the suit is filed.

The deposition process may sound innocuous but it isn't. Lawyers spend considerable time preparing defendants for it. The same goes for nurses who testify at depositions as fact witnesses (as opposed to named defendants). No one should ever go to a deposition without reviewing the medical record and without legal representation. If the case goes to trial, transcripts from the deposition may be introduced as evidence and compared with courtroom testimony for any discrepancies or contradictions.

Interrogatories

During the deposition, some attorneys use *interrogatories* (lists of written questions) to determine what evidence is available. The plaintiff's attorney may ask the health care facility for all records, policies, procedures, and committee minutes pertaining to the plaintiff. These documents may be protected from discovery under peer review acts, but each jurisdiction has different statutes governing what may be made available to opposing counsel. Some state and federal statutes provide confidentiality for these documents under quality assurance provisions.

Nurse's response

After being named in a malpractice suit, the nurse-defendant will need to devote considerable time to preparing her case. She'll work with her attorney to prepare for and respond to discovery requests from the plaintiff's attorney. In addition, the nurse's own attorney will rely on her to provide accurate information on the plaintiff's nursing care and other treatment issues. (For more information, see chapter 11, Malpractice Lawsuits.)

The attorney may also ask for the nurse's help in selecting the right type of expert witnesses for the defense and in developing probing questions to ask the plaintiff's expert witnesses.

Courtroom hearings

When the case finally goes to trial, the jury hears from a variety of witnesses. Fact witnesses include people with knowledge of the actual incident. Expert witnesses offer opinions about the case based on their expertise in a specific subject that's relevant to the case. Family members may attest to the plaintiff's pain and suffering.

In cases heard in a court, rather than by an arbitration panel, a jury weighs the credibility of the people testifying, listens to all the evidence, and then decides whose testimony it believes.

In malpractice cases, the parties involved almost always make contradictory statements. For example, a nurse may chart ominous changes in a patient's signs and symptoms (such as tachycardia or projectile vomiting) and document that the doctor was "notified." At trial, the doctor may admit having been called on the phone but deny learning of any problem requiring an immediate trip to the hospital. To avoid this kind of problem, you can write, "Doctor notified of these findings" and chart the doctor's response, such as "Will come to hospital" or "Doctor gave these telephone orders." This type of charting can prevent a "he said, she said" controversy.

Discrepancies in testimony sometimes arise not from deliberate deception but simply from a poor memory of events that may have occurred months or years earlier. Incomplete documentation only adds to the problem. For example, a nurse can testify that she always performs dressing changes a certain way, always observes for abnormal signs, and always notes changes in vital signs, but if she didn't chart the intervention, she has no proof that it occurred.

Role of documentation

Good documentation can save a nurse in a credibility dispute. In one case, a house doctor didn't respond to a nurse's calls about a patient's deteriorating neurologic condition for more than an hour. After repeated calls, the nurse finally notified the neurosurgeon directly. The patient had an epidural hematoma and left-sided hemiparesis. The house doctor claimed that he never received the calls, but the nurse had documented each one, noting the time and the doctor's responses. The jury decided against the house doctor.

Lack of documentation doesn't always imply negligence, but juries often believe it

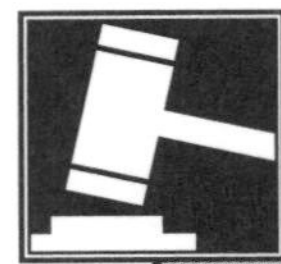

ON TRIAL

Not documented, not done

Even if you provide appropriate care, you risk a lawsuit if you fail to document. Consider the case of *Jarvis v. St. Charles Medical Center,* 713 P.2d 620 (Oregon 1986).

Concerned that his patient with a fractured leg was developing compartment syndrome, the patient's doctor spread the cast and instructed the nurses on duty to perform hourly tests (assessments and observations) and to notify him if problems developed.

Two days later, at 2030 hours, the doctor noticed that the patient's foot was white and pulseless. A nurse's entry on the progress notes at 1600 hours indicated no change in circulation, movement, or sensation.

Although emergency surgery was performed, the patient was left with restricted use of her leg.

Court's decision

In the malpractice suit that followed, the hospital argued that muscle death was gradual and that the doctor didn't manage the patient appropriately. The doctor claimed that a sudden change had occurred and that the nurses hadn't notified him.

The court ruled that the doctor was negligent and added that because the progress notes indicated only sporadic testing, the nurses had contributed to the doctor's negligence by failing to conduct regular examinations.

In this case, it didn't matter whether the nurses assessed the patient hourly and provided care as ordered. What mattered was that the records didn't demonstrate that the ordered care was provided. The result: a judgment of negligence.

does. You've probably heard the expression, "If it wasn't charted, it wasn't done." Juries may think that this statement applies to all situations, when in reality, you can't possibly document every word and action. Fair or not, this misconception can lead to a negative outcome in a malpractice case when no negligence occurred. (See *Not documented, not done.*)

Role of the judge

In a malpractice case, the judge's role is to monitor the testimony, to decide legal questions about how the evidence is presented, and to determine questions of law. After all the testimony has been presented, the judge discusses with the jury how the law should be applied.

Role of the jury

The jury decides whether negligence has occurred and, if so, what compensation should be awarded. At any point before the jury's decision, the opposing parties can decide to settle the case out of court. Out-of-court settlements are usually kept confidential.

Bioethical dilemmas and documentation

As a nurse, you routinely take part in decisions involving ethical dilemmas. These may range from "innocent" discussions of confidential patient information in hospital elevators to removing life support. Ethical dilemmas appear to have grown proportionately with increased technology. Years ago, nurses didn't have to ponder such issues as a patient's right to die or refuse treatment, terminating use of life-prolonging equipment, human experimentation and research, organ donation, and surrogate motherhood.

At the same time, nurses today have access to many excellent resources for addressing bioethical dilemmas, including professional conferences, textbooks, articles, and consultants. This material underscores the significance of documentation when facing bioethical dilemmas.

The JCAHO mandates that hospitals address ethical issues in providing patient care. The hospital must list specific patient rights and maintain a code of ethical behavior for the hospital. A few states have incorporated patient rights into their state statutes, and most have codified statutes for nursing home patients. The ANA and other nursing organizations have their own ethical codes of conduct for nurses. (See *Ethical codes for nurses,* pages 34 and 35.)

Health care facilities should have an established framework to support ethical decision making. Many have bioethics committees with multidisciplinary representation. Nurses serve on these committees and can present ethical dilemmas to the committees.

Your facility should have adopted policies to implement the JCAHO and state statutes regarding bioethical dilemmas. These policies can serve as guidelines that outline documentation needs. One significant document, a written statement of a patient's rights, should be delivered to every patient on admission.

Other bioethical issues involving documentation include the following:

- informed consent (including witnessing informed consent and informed refusal)
- advance directives (also known as living wills)
- power of attorney
- do-not-resuscitate orders
- withdrawal of treatment
- confidentiality of the medical record.

Informed consent

Required before most treatments and procedures, *informed consent* means that the patient understands the proposed therapy and its risks and agrees to undergo it by signing a consent form. The doctor (or other practitioner) who will perform the procedure is legally responsible for obtaining the patient's informed consent. In some situations, he may delegate the duty to a nurse; however, the responsibility remains with the doctor or practitioner. Depending on your facility's policy, you may be asked to witness the patient's signature.

Legal requirements

For informed consent to be legally binding, the patient must be mentally competent and the doctor must:

- explain the patient's diagnosis as well as the nature, purpose, and likelihood of success of the treatment or procedure
- describe the risks and benefits associated with the treatment or procedure
- explain the possible consequences of not undergoing the treatment or procedure
- describe alternative treatments and procedures

LEGAL AND ETHICAL IMPLICATIONS

Ethical codes for nurses

One of the most important ethical codes for registered nurses is the American Nurses Association (ANA) code. Licensed practical and vocational nurses (LPNs and LVNs) also have an ethical code, which is set forth in each state by the state's Nurses Association. The National Federation of Licensed Practical Nurses also has a code of ethics for its members. In addition, the International Council of Nurses, an organization based in Geneva, Switzerland, that seeks to improve the standards and status of nursing worldwide, has published a code of ethics. Summaries of these codes appear below.

ANA code of ethics

The ANA views both nurses and patients as individuals who possess basic rights and responsibilities and who should command respect for their values and circumstances at all times. The ANA code provides guidance for carrying out nursing responsibilities consistent with the ethical obligations of the profession. According to the ANA code, the nurse is responsible for the following actions:

- Provide services with respect for human dignity and the uniqueness of the patient unrestricted by considerations of social or economic status, personal attributes, or the nature of health problems.
- Safeguard the patient's right to privacy by judiciously protecting information of a confidential nature.
- Act to safeguard the patient and the public when health care and safety are affected by the incompetent, unethical, or illegal practice of any person.
- Assume responsibility and accountability for individual nursing judgments and actions.
- Maintain competence in nursing.
- Exercise informed judgment and use individual competence and qualifications as criteria in seeking consultation, accepting responsibilities, and delegating nursing activities to others.
- Cooperate in activities that contribute to the ongoing development of the profession's body of knowledge.
- Participate in the profession's efforts to implement and improve standards of nursing.
- Take part in the profession's efforts to establish and maintain conditions of employment conducive to high-quality nursing care.
- Share in the profession's efforts to protect the public from misinformation and misrepresentation and to maintain the integrity of nursing.
- Collaborate with members of the health care professions and other citizens in promoting community and national efforts to meet the health needs of the public.

Code for LPNs and LVNs

The code for LPNs and LVNs seeks to provide a motivation for establishing, maintaining, and elevating professional standards. It includes the following imperatives:

- Know the scope of maximum utilization of the LPN and LVN, as specified by the nurse practice act, and function within this scope.
- Safeguard the confidential information acquired from any source about the patient.
- Provide health care to all patients regardless of race, creed, cultural background, disease, or lifestyle.
- Refuse to give endorsement to the sale and promotion of commercial products or services.

- inform the patient that he has the right to refuse the treatment or procedure without having other care or support withdrawn; this includes withdrawing his consent after giving it
- identify who will perform the procedure
- identify who is responsible for the patient's care
- obtain consent without coercing the patient.

- Uphold the highest standards in personal appearance, language, dress, and demeanor.
- Stay informed about issues affecting the practice of nursing and delivery of health care and, where appropriate, participate in government and policy decisions.
- Accept the responsibility for safe nursing by keeping oneself mentally and physically fit and educationally prepared to practice.
- Accept responsibility for membership in the National Federation of Licensed Practical Nurses, and participate in its efforts to maintain the established standards of nursing practice and employment policies that lead to quality patient care.

International Council of Nurses code of ethics

According to the International Council of Nurses, the fundamental responsibility of the nurse is fourfold: to promote health, to prevent illness, to restore health, and to alleviate suffering.

The International Council of Nurses further states that inherent in nursing is respect for life, dignity, and human rights and that nursing is unrestricted by considerations of nationality, race, creed, color, age, sex, politics, or social status. The key points of the code appear below.

Nurses and people

- The nurse's primary responsibility is to those who require nursing care.
- The nurse, in providing care, respects the beliefs, values, and customs of the individual.
- The nurse holds in confidence personal information and uses judgment in sharing this information.

Nurses and practice

- The nurse carries personal responsibility for nursing practice and for maintaining competence by continual learning.
- The nurse maintains the highest standards of nursing care possible within the reality of a specific situation.
- The nurse uses judgment in relation to individual competence when accepting and delegating responsibilities.
- The nurse, when acting in a professional capacity, should at all times maintain standards of personal conduct that would reflect credit upon the profession.

Nurses and society

- The nurse shares with other citizens the responsibility for initiating and supporting action to meet the health and social needs of the public.

Nurses and coworkers

- The nurse sustains a cooperative relationship with coworkers in nursing and other fields.
- The nurse takes appropriate action to safeguard the individual when his care is endangered by a coworker or any other person.

Nurses and the profession

- The nurse plays a major role in determining and implementing desirable standards of nursing practice and nursing education.
- The nurse is active in developing a core of professional knowledge.
- The nurse, acting through the professional organization, participates in establishing and maintaining equitable social and economic working conditions in nursing.

Informed consent has two elements, the information and the consent. To be *informed*, the patient must be provided with a description of the treatment or procedure, the name and qualifications of the person who will perform it, and an explanation of risks and alternatives — all in language the patient can understand. Based on this, the patient may *consent* to the treatment or procedure.

The JCAHO mandates the elements of informed consent. In addition, most states have statutes that set out specific elements of informed consent. In a few states, the doctor can explain the procedure and simply ask if the patient has any questions. If the patient has none, the doctor is not obligated by state law to discuss alternatives and risks unless the patient requests the information. Although this policy is inconsistent with JCAHO guidelines, keep in mind that those guidelines are not the law; they're a set of requirements for licensure and accreditation.

In life-threatening emergencies, informed consent may not be required. In such cases, the law assumes that every individual wants to live and allows the doctor to intervene to save life without obtaining consent.

In many cases, a patient may attempt to clarify issues with a nurse after giving the doctor his informed consent. If you are questioned in this way, be aware that you're not obligated to answer the patient's questions; however, if you do, be careful to document your answers. You should also notify the doctor and document that you have done so, including the date and time.

Witnessing informed consent

When you witness the patient signing an informed consent document, you are *not* witnessing that he received or understood the information. You are simply witnessing that the person who signed the consent form is in fact the person he says he is. For this, check the patient's armband to ensure that he is in fact the correct patient. You don't need to be present when the doctor gives the information because you are only witnessing that the patient is signing the document, not that the information was given.

Before a procedure is performed, make sure the patient's record contains a signed informed consent form. If the patient appears to be concerned about the procedure or the doctor's explanation of it, notify your supervisor or the doctor, and chart that you've done this. If the patient wants to change his mind, contact the doctor as soon as possible and chart the patient's comments, the date and time you contacted the doctor, and the doctor's response.

Informed refusal

Just as the patient has a right to consent to medical treatment based on relevant information, he also has the right to refuse treatment based on knowledge of the outcomes and risks. The JCAHO requires (and federal statutes mandate) that health care facilities (both acute and long-term care) inform patients soon after admission about their treatment options.

Discuss the patient's wishes with him, and document the discussion for use later, in case the patient becomes unable to participate in decision making. With a few exceptions, a *competent* patient has a right to refuse mechanical ventilation, tube feedings, antibiotics, fluids, and other treatments that will clearly result in his death if they're withheld.

Legal competence differs from the medical or psychiatric concept of competence. The law presumes all individuals to be competent unless deemed otherwise through a court proceeding. The patient must also have *capacity* —that is, be legally considered an adult for consent purposes under state law.

BETTER CHARTING

Witnessing refusal of treatment

If a patient refuses treatment, the doctor must first explain the risks involved in making this choice. Then the doctor asks the patient to sign a refusal-of-treatment release form, such as the one below, which you may be asked to sign as a witness. Your signature only validates the identity of the patient signing the form — not that the patient received sufficient information or understood that information.

REFUSAL-OF-TREATMENT RELEASE FORM

I, Brenda Lyndstrom refuse to allow anyone to
(patient's name)

administer I.V. medication.
(insert treatment)

The risks attendant to my refusal have been fully explained to me, and I fully understand the benefits of this treatment. I also understand that my refusal of treatment seriously reduces my chances for regaining normal health and may endanger my life.

I hereby release Mercy General,
(name of hospital)

its nurses and employees, together with all doctors in any way connected with me as a patient, from liability for respecting and following my express wishes and direction.

Susan Reynolds, RN
(witness's signature)

Brenda Lyndstrom
(patient's or legal guardian's signature)

1/2/99
(date)

Some health care facilities have informed refusal forms. It is important to chart in the medical record progress notes that the information was given and the patient refused the treatment. (See *Witnessing refusal of treatment.*)

Exceptions to the right to informed refusal may include pregnant women (because the life of the unborn child is at risk) and parents' wishes to withhold treatment for their child.

Advance directives

The U.S. Constitution and case law have established that the patient has the right to determine what happens to his body. The JCAHO mandates that patients have the right to participate in decisions regarding their care and that health care facilities have a policy or procedure in place addressing how they'll implement the requirement. The JCAHO also requires that a facility address forgoing or withdrawing life-sustaining treatment and withholding resuscitative services and care at the end of life.

An *advance directive* (sometimes referred to as a *living will*) allows the patient to decide before he becomes terminally ill the type of care he'll be given at the end of life. The directive becomes effective only when the patient becomes terminally ill. It may be written or oral, but to comply with most state statutes, it must be written.

Some patients and health care providers have hesitated to accept the concept of advance directives, fearing that the patient won't be allowed to change his mind later. It's important to remember that an advance directive *can* be revoked. If a competent patient enters the hospital in a terminally ill state and decides that he wants all possible life-prolonging measures to be applied despite an existing advance directive to the contrary, his oral declaration that the advance directive be ignored effectively revokes the document. The patient's current wishes must be documented in the medical record. Some state statutes have guidelines for revoking a directive but the patient's oral wishes will suffice until those requirements can be met.

If an advance directive is in effect and the nurse or other health care provider fails to honor it, any subsequent care provided may be considered unconsented touching, assault and battery, negligence, or intentional infliction of emotional, physical, and financial distress and, as such, grounds for a malpractice suit.

Patient Self-Determination Act

The Patient Self-Determination Act of 1990 allows patients to use advance directives and to appoint a surrogate to make decisions if the patient loses the ability to do so. This act mandates that on admission, each patient be informed of his right to create an advance directive. The fact that the patient has been offered this information must be documented in the medical record. If the patient elects to create an advance directive, this document must be placed in the medical record and honored.

Power of attorney

An advance directive can be made by a friend or family member to whom the patient has given *power of attorney*. Power of attorney is a legal document in which a competent person designates another to act or conduct legally binding transactions (such as writing checks or signing legal documents) on his behalf. This power may encompass all of a person's affairs, including health and financial matters, or it may be limited to one specific area. If the power of attorney covers health matters, it allows the designated person to express an opinion and make decisions about the kind of health care the patient would want.

A power of attorney ceases if the patient becomes incompetent or revokes the document, unless he has executed a durable power of attorney.

A *durable power of attorney* is a legal document in which a competent person designates another person to act on his behalf if he should become incapable of managing his own affairs. Some states have created a durable power of attorney specifically for health care. This document ensures that the patient's wishes regarding treatment will be carried out if he should ever become incompetent or unable to make decisions because of illness.

A copy of the written power of attorney should be placed in a conspicuous place in the patient record. As with advance directives, failure to honor the power of attorney can result in litigation.

Do-not-resuscitate orders

The doctor writes a do-not-resuscitate (DNR) order when it is medically indicated—that is, when a patient is terminally ill and expected to die. In spite of the patient's autonomy and the requirement to honor the patient's wishes, the patient cannot mandate that a facility provide futile treatment. Thus, a DNR order may be written regardless of the advance directive, but ideally this decision should be thoroughly discussed with the patient or his legal surrogate. DNR orders should be reviewed as policy dictates or whenever a significant change occurs in the patient's clinical status.

Some facilities temporarily suspend DNR orders during surgery. Although the patient and doctor aren't seeking heroic measures at the end of life, they won't allow the patient to bleed to death if he should hemorrhage during a palliative surgical procedure. Another exception is the concept of partial or "a la carte" resuscitation codes. These are legally precarious since the standard of care is to attempt full resuscitation through all means available, not partial resuscitation.

The patient's family members or friends do not have the legal authority to write an advance directive or advise the doctor regarding a DNR order unless they have a legal power of attorney or durable power of attorney. The patient is presumed to be competent and has the sole right to state what care he wishes, unless that care isn't indicated from a medical standpoint.

Withdrawal of treatment

Although health care facilities are not required to provide medically futile treatment, they are reluctant to withdraw futile treatment unless the patient (or the patient's immediate family if the patient isn't legally competent) agrees. Bioethics committees at academic medical centers are struggling to find an ethical and practical way to approach withdrawal of medically futile and costly treatment without inviting an even more costly lawsuit brought by a dissenting family member. Whether treatment is withdrawn because of medical futility or the patient's wishes, as expressed through an advance directive or a legal surrogate, it's important to document the patient's condition and prognosis.

Confidentiality

One of your documentation responsibilities includes protecting the confidentiality of the patient's medical record. Usually, you can't reveal confidential information without the patient's permission. Besides your legal responsibilities, you also have professional and ethical responsibilities (as specified by the ANA, the JCAHO, and other professional

Confidentiality and computers

Computerization of medical records offers many advantages because entries can be made more easily and in a more timely manner. Computerized medical records must be backed up by hard-copy documents.

The Joint Commission on Accreditation of Healthcare Organizations requires health care facilities to have mechanisms in place for preserving confidentiality and safeguarding records against loss, destruction, and unauthorized access or use. These requirements apply to any form of record keeping, including computerized records.

Although computerized records facilitate the communication of patient information, they also present a serious risk of breach of confidentiality. They raise considerable concern not only about accidental disclosure by health care providers but also about inappropriate access by secondary users of the record, such as insurance companies or government agencies. Unauthorized disclosure can lead to criminal and civil penalties as well as civil lawsuits brought by patients or their families. Systems to avoid such disclosure include personal identification or user passcodes, encryption (scrambling of contents requiring a key to decipher), built-in safety devices to prevent tampering, and sophisticated programs to prevent sabotage.

Care must also be taken to protect patient information sent by fax machines. Policies and procedures should be established that dictate how to incorporate such information into the medical record.

bodies in their codes and standards) to protect your patient's privacy.

Nurse's role

Nurses assume a primary role in maintaining confidentiality and in safeguarding the privacy of medical records. Breaches in confidentiality can result from unintentional release of information, unauthorized entry into a patient's record, or even a casual conversation that's overheard by others. In fact, breaches of patient confidentiality on the part of nursing staff are more likely to occur through inadvertent conversations in cafeterias and elevators than through a specific request for a patient's chart. The best way to prevent such breaches is to avoid discussing patient concerns in areas where you can be overheard.

Most requests for copies of the medical record will go through the medical records department rather than through nursing staff. However, if you are asked for a copy of the record or an opportunity to view it, do not release the record without the documented consent of a competent patient. Increasing use of computers for documentation creates a new avenue for unauthorized release of patient information. (See *Confidentiality and computers.*)

All patient information is confidential, even information that may seem innocent. The release of certain information — for example, mental health records as well as information about drug and alcohol abuse and infectious diseases — is further constrained by state statutes.

In the case of *Anonymous v. Chino Valley Medical Center,* San Bernadino County, California Superior Court (1997), a 35-year-old disabled inpatient underwent a blood test for human immunodeficiency virus (HIV). He specifically told the doctor he did not want the results to be given to anyone but him. On the day of discharge, his sister was present in the hospital room. A nurse asked the sister to come into the hall so she could tell her about the patient's diet instructions upon discharge. Once in the hallway, the nurse told the sister that the patient had a positive HIV test. A few moments later, the doctor approached them and also conveyed the test results. No action was filed against the doctor. The nurse denied releasing the information. A trial court imposed a $5,000 statutory civil penalty against the medical center.

In the case of *Hobbs v. Lopes,* 645 NE 2d 1261, Ohio App. 4 DST. (1994), a 21-year-old Ohio woman was found to be pregnant after consulting a doctor for another medical problem. Options, including abortion, were discussed. The doctor instructed a nurse to call the woman to find out what option she had chosen. The nurse called the woman's parents' home and disclosed the fact that their daughter was pregnant and had sought advice about an abortion. The daughter sued for medical malpractice, invasion of privacy, breach of privilege, and infliction of emotional distress.

Both of these cases underscore the importance of documenting the patient's consent or nonconsent to release of information. The patient's consent to release information should be on an official facility form. This form is handled not by the nurse but by the medical records department or hospital attorney.

Keep in mind that the law requires you to disclose confidential information in certain situations — for example, in instances of alleged child abuse, matters of public health and safety, and criminal cases.

Right to information

As stated earlier, the patient has the right to the information in his medical record. Although the facility owns the actual record, the patient has a legal right to a copy of his chart, X-rays, and other reports. Many state statutes grant patients an express right to access the medical record. In the absence of a statute, some states have recognized the hospital's duty to allow the patient at least limited access to the medical record. Release of psychiatric records, records of minors, records with adoptive parent information, and records addressing drug and alcohol treatment or communicable diseases may be covered by special state statutes.

Patients treated in federal facilities also have right of access to their medical records, as mandated by the Freedom of Information Act of 1966 and the Privacy Act of 1974. Some states have freedom of information acts called public records or open records laws. Third-party access to medical records is controlled by these and other statutes dealing with criminal law, domestic abuse, and third-party payer or Medicare claims.

Selected references

Aiken, T.D. "Legal Update: Depositions and the Expert Witness," Part 2, *Pelican News* 53(3):7, July 1997.

Beckman, J.P. *Nursing Negligence: Analyzing Malpractice in the Hospital Setting.* Thousand Oaks, Calif.: Sage Publications, 1996.

Brazell, N.E. "The Significance and Application of Informed Consent," *AORN Journal* 65(2):377-82, February 1997.

Bunnell, T.P. "Self-Protection against Frivolous—and Expensive—Lawsuits," *Nursing Homes* 45(9):28-31, October 1996.

Carroll, R., ed. *Risk Management Handbook,* 2nd ed. Chicago: American Hospital Publishing, Inc., 1997.

Dowd, S.B., et al. "Maintaining Confidentiality: Health Care's Ongoing Dilemma," *Health Care Supervisor* 15(1):24-31, September 1996.

Guido, G.W. *Legal Issues in Nursing,* 2nd ed. Stamford, Conn.: Appleton & Lange, 1996.

Joint Commission on Accreditation of Healthcare Organizations (JCAHO). *Comprehensive Accreditation Manual for Hospitals: The Official Handbook.* Oakbrook Terrace, Ill.: JCAHO, 1998.

Morris, M.R. "The Legal Side: Falsifying an Incident Report, *AJN* 98(1):20, January 1998.

Nurse's Legal Handbook, 3rd ed. Springhouse, Pa.: Springhouse Corp., 1996.

Sardinas, J.L., Jr., et al. "Securing the Transmission and Storage of Medical Information," *Computers in Nursing* 16(3):162-70, May-June 1998.

Simpson, R.L. "Ethics and Privacy in a Technologically Driven Health Care Network," *Nursing Administration Quarterly* 21(1):81-84, Fall 1996.

3

Quality Management and Reimbursement

The impact of nursing documentation on the quality of patient care and the reimbursement for patient care extends throughout — and beyond — the patient's stay in a health care facility. What makes this documentation so important? In most cases, nursing documentation constitutes a major part of the medical record. It helps prove or disprove that a health care facility provides acceptable care and qualifies for reimbursement. This means that the various parties interested in quality health care, reimbursement standards, and legal practices will study a great deal of nursing documentation.

Quality watchdogs

Who are these parties? Typically, they include representatives of the Joint Commission on Accreditation of Healthcare Organizations (JCAHO), Medicare and Medicaid auditors, peer review organizations (PROs), quality management (also known as quality improvement) committees, and others, such as those involved in assigning patients to appropriate diagnostic groups and meeting legal requirements. These parties are directly charged with improving quality and justifying government and insurance company disbursements for health care.

To accomplish their mission, they scrutinize medical records to evaluate care that they can't observe firsthand. Because what you document or don't document either supports or challenges the quality standards and appropriateness of care, your notes directly affect your health care facility's accreditation, financial reimbursement, and legal security.

DOCUMENTATION AND QUALITY MANAGEMENT

The JCAHO, PROs, case managers, quality management committees, and the National Committee for Quality Assurance (NCQA) are just a few of the groups that will periodically evaluate your facility's quality of care and service and overall nursing competence. (For information on the NCQA, see chapter 7, Documentation in Home Care.)

JCAHO QUALITY STANDARDS

The JCAHO routinely surveys health care facilities in the United States to make sure that they meet its standards as accredited health care providers. Health care facilities submit to these surveys mainly to demonstrate that they provide high-quality, safe health care. They also seek JCAHO accreditation to qualify for reimbursement and other funding from governmental and private insurance agencies. These agencies require health care facilities to hold JCAHO accreditation before they're eligible to receive Medicare, Medicaid, or private funds. (For information on Medicare and Medicaid reimbursement benefits, see *Comparing Medicare and Medicaid.*)

Besides requiring that documentation demonstrate a facility's measurable overall quality care and service, the JCAHO also insists that the documentation itself meet certain quality standards. Specifically, reviewers examine medical records containing patient assessments, plans of care, and personnel records, such as clinical nurse competence evaluations, nursing licenses and credentials, and nursing assignments.

Because the JCAHO depends on nursing documentation to evaluate patient care, what

Comparing Medicare and Medicaid

Both Medicare and Medicaid were established in 1966 under the Social Security Act. As the following chart shows, the two organizations differ in their reimbursement policies, regulations, and documentation guidelines.

MEDICARE	MEDICAID
Federal health insurance benefits program for persons over age 65. Part A covers skilled nursing home and hospital care; Part B covers care by doctors, hospital equipment, and supplies.	Combined state and federal insurance and medical assistance plan for qualified needy individuals of any age; encourages home care as an alternative to institutional care
Benefits are uniform for eligible recipients nationwide.	Benefits differ from state to state.
Pays for skilled medical and nursing care only	Pays for home nursing care (not necessarily skilled care).
Patients must be confined to home to receive reimbursement for part-time or intermittent skilled nursing care.	Patients aren't required to be confined to home.
Documentation is required to support the need for skilled medical and nursing care and its delivery.	Documentation is required to ensure payment, but required content varies according to setting.
Doesn't pay for custodial care	Pays for custodial care in specified care settings
A doctor's order initiates service.	The patient's qualifying need initiates service.

QUALITY MANAGEMENT AND REIMBURSEMENT

and how you document plays a crucial role in the accreditation process. To be accredited by the JCAHO, a health care facility must have an organized, systematic, and ongoing method for documenting quality. (See *Documenting to reflect JCAHO standards,* page 46.) The JCAHO recommends a monitoring and evaluation process based on a 10-step model.

Step 1: Assigning responsibility

Ultimately, the responsibility for quality lies with a hospital's governing body—its board of directors. In general, the board charges the health care facility administrator to appoint someone to oversee monitoring and evaluation activities throughout the facility. In turn, this person assigns hands-on quality management responsibilities to the group responsible for each service. For example, the responsibility for monitoring and evaluating nursing care may pass through a long chain of command from the board to the administrator, to the quality management director, to the vice president of nursing, and to the nurse-manager.

Specifically, the medical staff monitors medical care, the nursing department evaluates nursing care, and pharmacists review

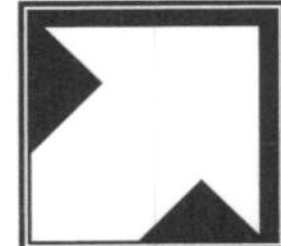

CHARTING GUIDELINES

Documenting to reflect JCAHO standards

When representatives of the Joint Commission on Accreditation of Healthcare Organizations (JCAHO) review medical records, they look for indications that the health care facility provides quality care.

Of particular interest to the JCAHO is evidence that the health care facility has an organized and systematic method for monitoring and evaluating patient care. And, of course, your documentation should reflect this method.

As you document care, keep in mind that your documentation can prove detrimental or beneficial to your facility during JCAHO reviews. Ideally, it should show that your facility:

- monitors and evaluates health care activities and caregivers
- defines the scope of care provided
- recognizes the most important aspects of care provided
- identifies indicators (a sign or symptom or set of signs or symptoms) and appropriate clinical criteria for monitoring the important aspects of care
- establishes thresholds (or limits) for the indicators to trigger evaluation of care
- collects and organizes data for each indicator to analyze and monitor the important aspects of care
- evaluates health care when thresholds are reached to identify problems or opportunities to improve care
- acts to correct identified problems or to improve care
- assesses the effectiveness of corrective actions and documents improvements in care
- communicates the results of the monitoring and evaluation to relevant individuals, departments or services, quality improvement administrators and, in general, the entire health care staff.

pharmacy service. The director of each group then appoints a committee or quality management team to identify indicators of key elements of patient care, collect data, evaluate care, and take corrective actions or initiate improvements.

Step 2: Delineating scope of care and service

As a basis for future monitoring, the team members of each service must clearly define their group's function. To do so, they consider the types and numbers of patients treated, the patients' diagnoses, the treatments performed, the staff members providing the service, and the locations and times of care.

Step 3: Identifying key aspects of care

To pinpoint where quality management activities will begin, team members identify their group's most important functions by considering the type of care their service provides and determining which kinds of care:

- occur most frequently
- affect the greatest number of patients
- carry the greatest current risk or have posed the most problems for patients or staff in the past.

Step 4: Identifying indicators

The team members evaluate the latest information presented by researchers, journals, and professional organizations in relation to local, state, and national standards of care.

They undertake these studies to identify indicators for each key aspect of care. Basically, indicators measure the structures, processes, and outcomes of care.

Step 5: Establishing a means to trigger evaluations

Before data collection, team members must establish a threshold — a boundary that alerts the team to the need for an intensive review. For example, a mental health unit may establish a threshold for individual treatment plans, requiring the staff to complete 95% of these plans within 24 hours of admission. If the actual compliance rate were 92%, the threshold would remain unmet, triggering an investigation. Depending on the threshold at issue, the staff may need to review resources, staff education, or even a doctor's response time.

Not all thresholds are, or should be, set at 100%. Such a target might be unrealistic and, possibly, counterproductive. However, certain crucial aspects of care, such as the requirement to type all blood before a transfusion, should always have a threshold of 100%. Failing to meet this threshold — or any threshold that would jeopardize a patient's survival — should trigger an immediate, extensive review.

Occasionally, failing to meet a threshold may be justifiable. However, a pattern of noncompliance points to a problem requiring correction.

Step 6: Collecting and organizing data

Once the team members establish thresholds, they can begin collecting and organizing data for each one. (See *Collecting and organizing data,* page 48.)

Step 7: Initiating evaluation

The team members study the data, looking for trends or patterns to determine whether a problem exists or whether they need to investigate further. If no problem exists or if the team members find acceptable care, they take no further action. If the team members find unacceptable care or if they identify a problem, they proceed with appropriate action.

Step 8: Taking action to improve care and service

If possible, the team members recommend and initiate corrective action themselves. However, if the required action is beyond their authority, they make their recommendations to the person or department that does have the authority to act. A corrective action plan should identify:

- who or what needs to change
- who is responsible for implementing the action
- the specific action required in view of the problem's cause and severity
- when the change should occur.

Step 9: Assessing the effectiveness of actions

After suggesting or taking action, the team members continue to monitor and evaluate the problem area to assess whether the action resulted in a measurable improvement in patient care and to ensure that improvement is maintained.

Step 10: Communicating results

Whatever the findings, the quality management team members must report their findings to the quality management program director and to relevant staff members, departments, and services. This allows the quality management personnel to trace trends and

Collecting and organizing data

To make sure that the data collected for evaluation accurately represent the patient care provided, a health care facility's evaluators must establish a procedure for collecting and tabulating information.

Searching resources
First, the evaluators must decide exactly which areas of care they need to know more about. Then they'll choose relevant resources for scrutiny. For example, they may collect data from parts of the medical record, such as the nurses' progress notes and laboratory reports, and from medication administration records or other documents, such as incident reports and logs.

Choosing a method
The evaluators must decide how to collect the information needed to review the quality of patient care. The methods used are retrospective, concurrent, or prospective.

Deciding on the sample size
Next, the evaluators must determine how many instances of care — procedures, treatments, or patients with the same diagnosis, for example — they'll need to study.

Typically they'll base their decision on frequency. For example, for an aspect of care that produces a rare complication, the evaluators may need a sample from only one source or a set of sources; on the other hand, for an aspect of care that produces problems consistently, they may need to collect much more data from many more sources.

Determining frequency
When deciding on the frequency of data collection, the evaluators must review such factors as the number of patients involved, the anticipated risk of the procedure or treatment being studied, the regularity of the care being studied, the extent to which the care measures have been problem-free, and so forth. However, they must collect data frequently enough for comparison with threshold data.

Evaluating results
Ideally, cumulative data for each indicator should be available for periodic comparison with corresponding thresholds. Evaluating indicators and thresholds in this way helps evaluators determine early on whether intensive reviews and corrective actions (or improvements) are needed.

issues between medical staff services and other departments.

Besides being used when the JCAHO reviews the health care facility for accreditation, data collected by the quality management team also helps justify third-party insurance reimbursement and assignment of medical staff privileges.

Other documentation models

In addition to the JCAHO's 10-step model, several other models exist to document quality management. (See *Other models for ensuring quality management.*)

PRO focus

Developed to assist in the utilization review process, PROs consist of groups of doctors and nurses required by the federal government to monitor and evaluate the quality and appropriateness of care given. In carrying out this task, PROs rely heavily on documentation in the medical record.

PROs evaluate a sample of a health care facility's medical records. They compare the data with specific screening criteria to assess the need for and appropriateness of medical services. Their screening criteria include basic standards or conditions that a comparable

Other models for ensuring quality management

Aside from the 10-step model developed by the Joint Commission on Accreditation of Healthcare Organizations, a number of other models have been developed to continuously evaluate and document the quality management process. The models listed below use mnemonics to show the steps in the process.

PDCA cycle
(Developed by Walter A. Shewart in the 1930s)
- **P**lan: Study a process by collecting data and evaluating results.
- **D**o: Carry out the plan on a small-scale pilot.
- **C**heck: Check results of the change. (Some now use "S" for "study.")
- **A**ct: Implement the change or abandon the plan and go through the cycle again.

FOCUS
(Developed by Hospital Corporation of America)
- **F**ind a process to improve.
- **O**rganize a team that knows the process.
- **C**larify current knowledge.
- **U**nderstand variation.
- **S**elect a potential process improvement.

FADE
(Developed by Organizational Dynamics, Inc.)
- **F**ocus: Narrow a list of problems to one.
- **A**nalyze: Collect data and determine influential factors.
- **D**evelop: Formulate a plan to solve the problem.
- **E**xecute: Gain an organizational commitment, put plan into action, and monitor effect.

IMPROVE
(Developed by Ernst and Young)
- **I**dentify and define the problem.
- **M**easure the impact on customers.
- **P**rioritize possible causes.
- **R**esearch and analyze root causes.
- **O**utline alternative solutions.
- **V**alidate that solutions will work.
- **E**xecute solutions and standardize.

group of health care facilities can reasonably be expected to meet. In studying a sample of the medical records, the PROs focus on the intensity of services and the severity of illnesses. (For more information on PROs, see chapter 1, Nursing Documentation and the Medical Record.)

Because a PRO's primary focus is quality patient care carried out within cost-containment guidelines, the reviewers also scrutinize documented care as a means for determining reimbursements. (See *How PROs screen specialized care,* page 50.)

Case management focus

Case management is a threefold process that consists of identifying individuals with specific health care needs, formulating and implementing a plan that efficiently uses health care resources, and measuring patient outcomes along a continuum of care.

A case management system provides an additional way for health care facilities to improve quality and contain costs. Case managers help to coordinate a patient's long-term care by using resources throughout the community. One of their primary goals is to control costs. In the process, they influence both the type of health care services a patient receives and where he receives them.

How PROs screen specialized care

When reviewing medical records, peer review organizations (PROs) use special screening criteria to evaluate the intensity of services and the severity of illness. These factors have a direct impact on Medicare and Medicaid reimbursement.

Being familiar with the PRO's criteria can help you document appropriately to demonstrate that patient care complies with Medicare and Medicaid standards. That, in turn, maximizes reimbursement.

Below are the monitoring, medication, and treatment screening criteria that a PRO looks for when verifying that care given in an alcohol or drug detoxification unit meets Medicare and Medicaid standards.

Monitoring criteria

A patient in an alcohol or drug detoxification unit should be monitored every 1 to 2 hours. Monitoring must be appropriate, needed, and ordered.

The caregiver needs to monitor:

- vital signs (pulse and respiratory rates and blood pressure every 1 to 2 hours; temperature at least every 4 hours)
- level of consciousness
- orientation to time and place
- fluid intake and output
- pupillary reaction to light and pupil size
- potential or actual signs and symptoms of withdrawal.

Medication criteria

Reimbursable medications include:

- I.V. medications (excluding vitamins and potassium unless potassium replacement was ordered and administered for documented hypokalemia)
- oral or I.M. medications to control acute withdrawal signs and symptoms (including chlordiazepoxide, magnesium sulfate, and thiamine).

Treatment criteria

Besides medication administration, treatment may include:

- I.V. therapy to replace or maintain the patient's fluid volume; the flow rate needs to exceed a keep-vein-open rate and be appropriate for the patient's body mass and condition
- initial need, continuing need, or both, as documented by the doctor, for inpatient detoxification to stabilize the patient's mental and physical condition.

Case management began as an offshoot of the Medicare and Medicaid waiver-demonstration projects, which made exceptions to usual federal Medicare and Medicaid eligibility requirements. The exceptions (or waivers) extended health care coverage to certain patients who could use community and nursing services at home. The intent was to prevent unnecessary nursing home admissions; the result is an expanded role for many nurses.

Nurses as case managers

Case managers direct patient care to the most cost-effective health care setting while still meeting quality standards. Today's case manager must ensure that the patient's care and reimbursement for care are appropriate for his diagnosis — or diagnosis-related group (DRG).

The case management system forces health care facilities to deliver care economically without compromising quality. If you become a case manager, your role will change from giving hands-on nursing care to coordinating cost-effective health care in various settings. You'll manage a closely monitored and controlled system of multidisciplinary care. You'll be responsible for outcomes, length of stay, and use of resources throughout the patient's illness — not just during your shift. And you'll become an expert at scrutinizing and interpreting nursing documentation. These records play a key role in the effect case managers have on a hospital.

Case managers scrutinize the medical record — especially the nursing documentation — to determine whether a patient's continued hospital and other health care costs and treatment are justified.

Case management is one of the services listed under the Comprehensive Omnibus Budget Reconciliation Act (commonly known as COBRA). This federal law permits states to apply for waivers and offer community services for patients eligible for nursing home care.

Outside of the health care facility, case managers may be in private practice or employed by home care agencies, family service agencies, hospitals, area agencies on aging, and health maintenance organizations (HMOs).

Quality management team efforts

Required for JCAHO accreditation and mandated by COBRA, quality management teams (or committees) are another means by which an organization monitors and evaluates the quality and appropriateness of patient care. Both acute care and long-term care facilities can use the JCAHO 10-step model as a guideline for quality management activities.

Quality management teams perform the following functions:

- They generate documentation to confirm that the care provided meets accepted standards.
- They identify areas that need improvement.
- They draw attention to problems.

Ongoing monitoring and evaluation provide information on the outcome of high-volume and high-risk services, which is required for budget and strategic planning. And examining areas of frequent and infrequent use helps the health care facility assess various needs. For example, an operating area that handles fewer than five elective neurosurgical cases yearly may use quality management data to evaluate the cost-effectiveness of continuing this service.

Other data may provide information that is useful to the community. For example, the health care facility may learn that it's located in a community experiencing a sudden increase in the number of school-age children. Such demographic data may serve to justify expansion of pediatric health services.

For nurses, especially, ongoing quality management activities, such as monitoring of medication administration, serve two purposes: They identify problems and track trends or patterns, and they also evaluate the performance of individual nurses, who are identified in the data by a numerical code. This enables nurse-managers to assess the performance and competence of the nurses they supervise. (See *Completing a quality management report,* page 52.)

What's more, the documentation gathered by quality management teams serves as a self-review for reimbursement eligibility. By applying the screening criteria used by third-party payers, an organization can estimate its projected revenues. Documentation

BETTER CHARTING

Completing a quality management report

Once you've identified troublesome issues or events, your next step is to complete a report similar to the one below. The quality management team may then use it to confirm that patient care meets accepted standards and to identify areas for improvement.

EVALUATION PERIOD: 1/99 **TO** 6/99
DEPARTMENT: Nursing 3 North
REPORT WRITER: Sharon Neilson, RN, BSN, Nurse Manager, 3 North

Date	January 1999	March 1999
Issue	Patients late for physical therapy appointments. Statistic provided by Rehab Dept.: 252 appointments scheduled for 3 North patients in November, December, and January; 104 (41%) were late for appointments. 59% were on time.	Orders for one-time doses of medication are inconsistently documented on both the physician order sheet and the medication administration record. Rate of compliance for January, February, and March is 62%.
Action	Met with department manager of physical therapy and 3 North nurses. Plan: Rehab Dept. will send schedule of appointments to 3 North by 1800 hours the previous day. Physical therapy appointment will be incorporated into the daily nurse assignment.	Reviewed policy with all nurses. Each shift assigned to monitor and submit results to Mary Lake, RN, who is the quality management coordinator for 3 North.
Follow-up	Compliance monitored for February, March, and April. Results: 231 appointments were scheduled. Patients were late for 26 (11%) of the appointments. 89% were on time. Results reflect a 30% improvement.	Compliance monitored for April, May, and June. Results: 81% compliance rate. Results reflect a 19% improvement.
Resolution	Continue to monitor for the next quarter. 90% of patients on time for appointments is an acceptable threshold based on the cooperation level of patients, the transport system, and emergencies on 3 North.	Continue to monitor for next quarter. A compliance rate of 100% is the goal, based on safety and billing issues. Quality management coordinator will track by nursing staff.

Using JCAHO indicators to improve quality of care

The Joint Commission on Accreditation of Healthcare Organizations (JCAHO) publishes a series of indicators for health care facilities to use in monitoring patients. These indicators cover perioperative, obstetric, oncologic, cardiovascular, and trauma care; medication use; and infection control. Carrying out and documenting these indicator actions helps a facility accumulate data to measure its performance, compare its performance with that of similar health care facilities, monitor trends, and enlist feedback from the JCAHO.

The following chart presents four JCAHO indicators and the corresponding patient populations being monitored.

INDICATOR	PATIENT POPULATION
Preoperative patient evaluation, intraoperative and postoperative monitoring, and timely clinical intervention	Patients who develop a central nervous system (CNS) complication within 2 days of procedures involving anesthesia administration, subcategorized by the American Society of Anesthesiologists' physical status class, patient age, and CNS- versus non–CNS-related procedures
Preoperative patient evaluation, appropriate surgical preparation, intraoperative and postoperative monitoring, and timely clinical intervention	Patients who develop a peripheral neurologic deficit within 2 days of procedures involving anesthesia administration
Prenatal patient evaluation, education, and treatment selection	Patients who undergo a vaginal birth after cesarean section
Prenatal patient evaluation, intrapartum monitoring, and clinical intervention	Live-born infants with a birth weight less than 2,500 g

compliance increases the likelihood of reimbursement for services provided.

Comparing data against national standards

In today's increasingly competitive health care market, there is a greater focus on comparing outcome data to other health care facilities' data. Such data help a facility identify areas needing improvement and gauge how it measures up to the competition. In addition, more and more health care consumers are demanding comparative performance results in order to make sure they get their money's worth from the health care system.

The JCAHO publishes a series of quality management indicators for use in monitoring perioperative, obstetric, oncologic, cardiovascular, and trauma care; medication use; and infection control. (See *Using JCAHO indicators to improve quality of care.*)

Further oversight needed

Although there are a number of quality-measurement tools that enable health care facilities to evaluate their performance, there is as yet no national quality oversight system to guarantee that quality management objectives are met. Such a system would need to offer four major features:

- an adaptable standards-based evaluation framework that relates processes to desirable patient outcomes
- a group of mature, user-friendly, cost-effective measurement systems
- capability to evaluate all levels of the delivery system
- achievement of consensus on the best evaluation tools and effective coordination of evaluation activities among all major evaluators in the public and private sectors.

Nursing staff quality

The paper trail accumulated in the medical record and elsewhere in the health care facility describes not only the patient's progress but also the nurse's performance. Data sources, such as indicators that measure clinical outcomes, personnel records, nursing credentials, and other documents, contribute to a full assessment of the quality of the nurse's care and qualifications.

A JCAHO quality standard for nursing care in specialty units states: "The supervision of nursing care in the unit is provided by a designated registered nurse (RN) who has relevant education, training, and experience and who has demonstrated current competence." Typically, the JCAHO auditors, quality management teams, and others judge compliance with this standard by evaluating various kinds of documentation.

Documentation of standards

To confirm the RN requirement, reviewers look for a valid RN license. They also survey staffing schedules and assignment sheets to verify that an RN is designated to supervise nursing care. They confirm relevant education, training, and experience by checking references and reviewing the nurse's continuing education units.

The reviewers assess a nurse's competence by following the intent of JCAHO nursing care standards (NC.2 through NC.2.4.1.1). These standards outline the documentation required to assess the clinical competence of nursing staff members, nursing personnel from outside agencies, and specialty unit nursing staff.

For example, expanded standards for nurses in a special care unit require the nurse to be knowledgeable about the emotional and rehabilitative needs of her patients and able to provide appropriate interventions. Reviewing documentation and patient outcomes enables supervisory personnel to evaluate the competence of nursing staff members. (See *Using documentation to assess specialty nursing ability.*)

All nurses — not just those in special care units — must perform their assigned duties competently. Again this requirement is defined by the JCAHO. A starting point for defining and documenting the scope of any nurse's responsibilities is a thorough job description.

Specific strategies to achieve quality nursing documentation center on the medical record. Nursing entries verify the quality of patient care, assist caregivers in coordinating treatment, and provide legal protection for the nurse and the employer.

Other resources to consult regarding quality nursing and documentation include the health care facility's risk management office, the medical records department, and the utilization management staff.

CHARTING GUIDELINES

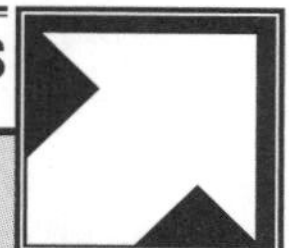

Using documentation to assess specialty nursing ability

The Joint Commission on Accreditation of Healthcare Organizations (JCAHO) publishes standards outlining the documentation needed to verify that a nurse assigned to a special care unit performs competently, thereby ensuring quality care.

According to JCAHO standards, documentation should demonstrate that the nurse can:

- interpret electrocardiograms and recognize significant arrhythmias
- interpret abnormal laboratory test values
- administer routinely used and emergency drugs
- initiate cardiopulmonary resuscitation and other patient safety measures as defined by facility policy
- perform defibrillation, as appropriate
- administer parenteral fluids, blood, and blood components
- provide respiratory and ventilatory care
- coordinate multidisciplinary care
- provide for patient and staff safety
- adhere to infection control policies and procedures.

FISCAL IMPLICATIONS OF DOCUMENTATION

What the nurse documents in the medical record — and how she documents it — has a direct impact not only on the quality of patient care but also on the health care facility's revenues. The nurse's progress notes, flowcharts, plans of care, and medication administration records are scrutinized by Medicare, Medicaid, and insurance company reviewers in addition to peer reviewers, case managers, and caregiving staff, among others.

The quality of care, patient outcomes, and the need for continued treatment are judged according to the documentation. For example, vital signs, level of consciousness, infusion rates, and administration of injectable medications are all parameters used to determine whether the patient should continue his stay in a health care facility. Failure to provide sufficient documentation may result in denial of reimbursement or transfer of the patient to an alternative health care setting. Unsatisfactory but avoidable outcomes may result in denial of payment.

Specific and complete nursing records are the key to ensuring financial reimbursement. Your records must be clear and concise. They must validate not only care and treatment but also the items that are billed. For example, a bill for 20 suction catheters used in a 24-hour period is unlikely to be paid if nursing documentation indicates that the patient was suctioned as needed during that time.

Reimbursement structures

Today's health care system includes multiple, complex structures with multiple, complex requirements for receiving reimbursement. Caregivers and health care facilities must deal not only with internal quality management teams, case managers, and required reimbursement structures (such as DRGs and COBRA requirements) but also with federal and state agencies, HMOs, preferred provider organizations (PPOs), and independent practice associations (IPAs), among others.

Reviewers from these groups examine the medical record for discrepancies. They look for differences in the treatment ordered and the treatment provided. If a discrepancy can't be explained satisfactorily or reconciled reasonably, payment may be denied.

DRGs

The basis for federal health care reimbursements, the DRG system groups diseases and disorders into specific categories. A DRG includes information about the principal and secondary diagnoses, surgical procedures, and the patient's age, sex, and discharge status.

When Medicare adopted a prospective payment system (PPS), reimbursement regulations changed. Before PPS, Medicare reimbursed a health care provider according to a cost-per-case formula. After PPS, Medicare computed reimbursements prospectively, using a formula adjusted for diagnostic groups, signs and symptoms, hospital, region, wage levels, and other relevant factors — the DRG system.

Today, health care facilities must ensure meticulous compliance with DRG preadmission and continued-stay criteria to ensure reimbursement. Likewise, they must adhere to the details of the DRG coding process.

The medical record must contain documentation verifying the DRG and supporting the appropriateness of care given in the health care facility. What's more, nursing documentation needs to support the diagnoses and indicate that appropriate patient and family teaching and discharge planning were provided.

COBRA

The federal law known as COBRA allows employees to temporarily be covered under their employer's health insurance when they would otherwise lose this benefit because of terminated employment or another qualifying event, such as a reduction in work hours or retirement.

Precise documentation is essential when providing care for patients insured under COBRA. The law requires health care facilities receiving federal funds to evaluate any patients admitted to the emergency department. Specifically, it states that a patient's condition must be stable before he's transferred to another health care facility. If the patient is in labor, her labor must be controlled before she is transferred to another health care facility.

To make sure that health care facilities comply with the law, COBRA and the JCAHO both require that all facilities thoroughly document their actions concerning patient transfers. This documentation must include the chronology of the event, measures taken or treatment implemented, the patient's response to treatment, and the results of the measures taken to prevent the patient's condition from worsening.

HMOs

An HMO is an organized system that provides an agreed-upon set of comprehensive inpatient and outpatient health services to a voluntarily enrolled population in exchange for a predetermined, fixed, and periodic payment.

An HMO may contract for beds and services and may build or buy hospitals. Many HMOs feature doctors who work for a salary or in a partnership arrangement. Or, the HMO may contract for medical services from individual doctors and may function as either a profit-making or nonprofit organization.

IPAs

Consisting of an independent group of doctors, an IPA offers services to a specified group of patients. Many HMOs contract with IPAs for medical services.

PPOs

A PPO contracts with health care providers, including hospitals, doctors, therapists, pharmacies, and other professional services. The contracted fees are typically lower than customary, with the understanding that PPOs will channel patients into empty hospital beds and underutilized services.

Medicare and Medicaid payments

Payments by Medicare and Medicaid are sources of operating revenue for hospitals. Both have specific requirements for participation and reimbursement.

Initially, a state agency determines whether a health care facility is eligible to participate in the Medicare program. In doing so, the state agency certifies that the hospital:

- holds JCAHO or American Osteopathic Association accreditation
- uses an adequate utilization review plan that is, or will be, in effect on the first day of the hospital's participation
- meets statutory requirements or, if not, proposes reasonable plans to correct deficiencies and demonstrates evidence of adequate patient care despite any shortcomings.

Medicare certifies hospitals for a 2-year period. Certification guidelines can be used to evaluate the function of all hospital services. Medicare and Medicaid also examine compliance with state and local laws and JCAHO standards. Health care facilities can use the steps for Medicare certification as preparation for JCAHO accreditation.

How documentation affects costs

Nursing documentation provides the data that examiners need to justify reimbursement for health care expenses. Besides studying the records to estimate revenues, examiners use the records to calculate nursing care costs.

Calculating nursing care costs

Traditionally, the cost of nursing care was included in the patient's daily room rate. Now, however, health care facilities are applying standard cost-accounting techniques to nursing care.

First, nurses estimate the number of nursing hours required to provide a quality patient outcome. Then, financial management personnel estimate the cost of that nursing time. A major component in providing patient care, the cost of nursing care is directly related to the type and level of care provided. Health care facilities typically factor nursing care costs into the financial and strategic planning process.

Some facilities bill patients separately for nursing care, using pricing systems that charge only for care the patient actually receives. Determining the cost of nursing time requires detailed documentation so that appropriate charges can be billed and validated. Nursing documentation then becomes a detailed financial record.

Calculating skilled care costs

Provided by RNs or by licensed practical nurses under an RN's supervision, skilled nursing care involves continuous use of the nursing process, technologically complex monitoring, and patient teaching. It also includes planning, organizing, and managing the plan of care with the doctor and other health care professionals.

Skilled nursing care requires specialized education and the ability to document competently. It differs from custodial care, which focuses on assistance with activities of daily living, such as eating, dressing, bathing, and walking, and which may be provided by nonskilled personnel.

Examples of skilled nursing care activities include the following:

- managing central venous lines
- administering I.M., S.C., or I.V. fluids or medications
- treating infected or extensive pressure ulcers
- administering oxygen
- providing nasopharyngeal suctioning
- managing enteral feedings
- changing sterile dressings.

How documentation affects revenues

Medicare Part A provides coverage for skilled nursing care; Part B, for durable medical equipment and supplies. Payment for services to patients insured by Medicare is based on their documented need for skilled nursing care and covers supplies and equipment used during that care.

Continued payment depends on *daily* documentation demonstrating the patient's ongoing need for skilled care. The quality of documentation in this area directly affects the amount of Medicare payments and other insurance reimbursements.

Documentation must confirm that the nursing staff meets various care standards, such as:

- adhering to the nursing process
- timely recording of changes in the patient's condition and care needs
- using medical equipment (such as bedpans, nebulizers, indwelling catheters, and walkers) judiciously and appropriately to meet the patient's needs
- adequately teaching the patient about his condition and treatment plan.

Finally, examiners search the documentation carefully for any inconsistencies that may hinder reimbursement. (See *Avoiding inconsistent documentation.*)

Importance of the nursing process

The nursing process involves the problem solving and decision making that nurses do to provide patient care. It's a simple, systematic process made up of five steps: assessment, nursing diagnosis, planning, implementation, and evaluation. The steps are always sequential and the process is cyclical. The completion of the fifth step returns you to the first step for reassessment. The nursing process stops when the patient is discharged.

Correctly used, the nursing process permeates every aspect of nursing documentation. Every patient event and assessment is recorded. The five-step process ensures compliance with plan of care requirements mandated by both acute care and long-term care standards. The nursing process is also evident throughout JCAHO requirements and regulations. (For more information, see chapter 8, Documentation of the Nursing Process.)

CHARTING GUIDELINES

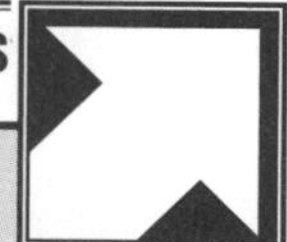

Avoiding inconsistent documentation

Inconsistencies in documentation leave both you and your health care facility open to accusations of incompetence and fiscal irresponsibility. What's more, a medical record containing inconsistencies can be difficult or impossible to defend in court. To avoid inconsistencies, follow these guidelines.

Be precise
For example, describing the exact size and location of a pressure ulcer (such as "2.5 cm × 2 cm × 3 cm deep, right elbow") minimizes guesswork when reviewing the patient's progress, whereas an approximation (such as "small, deep pressure ulcer on the patient's arm") may be judged inconsistent if previous or later descriptions differ.

Be specific
For example, describing an object or process in quantifiable terms, such as "500 ml of tea-colored urine" clearly specifies characteristics, whereas "about 400 to 500 ml of discolored urine" leaves room for later misinterpretation and inconsistencies.

Be thorough — and avoid summarizing
For example, a reviewer who encounters a complete outcome evaluation of teaching effectiveness, such as "Patient can correctly remove the colostomy bag, clean the ostomy site, and apply a new bag without assistance," is less likely to question your patient-teaching performance than a reviewer who encounters an evaluation stating "Patient handles his own colostomy care."

Changes in condition and care

When a patient's condition changes, documentation becomes a quality, reimbursement, and legal issue. An improvement in the patient's condition may signal a successful outcome and the need for discharge. A deterioration demands concise, factual recording of events.

A baseline assessment is recorded when each patient is admitted to the facility. Later changes are evaluated against the presenting signs and symptoms, health history, physical examination, and ancillary test results.

Admission, transfer, and discharge notes must accurately reflect changes in the patient's condition. Condition changes justify changes in care and subsequent reimbursement. The appropriateness of admission, transfer, and discharge is also evaluated based on the patient's condition. JCAHO standards provide guidelines for recording changes in the patient's condition and care.

Use of equipment

Nursing documentation provides evidence that certain equipment is essential to patient care, verifies that the equipment has been used appropriately, and justifies reimbursement. For example, documentation of an order for bed rest supports a patient's need for a bedpan, and documentation of insulin-dependent diabetes supports a patient's need for a blood glucose monitor. Examiners require this documentation before approving reimbursement.

Patient education

JCAHO standards require comprehensive patient education. In addition to informing the patient about relevant tests, treatments, and procedures, patient teaching can verify that a patient is ready for discharge. Documented teaching outcomes can also protect a health care facility and its nurses from legal problems.

According to JCAHO guidelines, patient teaching is required for many topics, including:

- medication use
- medical equipment use
- potential food and drug interactions
- rehabilitation techniques
- community resources
- further treatment.

Patient teaching must be interdisciplinary and related to the plan of care. In addition, arrangements must be made to communicate all discharge instructions to the person or organization responsible for continuing the patient's care.

Inconsistencies

Nursing documentation must be consistent to maximize reimbursement. Charting based on a central problem list or an interdisciplinary plan of care produces uniform data. Inconsistencies occur when nurses use different baseline criteria or record imprecise information.

Keep in mind that Medicare and other insurance examiners will always request an explanation for conflicting data in the medical record and that accurate details may be difficult to obtain retrospectively. The result of inconsistent data could be denial of payment.

Selected references

Dewing, K.C. "Case Management Information Needs: Effective Tools in the Management of Patient Care and Cost Containment," *Nursing Case Management* 2(4):168-72, July-August 1997.

Herzlinger, R. *Market-Driven Health Care: Who Wins, Who Loses in the Transformation of America's Largest Service Industry.* Reading, Mass.: Addison-Wesley-Longman Publishing Co., 1997.

Huggins, C.M., and Phillips, C.Y. "Using Case Management with Clinical Plans to Improve Patient Outcomes," *Home Healthcare Nurse* 16(1):14-20, January 1998.

Joint Commission on Accreditation of Healthcare Organizations (JCAHO). *Comprehensive Accreditation Manual for Hospitals: The Official Handbook.* Oakbrook Terrace, Ill.: JCAHO, 1998.

Mitchell, E. "Medicaid, Medicare, and Managed Care," *Journal of Case Management* 6(1):8-12, Spring 1997.

Rieve, J.A. "Guidelines and Outcomes: Quality Management Tools," Part I. *Case Manager* 8(6):38-41, November-December 1997.

Rieve, J.A. "Guidelines and Outcomes: Quality Management Tools," Part II. *Case Manager* 9(1):22-24, January-February 1998.

4

Documentation Systems

Although each health care facility determines its own requirements for documentation and evaluation, those requirements must comply with legal, accreditation, and professional standards.

Similarly, a nursing department can select the documentation system it wants to use as long as the system demonstrates adherence to standards and care requirements. For example, the system known as charting by exception (CBE) requires you to document only significant or abnormal findings. If the standard requires all patients' vital signs to be taken every 4 hours, you needn't document that you performed this activity but you do need to document any abnormal vital signs.

Regardless of the documentation system used, specific policies and procedures for documentation must be in place and known. Understanding them will help you document care accurately. It will also serve you well when evaluating or modifying your documentation system or when selecting a new one.

SYSTEM SELECTION

As health care facilities strive for greater efficiency and quality of care, you may need to participate in the decision about whether your current documentation system needs a simple revision, a total overhaul, or no change at all. Your aim: a system that reflects not only the patient's response to care but also the quality of care (which must meet the profession's accepted standards).

MEASURING UP TO STANDARD

The committees that set up continuous quality improvement programs (mandated by state regulations and the Joint Commission on Accreditation of Healthcare Organizations [JCAHO]) choose well-defined, objective, and readily measurable indicators that help them assess the structure, process, and outcome of patient care. They use these indicators to monitor and evaluate the contents of a patient's medical record.

To verify that treatment was required and provided or that medical tests and supplies were used, third-party payers (the insurers) review nursing documentation carefully. As a result, nurses now document more than ever before, including such data as every I.V. needle used to start an infusion, each use of an I.V. pump to deliver a specific volume of medication, and every test that the patient undergoes. (See chapter 1, Nursing Documentation and the Medical Record, and chapter 3, Quality Management and Reimbursement, for more information about standards and regulations concerning nursing documentation.)

Both shorter hospital stays and the need to verify the use of supplies and equipment in patient care have placed greater emphasis on nursing documentation as a yardstick for measuring not only the provision of patient care but also its quality. As quality indicators change, facilities must change their documentation to remain in compliance. Therefore, documentation review must be ongoing.

EVALUATING YOUR CURRENT SYSTEM

In evaluating your documentation system, ask the following questions:

- What are the specific positive features of the current documentation system?
- What are the specific problems or limitations of the current documentation system? How can they be solved?

Evaluating your documentation system

When reviewing the usefulness of your current documentation system, consider the following questions. If you answer no to any of them, you might recommend a closer evaluation of your system.

Documenting interventions and patient progress

- Does your current system reflect the patient's progress and the interventions based on recorded evaluations? Look for records that describe the patient's progress, actual interventions, and evaluations of provided care.
- Does the record include evidence of the patient's response to nursing care? For example, does it report the effectiveness of analgesics or the patient's response to I.V. medications? Does it show that care was modified according to the patient's response to treatment? For example, does it show what action was taken if the patient tolerated only half of a prescribed tube feeding?
- Does the record note continuity of care or exhibit unexplained gaps? If gaps appear, are notes entered later that document previous interventions? If late entries appear in the nursing notes on subsequent days, do you have to check the entire record to validate care?
- Are daily activities documented? For example, do the notes include evidence that the patient bathed himself or indicate that the patient could independently transfer himself to a wheelchair?

Documenting the health care team's actions

- Does the record portray the nursing process clearly? Look for actual nursing diagnoses, written assessments, interventions, and evaluation of the patient's responses to them.
- Does the current documentation system facilitate and show communication among health care team members? Check for evidence that telephone calls were made, that doctors were paged and notified of changes in a patient's condition, and that actions reflected these communications.
- Is discharge planning clearly documented? Do the records show evidence of interdisciplinary coordination, team conferences, completed patient teaching, and discharge instructions?
- Does the record reflect current standards of care? Does it indicate that caregivers and administrators follow hospital policies and procedures? If not, does the system provide for explanations of why a policy wasn't implemented or was implemented in an alternative manner?

Checking for clarity and comprehensiveness

- Are all portions of the record complete? Are all flow sheets, checklists, and other forms completed according to hospital policy? Are all necessary entries apparent on the medication forms? If not, does the record describe why a medication wasn't given as ordered and who was informed of the omission if necessary?
- Does the documentation make sense? Can you track the patient's care and hospital course on this record alone?
- Can you read your patient's record for the previous 24 hours of documentation and determine his problem, the interventions provided, and the outcomes obtained?

- How much time will be needed to develop a new system, educate staff, and implement changes?
- How much will changing the current system cost? (Consider the costs of time, staff education, and new equipment.) Will the result eventually save money?
- How will changing the documentation system affect other members of the health care team, including the business office, personnel, and medical staff? How will they handle resistance to the proposed changes? (See *Evaluating your documentation system.*)

(Text continues on page 66.)

Comparing charting systems

This chart summarizes the main features of the most commonly used documentation systems, which are discussed later in this chapter.

SYSTEM	USEFUL SETTINGS	PARTS OF RECORD	ASSESSMENT
Narrative	■ Acute care ■ Long-term care ■ Home care ■ Ambulatory care	■ Progress notes ■ Flow sheets to supplement plan of care	■ Initial: history and admission form ■ Ongoing: progress notes
POMR	■ Acute care ■ Long-term care ■ Home care	■ Database ■ Plan of care ■ Problem list ■ Progress notes ■ Discharge summary	■ Initial: database and plan of care ■ Ongoing: progress notes
PIE	■ Acute care	■ Assessment flow sheet ■ Progress notes ■ Problem list	■ Initial: assessment form ■ Ongoing: assessment form every shift
Focus	■ Acute care ■ Long-term care	■ Progress notes ■ Flow sheets ■ Checklists	■ Initial: patient history and admission assessment ■ Ongoing: assessment form
CBE	■ Acute care ■ Long-term care	■ Plan of care ■ Flow sheets, including patient-teaching records and patient discharge notes ■ Graphic record	■ Initial: database assessment sheet ■ Ongoing: nursing-medical order flow sheet
FACT	■ Acute care ■ Long-term care	■ Assessment sheet ■ Flow sheets ■ Progress notes	■ Initial: baseline assessment ■ Ongoing: flow sheet and progress notes
AIR	■ Acute care ■ Long-term care	■ Flow sheets ■ Plan of care ■ Progress notes	■ Initial: baseline assessment ■ Ongoing: flow sheet and progress notes

Selecting a new system

If assessing your current system indicates the need for a new system, begin by organizing a committee (or task force) composed of members from all departments that the change will affect. Having interdisciplinary representatives on this committee will facilitate acceptance of the new system when it's put into ef-

PLAN OF CARE	OUTCOMES AND EVALUATION	PROGRESS NOTES FORMAT
■ Plan of care	■ Progress notes ■ Discharge summaries	■ Narration at time of entry
■ Database ■ Nursing plan of care based on problem list	■ Progress notes (section E of SOAPIE and SOAPIER)	■ SOAP, SOAPIE, SOAPIER
■ None; included in progress notes (section P)	■ Progress notes (section E)	■ Problem ■ Intervention ■ Evaluation
■ Nursing plan of care based on problems or nursing diagnoses	■ Progress notes (section R)	■ Data ■ Action ■ Response
■ Nursing plan of care based on nursing diagnoses	■ Progress notes (section E)	■ SOAPIE or SOAPIER
■ Nursing plan of care based on nursing diagnoses	■ Flow sheet (section R)	■ Data ■ Action ■ Response
■ Nursing plan of care	■ Progress notes (section R)	■ Assessment ■ Intervention ■ Response

(continued)

fect. The committee should research all available systems; consult other health care facilities about systems that work or don't work for them; assess the change's likely costs, time commitment, and effects on staff members; and evaluate each system for how well it satisfies professional standards and regulation requirements. (See *Comparing charting systems.*)

Comparing charting systems *(continued)*

SYSTEM	USEFUL SETTINGS	PARTS OF RECORD	ASSESSMENT
Core (with DAE)	■ Acute care ■ Long-term care	■ Kardex ■ Flow sheets ■ Progress notes	■ Initial: baseline assessment ■ Ongoing: progress notes
Outcome	■ Acute care ■ Long-term care ■ Home care ■ Ambulatory care	■ Progress notes ■ Flow sheets ■ Nursing plan of care ■ Database ■ Teaching plan	■ Initial: baseline assessment ■ Ongoing: progress notes

Once the committee selects a new system, the next step is to initiate training sessions to familiarize staff members with it. Consider implementing change in one unit or area at a time.

Then select or design the appropriate forms, and allow enough time for the transition to take place. Participants should be encouraged to alert the committee to any problems that arise during implementation of the new system.

Revising an existing system

Altering a documentation system usually involves changing the way you collect, enter, and retrieve information, but it rarely affects the content of the information. If the content of your existing system is deficient in some way, changing formats probably won't solve the problem.

Content problems usually stem from sources outside the system — for example, inadequate objectives or guidelines or insufficient time to document properly. In such cases, it may be preferable to amend the existing system instead of selecting a new one.

Following the system format

Depending on the policies of your health care facility, you'll use one or more documentation systems to record your nursing interventions and evaluations and the patient's response.

Some health care facilities elect to use traditional narrative charting systems or newer narrative methods (such as AIR). Others choose alternative systems, such as problem-oriented medical record (POMR), problem-intervention-evaluation (PIE), focus, charting-by-exception (CBE), FACT, core, and outcome documentation systems. In addition, many health care facilities are using computerized charting systems.

Of the many systems in current use, each has special features and distinct advantages and disadvantages.

PLAN OF CARE	OUTCOMES AND EVALUATION	PROGRESS NOTES FORMAT
■ Plan of care	■ Progress notes (section E)	■ Data ■ Action ■ Evaluation
■ Data base ■ Plan of care	■ Outcome-based plan of care	■ Evaluative statements ■ Expected outcomes ■ Learning outcomes

Traditional narrative charting

Traditional narrative charting systems document ongoing assessment data, nursing interventions, and patient responses in chronological order. Today, few facilities rely on the narrative system alone; most combine it with other systems.

Format and components

Narrative charting consists of a straightforward chronological account of the patient's status, the nursing interventions performed, and the patient's response to those interventions. The nurse usually records the data on the progress notes, with flow sheets commonly supplementing the narrative notes.

Knowing when to document, what to document, and how to organize the data are the key elements of effective narrative notes. (See *Charting with the narrative format,* page 68.)

When and what to document

Current JCAHO standards direct all health care facilities to establish policies about the frequency of patient reassessment. You must assess your patient as often as required by your facility's policy, if not more often, and then document your findings.

If you find yourself writing repetitious, meaningless notes, you may be documenting too often. In such a case, double-check your facility's written policy. You may find that you're following a time-consuming, unwritten standard initiated by staff members, not by your facility. To guard against this, review the policy at least every 6 months.

Besides documenting simply according to policy, be sure to record specific and descriptive narrative notes whenever you observe any of the following:

- a change in the patient's condition (progression, regression, or new problems). For example, write, "The patient can walk 300 feet assisted by one person."
- a patient's response to a treatment or medication. For example, write, "The patient

BETTER CHARTING

Charting with the narrative format

This progress note provides an example of the narrative documentation format.

Date	Time	Notes
2/5/99	1100	Removed three 4" x 4" gauze pads saturated with blood-tinged, nonodorous drainage from Ⓛ lower leg wound. Wound measures 6 cm x 6 cm wide x 1 cm deep. Surrounding skin reddened and tender. Redressed wound with four 4" x 4" dressings and one 4" x 8" dressing and hypoallergenic tape. Will check wound q 1 hr to assess for continued drainage. Will monitor pt.'s T q 4 hr. T-98.8R; BP-122/84; P-86; R-22. Pt. reports pain in Ⓛ lower leg at 8 on scale of 1 to 10, with 10 being the worst he can imagine. Administered two Percocet tablets and repositioned pt. from back to Ⓛ side. Will give Percocet 1/2 hour before subsequent dressing changes. Instructed pt. in dressing change procedure. Pt. stated "I know that it's important to wash my hands before I do anything so I don't get germs in my wound." Pt. demonstrated sufficient manual dexterity to put on gloves and handle all dressing supplies. Instructed pt. in proper hand-washing technique, dressing removal and disposal, opening and positioning dressing supplies, and signs and symptoms of wound infection and the importance of reporting them. Pt. demonstrated acceptable hand-washing technique and ability to remove dressings but needed instruction on positioning the leg so he could reach the wound. ——— Carol Witt, RN
2/5/99	1200	Ⓛ lower leg wound dressing dry and intact. Pt. reports pain in leg at 2 on scale of 1 to 10. ——— Carol Witt, RN

states that right leg pain is unrelieved 1 hour after receiving medication. He's still grimacing and rubbing the site."

- a lack of improvement in the patient's condition. For example, write, "No change in size or condition of leg wound after 5 days of treatment. Dimensions and condition remain as stated in 12/15/98 note."
- a patient or family member's response to teaching. For example, write, "The patient performed a return demonstration of wound care and correctly stated that he should do it three times a day."

Document exactly what you hear, observe, inspect, do, or teach. Include as much specific, descriptive information as possible. For example, if your patient has lower leg edema, include ankle and midcalf measurements and skin characteristics. Always document how the patient responds to your care and the extent of his progression toward a desired outcome.

How to write meaningful notes

- Read the narrative notes written by other health care professionals before you write your own.
- Read the notes recorded by nurses on other shifts and make additional comments on their findings. This demonstrates continuity of care.
- If policy permits, use flow sheets to document repetitious procedures or measurements and summarize the information in the narrative notes.
- Include specific information when you observe a change in your patient's condition, a lack of progress in his condition, or a response to treatment, medication, or patient teaching. Also record the exact time these events occurred. (See *Using military time.*)
- When possible, document an event immediately after it occurs. If you wait until the end of your shift, you may forget some important information. If you can't document at the time of an event, make notes on a piece of paper to help you remember details.

CHARTING GUIDELINES

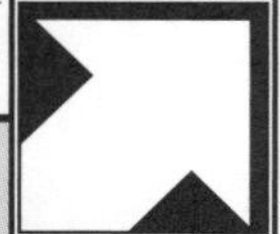

Using military time

To promote accurate charting, many institutions use military time equivalents. Such use avoids confusion over a.m. and p.m. entries.

0100 =	1 a.m.	1300 =	1 p.m.
0200 =	2 a.m.	1400 =	2 p.m.
0300 =	3 a.m.	1500 =	3 p.m.
0400 =	4 a.m.	1600 =	4 p.m.
0500 =	5 a.m.	1700 =	5 p.m.
0600 =	6 a.m.	1800 =	6 p.m.
0700 =	7 a.m.	1900 =	7 p.m.
0800 =	8 a.m.	2000 =	8 p.m.
0900 =	9 a.m.	2100 =	9 p.m.
1000 =	10 a.m.	2200 =	10 p.m.
1100 =	11 a.m.	2300 =	11 p.m.
1200 =	12 p.m.	2400 =	12 a.m.

How to organize your notes

Before you write anything, organize your thoughts so your paragraphs will be coherent. If you have difficulty deciding what to write, refer to the patient's plan of care to review unresolved problems, prescribed interventions, and expected outcomes. Then comment on the patient's progress in relation to these items.

If you still have trouble organizing your thoughts, use this sequence of questions to order your entry:

- How did I first become aware of the problem?
- What has the patient said about the problem that's significant?
- What have I observed that's related to the problem?
- What's my plan for dealing with the problem?
- What steps have I taken to intervene?
- How has the patient responded to my interventions?

To make your notes as coherent as possible, discuss each of the patient's problems in a separate paragraph.

Alternatively, you may use a head-to-toe approach to organize your information. Be sure to notify the doctor of significant changes that you observe. Then document this communication, the doctor's responses, any new orders to be implemented, and the patient's response to the intervention.

AIR: A narrative format

A charting format called AIR may help you organize and simplify your charting. The AIR format synthesizes major nursing events while avoiding repetition of information found elsewhere in the medical record. Combined with nursing flow sheets and the nursing plan of care, the AIR format can document your care clearly and concisely.

Here's how it works:

Assessment

Summarize your physical assessment findings. Rather than simply describing the patient's current condition, document trends and record your impression of the problem. Begin by titling each specific issue that you address, such as nursing diagnosis, admission note, and discharge planning.

Intervention

Summarize your actions and those of other caregivers in response to the assessment data. The summary may include a condensed nursing plan of care or plans for additional patient monitoring.

Response

Summarize the outcome or the patient's response to the nursing interventions. Because a response may not be evident for hours or even days, this documentation may not immediately follow the entries. In fact, it may be recorded by another nurse, which is why titling each of your assessments and interventions is so important.

Advantages

The most flexible of all the documentation systems, narrative charting suits any clinical setting and strongly conveys your nursing interventions and your patients' responses.

Because narration is the most common form of writing, the training time needed for new staff members is usually brief. Also, because narrative notes are in chronological order, other team members can review the patient's progress on a day-to-day basis.

The narrative format easily lends itself to presenting information collected over an extended period. Furthermore, the ease with which narrative notes combine with other documentation devices, such as flow sheets, helps to decrease charting time.

Disadvantages

Narrative charting can be weak when it comes to recording patient outcomes because you must read the entire record to arrive at the outcome. Even then, you may have trouble determining the outcome of a particular problem because the same information may not be consistently documented.

Tracking problems and identifying trends in the patient's progress can also be difficult and time consuming for the same reason: You have to read the entire record to arrive at an overall impression of the patient's condition and a complete account of his treatment course.

Because the narrative format offers no inherent guide to what's important to document, the tendency is to document everything; the result is a long, rambling, repetitive, subjective, and time-consuming record.

This system also makes it difficult to retrieve specific information, such as the patient's previous hospitalizations or surgeries, without reading the entire record.

The narrative format also lends itself to vague or inaccurate language, such as "appears to be bleeding" or "small amount." In addition, some problems may be documented briefly and others may be documented at length for no clear reason. (See *AIR: A narrative format.*)

Problem-oriented medical record system

Originally developed by doctors and later adapted by nurses, the problem-oriented medical record (POMR) system (also called the problem-oriented record), focuses on specific patient problems. In this documentation system, you'll describe each problem on multidisciplinary patient progress notes, not on progress notes containing only nursing information. (See *Writing a problem-oriented progress note,* page 72.)

Format and components

The POMR has five components: database, problem list, initial plan, progress notes, and discharge summary. You'll record your interventions and evaluations in the progress notes and the discharge summary only. To gain a full understanding of the POMR, briefly review all five components.

Database

Usually completed by a nurse, the database (or initial assessment) is a collection of subjective and objective information about the patient that forms the foundation for the patient's plan of care. This initial assessment includes the reason for hospitalization, medical history, allergies, medication regimen, physical and psychosocial findings, self-care ability, educational needs, and other discharge planning concerns. This information becomes the foundation for a problem list.

Problem list

After analyzing the database, you, the doctor, and other relevant health care team members will identify and list the patient's current problems in chronological order according to the date each was identified, not in order of acuteness or priority. Originally, this system called for one interdisciplinary problem list. You may still see this format used, but nurses and doctors usually keep separate problem lists with problems stated as either nursing or medical diagnoses. This problem list provides an overview of the patient's health status.

Try to number each problem so you can use the numbers to refer to the problems in the rest of the POMR. Make sure that every entry on the patient's initial plan, progress notes, and discharge summary corresponds to a number, and file the numbered problem list at the front of the patient's chart. Keep the problem list current by adding new numbers as new problems arise.

As soon as a problem is resolved, draw a line through it, or show that it's inactive by retiring the problem number and highlighting the problem with a colored felt-tip pen. Don't use that problem number again for the same patient.

Initial plan

After constructing the problem list, write an initial plan for each problem. This plan

BETTER CHARTING

Writing a problem-oriented progress note

Here's the nursing portion of a problem-oriented progress note. The nurse used the SOAP framework in the sample below.

Date	Time	Notes
3/20/99	1000	#1 Altered cerebral tissue perfusion R/T transient decrease in blood flow.
		S: Pt.: "I can't remember from one minute to the next."
		O: Pt. states she has no idea what day or time it is.
		Ⓡ pupil 3 mm and sluggish to react. Ⓛ pupil 3 mm and reacts briskly to light. Unsteady gait noted. Otherwise neurologic assessment normal.
		A: Pt. disoriented to time and has abnormal pupillary reaction in response to light.
		P: Notify the Dr. Orient pt. to time, place, and person q h. Assess the pt.'s ability to retain bilaterally equal motor function q h. Assess the patient for sensory deficits q h. Assess pupillary reaction to light q h. Assess the pt.'s BP q h. Assess pt.'s speech and memory for deficits q h. Marianne Evans, RN
		#2 High risk for injury R/T sensory and motor deficits.
		S: Pt.: "I feel dizzy and off balance."
		O: Pt.'s eyes fluttering; pt. holding onto bedside table.
		A: Pt. experiencing dizziness and loss of balance similar to previous episode of TIA.
		P: Assist pt. back to bed and place side rails up. Modify environment to prevent injury. Marianne Evans, RN
		#3 Anxiety R/T possible CVA.
		S: Pt. reports being scared of what will happen to her if she has a stroke — who will take care of her?
		O: Pt. clutching onto siderails and hyperventilating.
		A: Pt. becoming increasingly anxious.
		P: Discuss pt.'s anxiety and feelings about her illness. Help pt. identify the source of her anxiety. Identify and use effective coping mechanisms with the pt. Assure pt. that she will be monitored closely.
		Marianne Evans, RN

should include the expected outcomes, plans for further data collection (if needed), and patient care and teaching plans. Mutual goal setting is essential to ensure patient compliance and the effectiveness of your interventions.

Progress notes

One of the most prominent features of the POMR system is the structured way in which narrative progress notes are written by all team members, using the SOAP, SOAPIE, or SOAPIER format.

SOAP format

If you use the SOAP format, you'll document the following information for each problem:

- **S**ubjective data: information the patient or family members tell you, such as the chief complaint and other impressions
- **O**bjective data: factual, measurable data you gather during the assessment, such as observed signs and symptoms, vital signs, and laboratory test values
- **A**ssessment data: conclusions based on the collected subjective and objective data and formulated as patient problems or nursing diagnoses (This dynamic and ongoing process changes as more or different subjective and objective information becomes known.)
- **P**lan: your strategy for relieving the patient's problem (including both immediate or short-term actions and long-term measures).

SOAPIE format

Some facilities use the SOAPIE format, adding:

- **I**ntervention: measures you've taken to achieve an expected outcome (As the patient's health status changes, you may need to modify these interventions. Be sure to document the patient's understanding and acceptance of the initial plan in this section of your notes.)
- **E**valuation: an analysis of the effectiveness of your interventions. (If expected outcomes fall short, use the evaluation process as a basis for developing alternative interventions.)

SOAPIER format

The SOAPIER format allows for the documentation of alternative interventions by including:

- **R**evision: any changes from the original plan of care. (Interventions, outcomes, or target dates may need to be adjusted to reach a previous goal.)

Typically, you must write a complete SOAP, SOAPIE, or SOAPIER note every 24 hours on any unresolved problem or whenever the patient's condition changes. When doing so, be sure to specify the appropriate number of the problem you're discussing. Keep in mind that you don't need to write an entry for each SOAP or SOAPIE component every time you document. If you have nothing to record for a component, either omit the letter from the note or leave a blank space after it, depending on your facility's policy.

If your facility uses the SOAP format, record your nursing interventions and evaluations on flow sheets. If you use the SOAPIE format, provide explanations as needed in your progress notes under I and E.

Discharge summary

Completing the POMR format, the discharge summary covers each problem on the list and notes whether it was resolved. Discuss any unresolved problems in your SOAP or SOAPIE note, and specify your plan for dealing with the problem after discharge. Note any communications with other facilities, home health care agencies, and the patient.

Advantages

POMR documentation organizes information about each problem into specific categories understandable to all health care team members, thereby promoting interdisciplinary communication and data retrieval. The problems serve as an index to the medical record.

POMR documentation also illustrates the continuity of care, unifying the plan of care and progress notes into a full record of the care actually planned and delivered. This information is easily incorporated into care planning because the caregiver addresses each problem or nursing diagnosis in the nursing notes.

The POMR format also promotes documentation of the nursing process, facilitates more consistent documentation, and eliminates documentation of nonessential data, thereby eliminating the need for task documentation. It can also serve as a checklist that draws attention to problems requiring interventions. The POMR format is most effective in acute care or long-term care settings.

Disadvantages

A drawback of POMR documentation is its emphasis on the *chronology* of problems rather than their *priority*. Analyzing trends with this format can be difficult because information may be buried in the daily narrative.

The POMR format commonly produces repetitious charting of assessment findings and interventions, especially with the SOAPIE format, because both your assessments and interventions commonly apply to more than one problem. The resulting overlap makes the POMR system time-consuming to perform and to read. In addition, because the format emphasizes problems, routine care may remain undocumented unless flow sheets are used.

Furthermore, difficulties may arise if teammates fail to update the problem list regularly or if they're confused about which problems should be listed. The considerable time and cost of training new personnel to use the SOAP, SOAPIE, or SOAPIER method may also be a disadvantage.

The POMR format isn't well suited for settings with rapid patient turnover, such as the postanesthesia care unit, short procedure unit, or emergency department.

Problem-intervention-evaluation system

The problem-intervention-evaluation (PIE) documentation system was developed to simplify the documentation process. PIE charting organizes information according to patients' problems as defined by a group of nurses at Craven Hospital in New Bern, N.C., in 1985. As its name indicates, this problem-oriented documentation approach considers three categories: problem (P), intervention (I), and evaluation (E). To follow this format, you'll need to keep a daily patient assessment flow sheet and progress notes.

By integrating the plan of care into the nurses' progress notes, the PIE format eliminates the need for a separate plan of care. The intention is to provide a concise, efficient record of patient care that has a nursing—rather than medical—focus.

Format and components

To implement the PIE documentation system, first assess the patient and document your findings on a daily patient assessment flow sheet. This flow sheet lists defined assessment terms under major categories (such as respiration), along with routine care and monitoring (such as providing hygiene and monitoring breath sounds). The flow sheet typically includes space to record pertinent treatments.

Initial only the assessment terms on the flow sheet that apply to your patient and mark abnormal findings with an asterisk. Record detailed information in your progress notes.

Problem

After performing and documenting an initial assessment, use the collected data to identify pertinent nursing diagnoses. You can use the list of nursing diagnoses accepted by your facility, which usually corresponds to those approved by the North American Nursing Diagnosis Association (NANDA).

If you can't find a nursing diagnosis on an approved list, write the problem statement yourself using accepted criteria. Document all nursing diagnoses or problems in the progress notes, labeling each as "P" with an identifying number (for example, P#1).

This labeling system allows you to refer later to a specific problem by label only, eliminating the need to redocument the problem statement. Some facilities also use a separate problem-list form to keep a convenient running account of the nursing diagnoses for a particular patient. (See *Using the PIE format,* page 76.)

Intervention

In this step, document the nursing actions taken for each nursing diagnosis. Document each intervention on the progress sheet, labeling each as "I" followed by the assigned problem number. (To refer to an intervention for the first nursing diagnosis, for instance, you'd use IP#1.)

Evaluation

After charting your interventions, document the related effects in your progress notes. Use the label "E" followed by the assigned problem number (for example, EP#1).

Make sure that you or another nurse evaluates each problem at least every 8 hours. After every three shifts, review the notes from the previous 24 hours to identify the patient's current problems and responses to interventions.

Document continuing problems daily, along with relevant interventions and evaluations. Cross out any resolved problems from the daily documentation.

Advantages

Using the PIE format ensures that your documentation includes nursing diagnoses, related interventions, and evaluations. This format also encourages you to meet JCAHO requirements, provides an organizing framework for your thoughts and writing, and simplifies documentation by incorporating your plan of care into your progress notes.

The PIE format promotes continuity of care because it facilitates tracking the patient from admission to discharge. This method also improves the quality of progress notes by highlighting care interventions and requiring a written evaluation of the patient's response to those interventions.

Disadvantages

The PIE format may require in-depth training for staff members. The requirement that you reevaluate each problem during each shift is time consuming and leads to repetitive entries; some problems simply don't need such frequent evaluation.

BETTER CHARTING

Using the PIE format

This sample shows how to write progress notes using the problem-intervention-evaluation (PIE) format.

Date	Time	Notes
2/22/99	1600	P#1: High risk for ineffective breathing pattern related to possible smoke inhalation.
		IP#1: Assessed respiratory rate and breath sounds q h to R/O pulmonary edema and bronchospasm. Taught pt. how to perform deep-breathing and coughing exercises and taught use of incentive spirometer. O_2 applied @ 2 L/min via nasal cannula.
		EP#1: Pt. maintains patent airway and normal RR and depth. Pt. understands the importance of performing deep-breathing and coughing exercises q h. Pt. has normal ABG levels.
		Deborah Ryan, RN
		P#2: High risk for decreased CO R/T reduced stroke volume as a result of fluid loss through burns.
		IP#2: Teach pt. to report any restlessness, diaphoresis, or light-headedness, which may indicate shock. Evaluate VS and hemodynamic readings at least q 2 hr. Monitor urine output q h. Monitor ABG levels. Provide and monitor I.V. therapy.
		EP#2: Pt. maintains normal VS and stable hemodynamic status. ABGs WNL. Pt. has adequate urine output. Pt. verbalizes signs and symptoms of shock. Pt. receiving adequate replacement through I.V. therapy.
		Deborah Ryan, RN
		P#3: Pain related to second-degree burns over 20% of body.
2/22/99	1630	IP#3#: Assess pain q 2 hr and medicate q 3 to 4 hr with morphine, as ordered.
		EP#3: Pt. reports a decrease in pain rating from 8 to 2 on a scale of 1 to 10, with 10 being the worst pain imaginable. Deborah Ryan, RN

The PIE format omits documentation of the planning step in the nursing process. This step, which addresses expected outcomes, is essential to evaluating the patient's responses. Finally, PIE charting doesn't incorporate multidisciplinary charting.

FOCUS CHARTING

Developed by nurses at Eitel Hospital in Minneapolis who found the SOAP format awkward, focus charting encourages you to organize your thoughts into patient-centered topics, or foci of concern, and then to document precisely and concisely. This format encourages you to use assessment data to evaluate these patient care concerns. It also helps you identify necessary revisions to the plan of care as you document each entry. Focus charting works well in acute care settings and in areas where the same care and procedures are repeated frequently.

Format and components

To implement focus documentation, use a progress sheet with categories for date, time, focus, and progress notes. (See *Using focus charting*, page 78.) Then identify the foci by reviewing your assessment data.

Foci

Typically, you'll write each focus as a nursing diagnosis (such as decreased cardiac output or fluid volume deficit). However, the focus may also refer to a sign or symptom (such as hypotension or chest pain), a patient behavior (such as inability to ambulate), a special need (such as a discharge need), an acute change in the patient's condition (such as loss of consciousness or increase in blood pressure), or a significant event (such as surgery).

Progress notes

In the progress notes column, you'll organize information using three categories: data (D), action (A), and response (R). In the data category, include subjective and objective information that describes the focus.

In the action category, include immediate and future nursing actions based on your assessment of the patient's condition. This category also may encompass any changes to the plan of care you deem necessary based on your evaluation.

In the response category, describe the patient's response to any aspect of nursing or medical care.

Using all three categories ensures complete documentation based on the nursing process. Be sure to record routine nursing tasks and assessment data on your flow sheets and checklists.

Advantages

Focus charting is flexible and can be adapted to fit any clinical setting. It centers on the nursing process, and the data-action-response format provides cues that direct documentation in a process-oriented way.

By separating the focus statement from the narrative of the progress notes, this format makes it easy to find information on a particular problem, thereby saving time and promoting communication among health care team members.

The format also highlights the nursing process in the documentation of daily patient care, encourages regular documentation of patient responses to nursing and medical therapy, and ensures adherence to JCAHO requirements for documenting patient responses and outcomes.

You can use this format to document many topics without being confined to those on the problem list or plan of care. The focus format also helps you organize your thoughts and document succinctly and precisely.

Disadvantages

Learning the focus documentation system may require in-depth training, especially for staff members familiar with other systems. Additionally, the system requires you to use

BETTER CHARTING

Using focus charting

This sample shows how to write progress notes using the focus charting format.

Date	Time	Focus	Progress notes
2/18/99	0900	Ineffective breathing R/T decreased energy.	D: Pt. dyspneic and diaphoretic after bathing at bedside. Skin reddened. T-99.0,R; P-94; BP-142/86. Pt. reports that the dyspnea disrupts her sleep and she has lost 20 lb in 3 months. Pt. states she feels hot and is having difficulty catching her breath. A: Auscultation reveals decreased vesicular breath sounds, prolonged expiration, and scattered expiratory wheezes in both lung bases. O_2 applied at 2 L/min via nasal cannula. Dr. Miller notified and will examine pt. within 10 min. Explained the purpose of patterned breathing to pt.; demonstrated correct breathing techniques and had the pt. demonstrate them. ——— Ellen Grimes, RN
2/18/99	1630	Anxiety R/T difficulty in breathing.	D: Pt. shaking and grabbing my hand and stating she is scared. ——— A: Spent time with pt. providing support. Discussed importance of and demonstrated diaphragmatic pursed-lip breathing techniques. Allowed pt. to verbalize feelings when dyspnea improved. R: Pt. states she feels less anxious and she appears calmer. ——— Adela Suarez, RN
2/18/99	2200	Knowledge deficit R/T disease process and its treatment.	D: Pt. reports smoking history of 40 pack years (2 packs x 20 years). Currently smokes one pack per day. Denies exposure to respiratory irritants. ——— A: Reviewed the most common signs and symptoms associated with the disease: dyspnea, especially with exertion; fatigue; cough; occasional mucus production; weight loss; rapid heart rate; irregular P and use of accessory muscles to help with breathing from limited diaphragm function. Provided information about smoking cessation groups. Urged pt. to avoid fumes, temperature extremes, and people with infections. ——— Marc Ponte, RN

many flow sheets and checklists, which can lead to inconsistent documentation and can cause difficulty in tracking a patient's problems. The focus format can become a narrative note if you neglect to include the patient's response to interventions.

CHARTING-BY-EXCEPTION SYSTEM

The charting-by-exception (CBE) documentation system was designed by nurses at St. Luke's Hospital in Milwaukee to overcome long-standing charting problems, such as lengthy and repetitive notes, poorly organized information, difficult-to-retrieve data, and a high risk of errors of omission. To avoid these pitfalls, the CBE format radically departs from traditional systems by requiring documentation of only significant or abnormal findings. These findings are documented in a narrative portion of the record. The CBE system also uses military time to help prevent misinterpretations.

FORMAT AND COMPONENTS

To use CBE documentation effectively, you must know and adhere to established guidelines for nursing assessments and interventions. The CBE nursing assessment format has printed guidelines for each body system; this format relies on written standards of practice that identify the nurse's basic responsibilities to patients. For example, care standards for patient hygiene might include your responsibility to ensure that a patient has a complete linen change every 3 days or sooner if necessary.

Because the standards are clear and concise, all charting related to routine nursing care — or any other care outlined in the standards — is eliminated. You document only deviations from the standards, thereby omitting repetitive charting of routine procedures.

Intervention guidelines for the CBE system stem from these sources:

- nursing diagnosis–based standardized plans of care — identification of patient problems, desired outcomes, and interventions
- patient care guidelines — standardized interventions established for specific patient populations, such as patients with a nursing diagnosis of pain, that outline the nursing interventions, treatments, and time frame for repeated assessments
- doctor's orders — prescribed medical interventions
- incidental orders — usually one-time, miscellaneous nursing or medical orders or interdependent interventions related to a protocol or a piece of equipment
- standards of nursing practice — definition of the acceptable level of routine nursing care for all patients (the essential aspects of nursing practice for a specific unit or for all clinical areas).

The CBE format includes a nursing diagnosis–based standardized plan of care and several types of flow sheets, including the nursing care flow sheet, graphic record, patient-teaching record, and patient discharge note. In certain cases, you may need to supplement your CBE documentation by using nurses' progress notes.

Nursing diagnosis–based standardized plans of care

Use these preprinted plans of care whenever you identify a nursing diagnosis, and use a separate form for each pertinent diagnosis. Keep in mind that the forms have spaces that allow you to individualize them as needed; for example, you can include expected outcomes and major revisions to the plan of care. Place the completed forms in the nurses' progress notes section of the clinical record.

Nursing care flow sheet

Use this form to document your assessments and interventions. Each flow sheet is designed for a 24-hour period of care for one patient.

After completing an assessment, compare your findings with the normal parameters defined in the printed guidelines on the form. If the findings are within normal parameters, place a check mark in the appropriate category box and add your initials. If the findings are not within the normal range, put an asterisk in the category box; then explain your findings in the comments section on the form.

Remember, a finding that's not defined in the guidelines may be normal for a particular patient; for example, unclear speech may be a normal finding in a patient with a long-standing tracheostomy. If the patient's condition hasn't changed from the last assessment, draw a horizontal arrow from the previous category box to the current one.

After assessing your patient, review the previous nurse's note and symbol to determine if the patient's condition changed. Indicate significant findings or abnormal patient responses with an asterisk, and write an explanation in the comments section. If the patient's response is unchanged, use an arrow.

After you document an entire column in the assessments and interventions section, initial it at the bottom. Also initial all your entries in the comments section, and sign the form at the bottom of the page.

Some facilities use a nursing care flow sheet that combines all the necessary sections, such as the graphic record, a daily nursing care activities checklist, and a patient care assessment section. (See *Using a combined nursing care flow sheet.*)

Graphic record

Use this flow sheet or section of a flow sheet to document trends in the patient's vital signs, weight, intake and output, and stool, urination, appetite, and activity levels. As with the nursing care flow sheet, use check marks to indicate expected findings and asterisks to indicate abnormal findings. Record information about abnormalities in the nurses' progress notes.

In the box labeled "Routine standards," check off the established nursing care interventions you performed, such as providing hygiene. Don't rewrite these standards as orders on the nursing care flow sheet. Refer to the guidelines on the back of the graphic record for complete instructions.

Patient-teaching record

Use this form or section on the form to identify the knowledge, psychomotor skills, and social or behavioral measures that your patient or his caregiver must learn by a predetermined date. The patient-teaching record includes teaching resources, dates of patient achievements, and other pertinent observations. You may use more than one form for a patient with multiple learning needs.

Patient discharge note

Similar to other discharge forms, the patient discharge note is a flow sheet for documenting ongoing discharge planning. Follow the instructions printed on the back of the form.

Progress notes

Another component of the CBE format, the progress notes are used to document revisions to the plan of care and interventions that don't lend themselves to the nursing care

(Text continues on page 84.)

BETTER CHARTING

Using a combined nursing care flow sheet

This sample shows a portion of a nursing care flow sheet that combines a graphic record, a daily nursing care activities checklist, and a patient care assessment form.

Name *Alejandro Mendoza*

Date *2/24/99*

Hour		**0700**	**0800**	**0900**	**1000**	**1100**	**1200**	**1300**	**1400**	**1500**	**1600**	**1700**	**1800**
Temperature													
C°	F°												
40.4	105												
40.0	104												
39.4	103												
38.9	102												
38.3	101												
37.8	100												
37.2	99												
36.7	98												
36.1	97												
35.6	96												
Pulse		*84*	*80*	*82*	*78*	*76*	*78*	*78*	*82*	*84*	*82*	*80*	*78*
Respiration		*16*	*20*	*20*	*22*	*24*	*24*	*18*	*20*	*22*	*20*	*18*	*24*
BP	Lying												
	Sitting	*136/82*	*130/80*	*126/74*	*132/82*	*132/80*	*140/82*	*136/74*	*130/70*	*138/78*	*140/80*	*132/78*	*136/76*
	Standing												
Intake	Oral	*400*					*300*						*100*
	Tube												
	I.V.												
	Blood												
8-hour total		*700*											
Output	Urine	*300*					*200*						
	Other												
	Other												
8-hour total		*500*											
Teaching		*Skin care, s/s of UTI, Safety*											
Signature		*Carol Witt, RN*									*Donald Baron, RN*		

(continued)

DOCUMENTATION SYSTEMS

Using a combined nursing care flow sheet *(continued)*

	Hour	0700	0800	0900	1000	1100	1200	1300	1400	1500	1600	1700
ACTIVITY	Bed rest	CW →								→	DB →	→
	OOB											
	Ambulate (assist)											
	Ambulatory											
	Sleeping											
	BRP											
	HOB elevated	CW →								→	DB →	→
	Cough, deep-breathe, turn		CW								DB	
	ROM: Active		CW								DB	
	ROM: Passive											
HYGIENE	Bath		CW									
	Shave		CW									
	Oral		CW									
	Skin care											
	Perianal care											
NUTRITION	Diet	Soft — no added salt										
	% Eating			90%				60%				90%
	Feeding											
	Supplemental											
	S=Self, A=Assist, F=Feed			S				S				S
BLADDER	Catheter	Indwelling urinary #18 Fr										
	Incontinent											
	Voiding	QS — clear, yellow urine										
	Intermittent cath.											
BOWEL	Stools (OB+, OB–)											
	Incontinent											
	Normal	Small, soft, formed brown stool										
	Enema											
SPECIAL TREATMENTS	Special mattress	Low-pressure airflow mattress applied 0900										
	Special bed											
	Heel and elbow pads											
	Antiembolism stockings											
	Traction: + = on, – = off											
	Isolation type											

Using a combined nursing care flow sheet *(continued)*

ASSESSMENT FINDINGS

Key:
√ = normal findings
* = significant finding

	Day	Evening	Night	
Neurologic	* CW	* DB		Limited ROM Ⓛ shoulder. Pt. states, "I have arthritis and my shoulder is always stiff." — CW
Cardiovascular	√ CW	√ DB		
Pulmonary	* CW	√ DB		Decreased breath sounds at Ⓡ base posteriorly at 0800 + 1400. Lungs clear at 1600 + 2000. — DB
Gastrointestinal	√ CW	√ DB		
Genitourinary	√ CW	√ DB		
Surgical dressing and incision	N/A	N/A		
Skin integrity	* CW DB	*		Poor skin turgor; dry, flaky skin. — CW 4 cm x 4 cm area of redness at sacral area. — CW
Psychosocial	√ CW	√ DB		
Educational	* CW	* DB		Taught pt. safety, skin care, and signs and symptoms of UTI — DB
Peripheral vascular	√ CW	√ DB		

NORMAL ASSESSMENT FINDINGS

Neurologic
- Alert and oriented to time, place, and person
- Speech clear and understandable
- Memory intact
- Behavior appropriate to situation and accommodation
- Active range of motion (ROM) of all extremities; symmetrically equal strength
- No paresthesia

CV
- Regular apical pulse
- Palpable bilateral peripheral pulses
- No peripheral edema
- No calf tenderness

Respiratory
- Resting respirations 10 to 20 per minute, quiet and regular
- Clear sputum
- Pink nail beds and mucous membranes

GI
- Abdomen soft and nondistended
- Tolerates prescribed diet without nausea or vomiting
- Bowel movements within own normal pattern and consistency

GU
- No indwelling catheter in use
- Urinates without pain
- Undistended bladder after urination
- Urine is clear yellow to amber color

Surgical dressing and incision
- Dressing dry and intact
- No evidence of redness, increased temperature, or tenderness in surrounding tissue
- Sutures, staples, Steri-Strips intact
- Sound edges well approximated
- No drainage present

Skin integrity
- Skin color normal
- Skin warm, dry, and intact
- Moist mucous membranes

Psychosocial
- Interacts and communicates in an appropriate manner with others

Educational
- Patient or significant others communicate understanding of the patient's health status, plan of care, and expected response
- Patient or significant others demonstrate ability to perform health-related procedures and behaviors as taught

Peripheral vascular
- Affected extremity pink, warm, and movable within average ROM
- Capillary refill time < 3 seconds
- Peripheral pulses palpable
- No edema: sensation intact without numbness or paresthesia
- No pain on passive stretch

flow sheet. Because the CBE format permits you to document most assessments and interventions on the nursing care flow sheet, the progress notes typically contain little assessment and intervention data.

Advantages

The CBE format has several advantages. By including only information that deviates from expected findings, it decreases the amount of documentation needed, eliminates redundancies, and clearly identifies abnormal data, thereby decreasing the time needed to document normal and abnormal findings. The use of well-defined guidelines and standards of care promotes uniform nursing practice. Also, the flow sheets let you easily track trends.

Guidelines, including normal findings, are printed on the forms for ready reference. Abnormal findings are highlighted to help you quickly pinpoint significant changes and trends in a patient's condition. Documentation of routine care is eliminated through the use of nursing care standards.

The fact that all flow sheets (which are part of the permanent record) are kept at the patient's bedside where they serve as a ready reference, encourages immediate documentation. Because patient data are written on the permanent record immediately, you don't have to keep temporary notes and later transcribe them to the patient's chart; in addition, other caregivers always have access to the most current data. Also, because assessments are standardized, all caregivers evaluate and document findings consistently.

Finally, information that has already been recorded isn't repeated; for instance, you don't have to write a long entry in a patient's chart each time you assess him if his condition remains the same.

Disadvantages

The chief drawback of the CBE format is the major time commitment needed to develop clear guidelines and standards of care. To ensure a legally sound patient record, these guidelines and standards must be in place and understood by all nursing staff members before the format can be implemented. This radical departure from traditional documentation systems takes time for people to learn, accept, and use correctly. Consistent use of the appropriate documenting procedures is vital.

If your health care facility uses multiple forms rather than one form that combines all the CBE components, the documenting process can be confusing and the records incomplete. Narrative notes may be too brief and an evaluation of a patient's response may not be fully described.

CBE documentation does not accommodate integrated or multidisciplinary charting. Also, be aware that unexpected events or isolated occurrences may not be fully documented; these events will require a narrative note.

The CBE system was developed for registered nurses. If licensed practical nurses will be using the system, it must be evaluated and modified to meet their scope of practice. CBE charting complies with legal principles, but it may be questioned in court until the system becomes more widely known.

FACT system

Named for its individual elements, the FACT documentation system incorporates many CBE principles. It was designed to avoid the documentation of irrelevant data, repetitive notes, and inconsistencies among departments and to reduce the amount of time spent charting.

Format and components

The FACT system has four key elements:

- **F**low sheets individualized to specific services
- **A**ssessment features standardized with baseline parameters
- **C**oncise, integrated progress notes and flow sheets documenting the patient's condition and responses
- **T**imely entries recorded when care is given.

The FACT system requires that you document only exceptions to the norm or significant information about the patient. It eliminates the need to chart normal findings. It also incorporates each step of the nursing process. (See *Documenting with FACT*, pages 86 and 87.)

FACT documentation begins with a complete initial baseline assessment on each patient using standardized parameters. This format uses an assessment-action flow sheet, a frequent assessment flow sheet, and progress notes. The content of the flow sheets and notes may be individualized to some extent. The flow sheets cover a 24- to 72-hour period, and you'll need to date, time, and sign all entries.

Assessment-action flow sheet

Use this form to document ongoing assessments and interventions. Normal assessment parameters for each body system are printed on the form along with planned interventions. The flow sheet may be individualized according to the patient's needs.

Frequent assessment flow sheet

Use this form to chart vital signs and frequent assessments. On a surgical unit, for example, this form would include a postoperative assessment section.

Progress notes

This form includes an integrated progress record where you'll use narrative notes to document the patient's progress and any significant incidents. As in focus charting, write narrative notes using the data-action-response method. Update progress notes related to patient outcomes every 48 hours.

Advantages

The computer-ready FACT charting system has several advantages. It eliminates repetition and encourages consistent language and structure. The system is outcome oriented and communicates patient progress to all health care team members. It permits immediate recording of current data and is readily accessible at the patient's bedside. The system also eliminates the need for many different forms and reduces the time spent writing narrative notes.

Disadvantages

FACT charting requires a major time commitment to develop standards and implement the system across all departments of the health care facility. Narrative notes may be too brief, and the nurse's perspective on the patient may be overlooked. The nursing process framework may be difficult to identify in this system as well.

(Text continues on page 88.)

BETTER CHARTING

Documenting with FACT

Developed in 1987 at Abbott Northwestern Hospital in Minneapolis, the FACT system records nursing assessment findings and interventions that are exceptions to the norm. This sample shows portions of an assessment flow sheet and a postoperative flow sheet using the FACT format.

ASSESSMENT AND ACTION RECORD

Date Time	2/18/99 1300	2/18/99 1800	2/18/99 2400
Neurologic Alert and oriented to time, place, and person. PEARL. Symmetry of strength in extremities. No difficulty with coordination. Behavior appropriate to situation. Sensation intact without numbness or paresthesia.	√	√	√
Orient patient.			
Refer to neurologic flow sheet.			
Pain No report of pain. If present, include patient statements about intensity (0 to 5 scale), location, description, duration, radiation, precipitating and alleviating factors.	Abdominal incision pain 8 — "severe pain"	√	2 — incision pain — "It hurts."
Location	RLQ		RLQ
Relief measures	Percocet 1 tablet P.O.		Percocet 1 tablet P.O.
Pain relief: Y = Yes N = No	Y		Y
Cardiovascular Apical pulse 60 to 100. S_1 and S_2 present. Regular rhythm. Peripheral (radial, pedal) pulses present. No edema or calf tenderness. Extremities pink, warm, movable within patient's ROM.	√	√	√
I.V. solution and rate	D5½NSS @ 125 ml/hr.	D5½NSS @ 125 ml/hr.	D5½NSS @ 125 ml/hr.
Respiratory Respiratory rate 12 to 20 at rest, quiet, regular, and nonlabored. Lungs clear and aerated equally in all lobes. No abnormal breath sounds. Mucous membranes pink.	√	↓BS RUL	√
O_2 therapy			
TCDB/Incentive spirometer	√	√	√
Musculoskeletal Extremities pink, warm, and without edema; sensation and motion present. Normal joint ROM, no swelling or tenderness. Steady gait without aids. Pedal, radial pulses present. Rapid capillary refill.	√	√	√
Activity (describe)	Bed rest	OOB in chair	Bed rest
Nurse's signature and title	Cindy Weir, RN	Dave Shaw, RN	Lynn Tate, RN

Key: √ = Meets assessment criteria

DOCUMENTATION SYSTEMS

Documenting with FACT *(continued)*

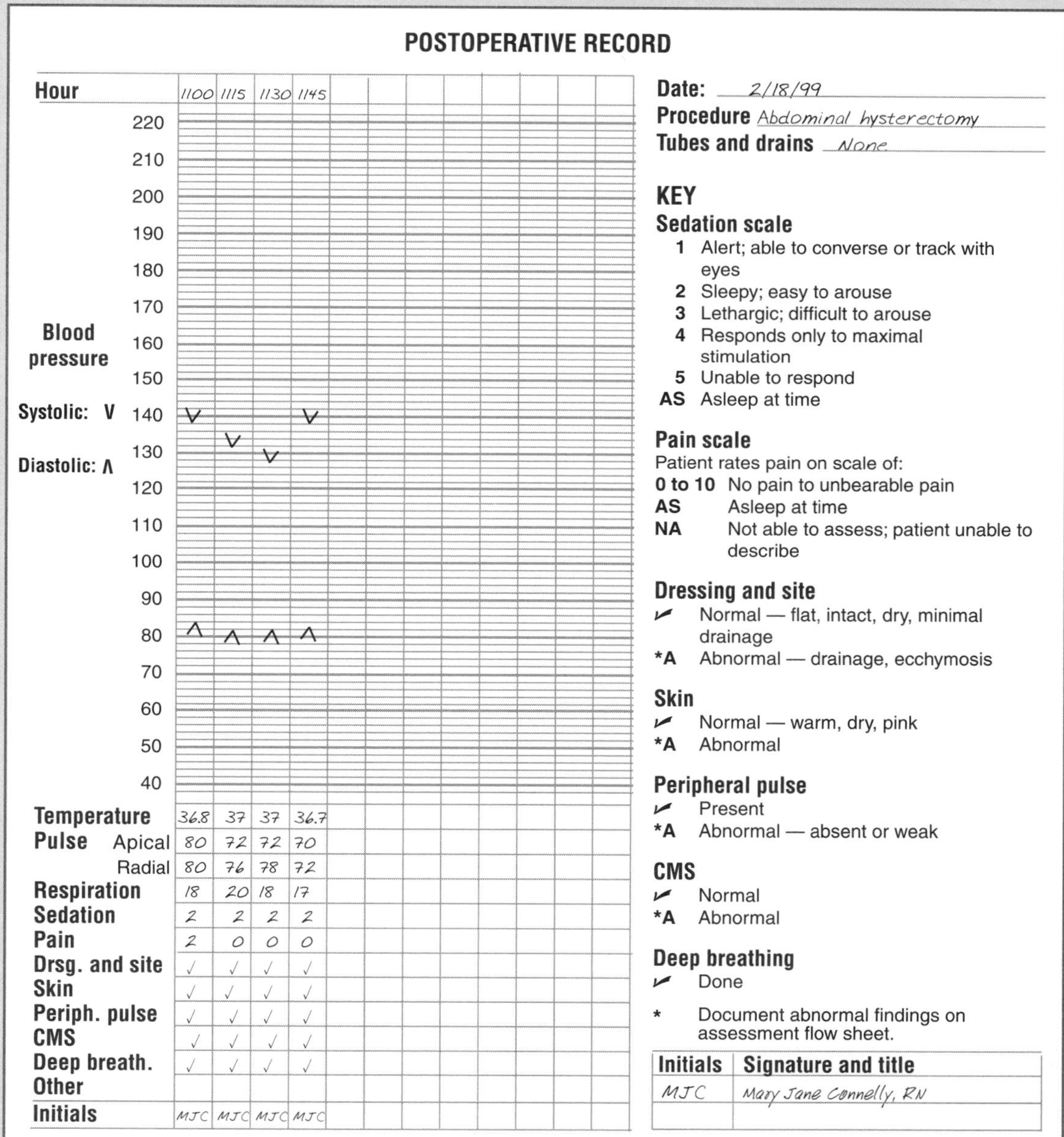

POSTOPERATIVE RECORD

Hour	1100	1115	1130	1145								
220												
210												
200												
190												
180												
170												
Blood pressure 160												
150												
Systolic: V 140	V			V								
130		V	V									
Diastolic: Λ 120												
110												
100												
90												
80	Λ	Λ	Λ	Λ								
70												
60												
50												
40												
Temperature	36.8	37	37	36.7								
Pulse Apical	80	72	72	70								
Radial	80	76	78	72								
Respiration	18	20	18	17								
Sedation	2	2	2	2								
Pain	2	0	0	0								
Drsg. and site	✓	✓	✓	✓								
Skin	✓	✓	✓	✓								
Periph. pulse	✓	✓	✓	✓								
CMS	✓	✓	✓	✓								
Deep breath.	✓	✓	✓	✓								
Other												
Initials	MJC	MJC	MJC	MJC								

Date: 2/18/99
Procedure Abdominal hysterectomy
Tubes and drains None

KEY

Sedation scale

1 Alert; able to converse or track with eyes
2 Sleepy; easy to arouse
3 Lethargic; difficult to arouse
4 Responds only to maximal stimulation
5 Unable to respond
AS Asleep at time

Pain scale

Patient rates pain on scale of:
0 to 10 No pain to unbearable pain
AS Asleep at time
NA Not able to assess; patient unable to describe

Dressing and site

✓ Normal — flat, intact, dry, minimal drainage
***A** Abnormal — drainage, ecchymosis

Skin

✓ Normal — warm, dry, pink
***A** Abnormal

Peripheral pulse

✓ Present
***A** Abnormal — absent or weak

CMS

✓ Normal
***A** Abnormal

Deep breathing

✓ Done

* Document abnormal findings on assessment flow sheet.

Initials	Signature and title
MJC	Mary Jane Connelly, RN

DOCUMENTATION SYSTEMS

Core system

The core documentation system focuses on the nursing process—the *core,* or most important part, of documentation.

Format and components

Consisting of a database, plans of care, flow sheets, progress notes, and discharge summary, core charting requires you to assess and record a patient's functional and cognitive status within 8 hours of admission. (See *Using core charting.*)

Database and plans of care

This initial assessment focuses on the patient's body systems and activities of daily living and includes a summary of the patient's problems and appropriate nursing diagnoses. The completed database and plan of care are then entered on the patient's medical record card (Kardex).

Flow sheets

Use flow sheets to document the patient's activities and response to nursing interventions, diagnostic procedures, and patient teaching.

Progress notes

In the progress notes, record the following information (DAE) for each problem:

- **D**ata
- **A**ction
- **E**valuation or response.

Discharge summary

This component of core documentation incorporates information related to nursing diagnoses and patient teaching. The discharge summary also includes recommended follow-up care.

Advantages

Core documentation incorporates the entire nursing process into one system. Complemented by the DAE component, this system groups nursing diagnoses and functional status assessments together, allowing various solutions to be considered. The system also promotes concise documentation with minimal repetition and encourages the daily recording of psychosocial information. Core charting is useful in acute care and long-term care facilities.

Disadvantages

Core documentation may require in-depth training for staff members who are familiar with other documenting systems. Developing forms may be costly and time consuming. The DAE format doesn't always present information chronologically, making it difficult to perceive the patient's progress quickly. What's more, the progress notes may not always relate to the plan of care, so you'll need to monitor your documentation carefully to ensure a record of quality care.

Outcome documentation system

Focused on the patient's behaviors and his responses to nursing care and patient teaching, outcome documentation is a process-oriented system. It presents the patient's condition in relation to predetermined outcomes on the plan of care, focusing on desired outcomes rather than problems.

(Text continues on page 93.)

BETTER CHARTING

Using core charting

Developed in 1986 by the nurses at St. Joseph's Hospital in Hamilton, Ontario, core charting focuses on the key elements of the nursing process. This sample shows the features of an initial assessment and plan of care.

INITIAL ASSESSMENT

General appearance	Physical	*Immobile and severe headache*		
	Skin	☑ Clear ☑ dry ☑ intact ☐ Other		
	Hygiene	*good*		
Cardiopulmonary		*Tachycardia and tachypnea*		
Mobility	*Unable to stand or walk*		Aided by	*Wheelchair*
Vision	*Good*		Aided by	
Hearing	*Good*		Aided by	
Speech	Language *English*			
	Impediment *None*		Aided by	
Appetite, diet	*Fair, regular*			
	Dentures	☐ Upper	☐ Lower	☐ Partial ☑ None
Urination	*Good – voids freely*		Aided by	*Urinal*
Bowel routine	*Daily*		Aided by	*Laxatives*
Sleep and rest	*Poor, secondary to pain*		Aided by	*Analgesics*
Pain and discomfort	*Severe pain Ⓡ temporal area*		Aided by	*Percocet*
Reproduction and sexuality		*Normal*		
Mental status (orientation, memory)		*Oriented x3*		
Emotional status (mood, attitude)		*Agitated*		
Religion	*Catholic*			
Nationality	*Irish*			
Lifestyle habits	☑ Alcohol *occasional beer*		☐ drugs *none*	
	☐ tobacco *none*		☐ other	
Occupation	*Construction worker*			
Hobbies	*Sports*			

Patient's concerns for discharge *Pt. states that he's concerned about when he will be able to return to work. States that if he requires surgery, no one will be home to help him because his wife works.*

Signature *Pam Watts, RN*

Date and time *1/8/99 0200*

(continued)

DOCUMENTATION SYSTEMS

Using core charting *(continued)*

VITAL SIGNS FLOW SHEET

Date		1/8/99						1/9/99						1/10/99					
Time		0200	0600	1000	1400	1800	2200	0200	0600	1000	1400	1800	2200	0200					
Temp	**Pulse**																		
41	170																		
	160																		
40	150																		
	140																		
39	130																		
	120			•															
38	110		X •	X			•	X											
	100					•		•		•	X			• X					
37	90				X •	X			•	X		X	X						
	80	X •					X		X		•	•	•						
36	70																		
	60																		
35	50																		
	40																		
Respirations		20	22	24	21	20	22	18	20	22	24	20	18	20					
Blood pressure																			
230																			
220																			
210																			
200																			
190																			
180																			
170																			
160									V										
150			V	V															
140		V			V	V		V		V	V	V	V	V					
130																			
120																			
110																			
100																			
90													Λ						
80			Λ	Λ	Λ	Λ		Λ	Λ	Λ	Λ	Λ		Λ					
70		Λ																	
60																			
50																			
Nurse's signature		Pam Watts, RN	Pam Watts, RN	Esther Blake, RN	Esther Blake, RN	Wendy Moss, RN	Wendy Moss, RN	Ann Jones, RN	Ann Jones, RN	Lois Caen, RN	Lois Caen, RN	John Smith, RN	John Smith, RN	Carol Davis, RN					

Key:
Temp = •
Pulse = X

Blood pressure, standing
Systolic = ∇
Diastolic = Δ

Blood pressure, lying
Systolic = V
Diastolic = Λ

DOCUMENTATION SYSTEMS

Using core charting *(continued)*

24-HOUR FLUID BALANCE FLOW SHEET

Date	INTAKE							OUTPUT						
1/8/99	Oral or tube feeding	Intravenous		TPN		Blood & blood products	Total	Urine	NG tube	Emesis	Stool	Drainage		Total
Time		D5 1/2 NSS		Travasol	Lipid									
0800	250							500						
0900	100													
1000	250													
1100								500						
1200	400													
1300														
1400	250							1000						
1500														
Subtotal	1250	800					2050	2000						2000
1600								400						
1700	300													
1800														
1900	100							500						
2000														
2100														
2200								400						
2300														
Subtotal	400	800					1200	1300						1300
2400														
0100								200						
0200	100													
0300														
0400								400						
0500														
0600								400						
0700	100													
Subtotal	200	800					1000	1000						1000
Total	1850	2400					4250	4300						4300

Nurse's signature				
	Day 0800-1500	Pam Watts, RN	**24-hour intake** 0800-0700	4,250 ml
	Evening 1600-2300	Esther Blake, RN	**24-hour output** 0800-0700	4,300 ml
	Night 2400-0700	Wendy Moss, RN	**Balance ±**	-50 ml

(continued)

Using core charting *(continued)*

PATIENT CARE PLAN

Date	Nurse's initials	NURSING DIAGNOSES	EXPECTED OUTCOMES	Deadline	Chart	NURSING INTERVENTIONS	Date resolved	Nurse's initials
						Monitor VS & neuro. VS q h. Monitor CSF output q h. Observe for signs of rebleeding.		
		Safety needs						
1/8/99	PW	High risk for injury related to altered LOC	Pt. will remain free from injury			Raise the bed side rails. Avoid using restraints, which may raise ICP.		
		Psychosocial needs						
		Fear related to unknown prognosis				Provide emotional support to pt. and family.	1/8/99	PW
		Spiritual, cultural needs						

PATIENT-TEACHING PLANS	DISCHARGE PLANNING
Teach pt. and family about condition.	Expected discharge date 1/12/99
Explain all tests, neurologic exams, treatments, and	Home situation
procedures to pt.	Discharge resources involved
Explain cerebral aneurysm precautions and their purpose.	Public health
Explain physical rehab. plan to pt. and family.	Home care
Provide nutrition guidelines to pt.	Social work
	Placement Cedar Crest Rehab.
	Other

Nurse's signature	Initials	Nurse's signature	Initials	Nurse's signature	Initials
Pam Watts, RN	PW				

DOCUMENTATION SYSTEMS

Format and components

This documentation system makes use of progress notes, flow sheets, and plans of care for documentation. Typically combined with another documentation system, it features three components: a database, a plan of care, and expected outcome statements.

Database

Obtain an initial information base that includes subjective and objective data identifying the patient's problems and learning needs. This collected information serves as a foundation for ongoing evaluations of the patient's status. The teaching sheet should include the patient's and family's problems, special learning needs, and any barriers to learning that have been identified. (See *Multidisciplinary patient-family education record,* page 94.)

Plan of care

Using the information in the initial database, develop a patient plan of care that establishes priorities, identifies expected outcomes and nursing interventions, and documents the plan. This plan gives the health care team a central source of information about the patient's needs and goals.

All of the following types of plans of care include expected outcomes:

- traditional handwritten plans of care for an individual patient
- standardized plans of care with preprinted categories, such as nursing diagnoses, outcome statements, and recommended interventions as well as blank spaces for individualization of the plan
- patient care guidelines that include specific sequential instructions for treating patients with a specific problem
- clinical pathways or health care maps that outline expected outcomes on a timeline and provide key interventions for a patient with a specific diagnosis.

Expected outcome statements

Also known as goals or objectives, expected outcome statements are drawn from the patient's nursing diagnoses. Expected outcomes describe the desired results of nursing care and serve as the basis for identifying nursing actions to help the patient achieve goals. They also provide a means to evaluate the effectiveness of nursing care and patient teaching.

Because a single nursing diagnosis may have many expected outcomes, be specific when stating an expected outcome. Then establish specific criteria to determine whether the outcome has been achieved. (See *Writing expected outcomes and outcome criteria, page 95.*)

Outcome criteria

The standards by which you objectively evaluate outcomes include these four components:

- specific behaviors that show the patient has progressed toward or reached his goal
- a standard for measuring the patient's behaviors, such as how much he does and for how long
- the conditions under which the behavior should occur
- a target date or time by which the behaviors should occur (short-term goals and long-term goals are identified by their target dates).

When writing outcome criteria, follow these guidelines:

- Make the statement specific. For example, don't write "within a short time" to target an outcome; rather, write "within 3 days."

BETTER CHARTING

Multidisciplinary patient-family education record

This sample shows the features of a typical multidisciplinary patient-family education record.

INITIAL EDUCATIONAL EVALUATION

Date/Time 3/15/99 1800

Motivational level: P = patient F = Family

P/F Asks questions
___ Uninterested
P/F Eager to learn
___ Denies need for education
P Very anxious
___ Not appropriate for education

Barrier to education:

X No barrier identified
___ Visual deficit
___ Auditory deficit
___ Physical deficit
___ Religious barrier
___ Cultural barrier
___ Dexterity deficit
___ Language barrier
___ Language spoken

Special learning needs Care after mastectomy

Community resources discussed:

___ Cardiac support
___ Twelve-step program
___ Diabetic support
___ Hospice
___ Achievement center
___ Other
X Cancer support

DATE/INITIAL	TOPIC	PT	FAM	RESPONSE CODE
3/15/99 GC	Pt. oriented to room postoperatively	✓	✓	2, 6
3/15/99 GC	Explained purpose of Jackson-Pratt drain	✓	✓	2, 6
3/15/99 GC	Instructed pt. on differences of PO vs IV pain meds	✓		
3/16/99 MD	Instructed pt. on postop exercises for mastectomy	✓	✓	1, 3, 5
3/16/99 DR	Pt. instructed to empty and record Jackson-Pratt drainage herself	✓		5, 6
3/16/99 DR	Pt. instructed on wound/tube care for home (Discharge)	✓		2, 6
3/16/99 LS	Pt. given discharge instructions for medications, exercises, limitations	✓		2, 6
5/19/99 LS	Physical therapy/OT consult for home care	✓	✓	7

Response codes:

1 Received literature
2 Communicates understanding
3 Requires reinforcement
4 Prior experience
5 Returned demo
6 Education achieved
7 Referral indicated
8 Refused/Uninterested
9 Inappropriate for education

Initials	Signature - Status	Initials	Signature - Status
MD	Mark Duncan, RN	GC	Ginny Clements, RN
DR	Daniella Reams, RN	LS	Linda Savio, RN

DOCUMENTATION SYSTEMS

CHARTING GUIDELINES

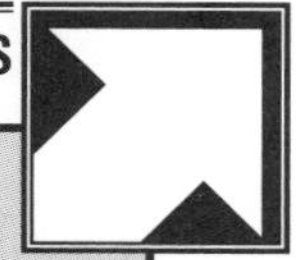

Writing expected outcomes and outcome criteria

Here are two examples of how to develop patient-focused outcomes and outcome criteria based on selected nursing diagnoses.

NURSING DIAGNOSIS	EXPECTED OUTCOMES	OUTCOME CRITERIA
Ineffective breathing pattern related to incisional pain	Patient will demonstrate an effective breathing pattern by the end of the shift.	■ Patient's respiratory rate is 16 to 20 breaths/minute and regular. ■ Patient uses no accessory muscles. ■ Patient demonstrates the ability to breathe easily.
Pain related to effects of surgery	Pain will be reduced by time of discharge.	■ Patient rates less pain using a numerical scale (for example, if patient had rated pain as 8 on scale of 1 to 10, any reduction in pain would be a rating of less than 8). ■ Patient expresses pain relief. ■ Patient can perform self-care activities without assistance. ■ Patient shows no facial mask of pain. ■ Patient doesn't guard incision site.

- Focus on the patient's behavior, not on a nursing action.
- Encourage the patient to participate in developing the outcomes.
- Adapt the outcome to the patient. For example, consider his age, developmental stage, and coping ability. (See chapter 8, Documentation of the Nursing Process, for more information on writing outcomes.)

Learning outcomes

The patient-teaching plan identifies what a patient needs to learn, how you'll teach him, and ways to evaluate what he has learned. Some teaching plans are part of the patient's plan of care. However, many health care facilities require a separate teaching plan because of the emphasis that JCAHO and other regulatory bodies place on the use of interdisciplinary patient teaching with documentation of the patient's learning response.

Learning outcomes should describe measurable and observable behavior and must focus on the patient. A patient's learning behaviors fall into three categories: cognitive (related to knowledge), affective (related to attitudes), and psychomotor (related to movement and coordination). (See *Writing a concise learning outcome,* page 96.)

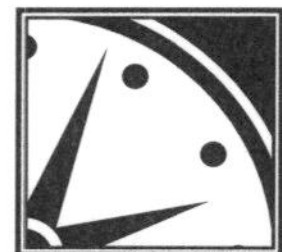

CHARTING TIMESAVER

Writing a concise learning outcome

When writing a learning outcome statement for your patient-teaching plan, save time by being concise and clear. Use the representative action verbs below to describe three kinds of learning behaviors and the desired outcomes.

DESCRIPTIVE VERBS	LEARNING OUTCOMES
Cognitive Recognize Describe State Discuss Identify List Explain	■ The patient will identify three signs of wound infection. ■ The patient will describe the relationship between a high-fat diet and coronary artery disease.
Affective Express Exhibit Relate Communicate Report Verbalize	■ The patient will verbalize his feelings regarding loss of independence. ■ The patient will exhibit positive interaction with family members.
Psychomotor Demonstrate Perform Practice Administer Measure Inject	■ The patient will correctly measure and record his apical-radial pulse rate before taking digoxin. ■ The patient will demonstrate the proper technique for dressing his wound.

Evaluation

Evaluating expected outcomes includes gathering assessment data, comparing the finding with the outcome criteria, determining the extent to which the goals were achieved (goals met, partially met, or not met), writing evaluation statements, and revising the plan of care. If the patient meets his goals and the problem is resolved, you can discontinue the plan of care or teaching plan. If not, continue the plan but set new target dates.

Factors that may work against successful goal completion include unrealistic outcome statements, unrealistic target dates, outcomes that are unacceptable to the patient, and ineffective strategies.

Advantages

With outcome documentation, you use and record all phases of the nursing process, making this system ideal for determining continuous quality improvement. Additionally, the system fosters mutual goal setting and clear documentation of patient teaching performed and learning achieved.

Disadvantages

If you fail to use the nursing process consistently, carrying out outcome documentation adequately will be difficult.

Computerized charting

Computerized charting can significantly reduce the amount of time you spend on documentation. Besides facilitating accurate and speedy documentation, computers can also help you complete nurse management reports, provide patient classification data, and make staffing projections. They can identify patient-teaching needs and supply data for nursing research and education. Some bedside terminals can track a patient's vital signs electronically.

A computer information system can be either a stand-alone unit or a subsystem of a larger, facility-wide network. Most health care facilities locate personal computers or terminals at workstations throughout the facility, allowing staff members quick access to vital information (such as lab results, designated times for scheduled tests and procedures, a list of all ordered medications and treatments, and changes in orders). Some facilities place terminals at patients' bedsides, making data even more accessible.

To call up a patient's computerized clinical record, a health care team member first must enter a special code or codes. Depending on the system, the code may even specify the type of information that a particular team member may have. For example, a dietitian may be assigned a code that allows her to see dietary orders and the patient's nutrition history but not the patient's physical therapy information. Although these codes are intended to maintain a patient's privacy, if they're misused, his rights can still be violated.

To use a computerized system for documentation, simply enter the special code and the patient's name or account number to bring the patient's electronic chart to the screen. Then choose the function you want to perform. For example, you can enter new data on the nursing plan of care or progress notes, or you may want to scan the record for vital signs data or intake and output records. With a computerized system, you can usually obtain information more quickly than you can from traditional documentation systems.

Systems and functions

Depending on which type of computer and software your health care facility has, you may access information by using a keyboard, a light pen, a touch-sensitive screen, a mouse, or even your voice.

Most computerized documentation systems provide a menu of words or phrases you can choose from to individualize documentation on standardized formats. Some systems permit you to use a series of phrases to quickly create a complete narrative note. You can then elaborate on a problem or clarify flow sheet documentation in the comment section of a computerized form by entering standardized phrases or typing in comments. (See *Computers and the nursing process,* page 98.)

Some current computerized systems are the Nursing Information System, the Nursing Minimum Data Set, the Nursing Outcomes Classification, and voice-activated systems.

Nursing Information System

Currently available Nursing Information System (NIS) software programs allow you to record nursing actions in the electronic record, making nursing documentation easier. These systems reflect most or all of the components of the nursing process so they can meet the standards of the American Nurses Association (ANA) and JCAHO. Each NIS provides different features and can be customized to conform to a facility's documentation forms and formats.

Currently, most NISs manage information passively — that is, they collect, transmit, organize, format, print, and display information that you can use to make a decision, but they don't suggest decisions for you. However, some of the newer systems can suggest nursing diagnoses based on predefined asses-

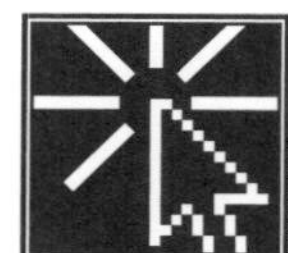

USING COMPUTERS

Computers and the nursing process

Nursing information systems (NISs) can increase efficiency and accuracy in all phases of the nursing process — assessment, nursing diagnosis, planning, implementation, and evaluation — and can help nurses meet the standards established by the American Nurses Association and the Joint Commission on Accreditation of Healthcare Organizations. In addition, an NIS can help you spend more time meeting the patient's needs. Consider the following uses of computers in the nursing process.

Assessment

Use the computer terminal to record admission information. As data are collected, enter further information as prompted by the computer's software program. Enter data about the patient's health status, history, chief complaint, and other assessment factors. Some software programs prompt you to ask specific questions and then offer pathways to gather further information. In some systems, if you enter an assessment value that's outside the usual acceptable range, the computer will flag the entry to call your attention to it.

Nursing diagnosis

Most current programs list standard diagnoses with associated signs and symptoms as references; you must still use clinical judgment to determine a nursing diagnosis for each patient. With this information, you can rapidly obtain diagnostic information. For example, the computer can generate a list of possible diagnoses for a patient with selected signs and symptoms, or it may enable you to retrieve and review the patient's records according to the nursing diagnosis.

Planning

To help nurses begin writing a plan of care, newer computer programs display recommended expected outcomes and interventions for the selected diagnoses. Computers can also track outcomes for large patient populations and general information to help you select patient outcomes. You can use computers to compare large amounts of patient data, help identify outcomes the patient is likely to achieve based on individual problems and needs, and estimate the time frame for reaching outcome goals.

Implementation

Use the computer to record actual interventions and patient-processing information, such as transfer and discharge instructions, and to communicate this information to other departments. Computer-generated progress notes automatically sort and print out patient data, such as medication administration, treatments, and vital signs, making documentation more efficient and accurate.

Evaluation

During evaluation, use the computer to record and store observations, patient responses to nursing interventions, and your own evaluation statements. You may also use information from other members of the health care team to determine future actions and discharge planning. If a desired patient outcome hasn't been achieved, record interventions taken to ensure such desired outcomes. Then reevaluate the second set of interventions.

ment data that you enter. The more sophisticated systems provide you with standardized patient status and nursing intervention phrases that you can use to construct your progress notes. These systems let you change the standardized phrases, if necessary, and allow room for you to add your own notes.

New developments

The most recent NISs interact with you, prompting you with questions and suggestions about the information you enter. Ultimately, this sequential decision-making format should lead to more effective nursing care and documentation. These systems require you to enter only a brief narrative. The questioning and diagnostic suggestions that the systems provide make your documentation thorough — and quick. Yet the programs allow you to add or change information so that your documentation fits your patient.

Nursing Minimum Data Set

The Nursing Minimum Data Set (NMDS) program attempts to standardize nursing information. It contains three categories of data: nursing care, patient demographics, and service elements. (See *Elements of the Nursing Minimum Data Set.*)

Elements of the Nursing Minimum Data Set

The Nursing Minimum Data set contains three elements — nursing care, patient demographics, and service. These elements are the core data needed to support decision making in clinical nursing and to implement the computerized patient record.

Nursing care elements

- Nursing diagnoses
- Nursing interventions
- Nursing outcomes
- Nursing intensity

Patient demographic elements

- Personal identification
- Date of birth
- Sex
- Race and ethnicity
- Residence

Service elements

- Unique facility or service agency number
- Unique health record number of patient
- Unique number of principal registered nurse providers
- Episode admission or encounter date
- Discharge or termination date
- Disposition of patient
- Expected payer for medical bills

Nursing benefits

The NMDS allows you to collect nursing diagnosis and intervention data and identify the nursing needs of various patient populations. It also lets you track patient outcomes and describe nursing care in various settings, including the patient's home. This system helps establish accurate estimates for nursing service costs and provides data about nursing care that may influence health care policy and decision making.

With the NMDS, you can compare nursing trends locally, regionally, and nationally, allowing you to compare nursing data from various clinical settings, patient populations, and geographic areas. But the NMDS does more than provide valuable information for research and policy making. It also helps you provide better patient care. For instance, examining the outcomes of patient populations will help you set realistic outcomes for an individual patient as well as formulate accurate nursing diagnoses and plan interventions.

The standardized format of the NMDS also encourages more consistent nursing documentation. All data are coded, making documentation and information retrieval faster and easier. Currently, NANDA assigns numerical codes to all nursing diagnoses so they can be used with the NMDS.

Nursing Outcomes Classification

The Nursing Outcomes Classification (NOC) system provides the first comprehensive standardized method of measuring nursing-sensitive patient outcomes. The NOC has major implications for nursing administrative practice and the patient care delivery system. This system allows the nurse to compare her patients' outcomes to the outcomes of larger groups according to such parameters as age, diagnosis, or health care setting.

NOC implementation is essential to support ongoing nursing research. This system makes possible the inclusion of patient data–related outcomes that have hitherto been absent from computerized medical information databases.

Voice-activated systems

Some hospitals have instituted voice-activated nursing documentation systems, which are most useful in hospital departments that have a high volume of structured reports, such as the operating room.

The software program uses a specialized knowledge base — nursing words, phrases, and report forms, combined with automated speech recognition (ASR) technology. This system allows the user to record prompt and complete nursing notes by voice. The ASR system requires little or no keyboard use; you simply speak into a telephone handset and the text appears on the computer screen.

The software program includes information on the nursing process, nursing theory, nursing standards of practice, report forms, and a logical format. The system uses trigger phrases that cue the system to display passages of report text.

Although voice-activated systems are designed to work most efficiently with these trigger phrases, they also allow word-for-word dictation and editing. The system increases the speed of reporting and frees the nurse from paperwork so that she can spend more time at the bedside.

Advantages

Computerized documentation systems make recording, storing, and retrieving information fast and easy. They allow for efficient and constant updating of information and help link diverse sources of patient information. The systems also store valuable data on patient populations that can help improve the quality of nursing care.

By using standard terminology, computerized documentation promotes better communication among health care disciplines and promotes more accurate comparisons. It also makes information legible. Finally, computerized documentation allows you to send request slips and patient information from one terminal to another quickly and efficiently.

Disadvantages

Used improperly, computerized systems can scramble patient information and threaten a patient's right to privacy if appropriate security measures are neglected. (See *Preventing breaches in patient confidentiality.*) They can also yield inaccurate or incomplete information if they use standardized, limited vocabulary or phrases.

Computer systems can break down, making information temporarily unavailable. Using the computer can take extra time if too many nurses are trying to chart on too few terminals. Finally, the cost of implementing a computerized documentation system may be prohibitive.

Preventing breaches in patient confidentiality

The chart below provides specific measures you can take to ensure that information about your patients remains confidential.

Type of breach	How to prevent it
Computers	
Displays Displaying information on a screen that's viewed by unauthorized users (especially for handheld computers)	Make sure display screens don't face public areas. For portable devices, install encryption software that makes information unreadable or inaccessible.
E-mail Sending confidential messages via public networks such as the Internet, where they can be read by unauthorized users	Use encryption software when sending E-mail over public networks.
Printers Sharing printers among units with differing functions and information (unauthorized people can read printouts)	Request that your unit have a separate printer not shared with another unit.
Copiers Discard copies of patient health information in trash cans adjacent to copiers	Use secure disposal containers (similar to mailboxes) adjacent to copiers.
Cordless and cellular phones Holding conversations vulnerable to eavesdropping by outsiders with scanning equipment	Use phones with built-in encryption technology
Fax machines Faxing confidential information to unauthorized persons	Before transmission, verify the fax number and that the recipient is authorized to receive confidential information.
Voice pagers Sending confidential messages that can be overheard on the pager	Restrict use of voice pagers to nonconfidential messages.

Adapted with permission from *In Confidence.* Chicago: American Health Information Management Association, July 1996.

Selected references

Barnes, L.P. "Patient Teaching: Documentation of Patient Teaching," *American Journal of Maternal Child Nursing* 21(2):111, March-April 1996.

Chase, S.K. "Charting Critical Thinking: Nursing Judgments and Patient Outcomes," *Dimensions of Critical Care Nursing* 16(2):102-11, March-April 1997.

Kobs, A. "Questions and Answers from the JCAHO: Common Questions about JCAHO Standards," *Nursing Management* 28(10):12, 14-15, October 1997.

McCloskey, J.C., and Bulechek, G.M. "Discharge Planning" in *Nursing Interventions Classification,* 2nd ed. St. Louis: Mosby–Year Book, Inc., 1996.

Mills, M.E., et al. *Information Management in Nursing and Health Care.* Springhouse, Pa.: Springhouse Corp., 1996.

North, S.D., and Serkes, P.C. "Improved Documentation of Initial Nursing Assessment," *Nursing Management* 27(4):30, 33, April 1996.

Parker, C.S. "Clinical Issues: Charting by Exception," *Caring* 16(3):36-44, March 1997.

Wesp, C.E., and Hartman, D.E. *Clinical Maps for Acute Care: Care Management through Collaborative Practice.* Gaitherburg, Md.: Aspen Publishers, Inc., 1996.

5

Documentation in Acute Care

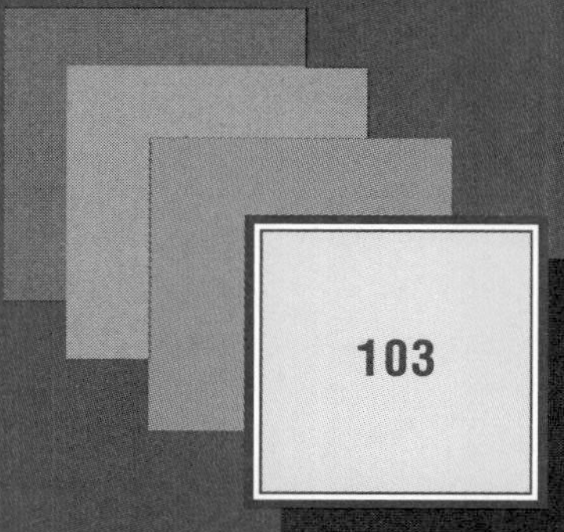

If you're like most nurses, you probably feel discouraged — even overwhelmed — by the number of forms you have to complete each day. Undeniably, paperwork takes time away from your chief priority—patient care. But being familiar with all the forms your health care facility requires and knowing how to use them efficiently bring major benefits.

A medical record with well-organized, completed forms will help you communicate patient information to the health care team, garner accreditation and reimbursements, and protect you and your employer legally. In the long run, taking the time initially to commit patient information to a standard, easy-to-use format will free you to spend more time providing direct patient care.

On the following pages, you'll find the charting forms and methods commonly used in hospital settings. Among the forms and notations you'll find in the medical record of a hospitalized patient are the nursing admission assessment form, progress notes, Kardexes, graphic forms, flow sheets, clinical pathways, patient-teaching documents, discharge summary–patient instruction forms, and others. Dictated documentation, patient self-documentation, and any adapted or newly developed forms may also be included. Let's look at each of these in turn.

Nursing admission assessment form

Also known as a nursing database, the nursing admission assessment form contains your initial patient assessment data. You'll take this step in the nursing process when you first meet the patient. Completing the form itself involves collecting relevant information from various sources and analyzing it to assemble a complete picture of the patient. (For more information on documenting nursing assessments, see Chapter 8, Documentation of the Nursing Process.)

The nursing admission assessment form may be configured in various ways. Some facilities use a form organized by patient responses, such as relating, choosing, exchanging, communicating, and so on, while others organize the form by body systems.

The nursing admission assessment form records your nursing observations, the patient's health history, and your physical examination findings. It includes data on the patient's medications; known allergies to foods, drugs, and other substances; nursing findings related to activities of daily living (ADLs); impressions of the patient's support systems; and documentation of the patient's advance directives, if any.

How you complete this form depends on your health care facility. You may need to fill in blanks, check off boxes, or write narrative notes. (See *Completing the nursing admission assessment.*)

Advantages

Carefully completed, the form provides pertinent physiologic, psychosocial, and cultural information. It contains subjective and objective data about the patient's current health status and clues about actual or potential health problems. It reveals the patient's ability to comply with treatments, his expectations for treatment, and details about lifestyle, family relationships, and cultural influences.

Using this information can guide you through the nursing process by helping you readily formulate nursing diagnoses, create pa-

BETTER CHARTING

Completing the nursing admission assessment

Most health care facilities use a combined checklist and narrative admission form such as the one below. The nursing admission assessment becomes a part of the patient's permanent medical record.

ADMISSION DOCUMENT

(To be completed on or before admission by admitting RN)

Name: *Raymond Bergstrom*
Age: *70*
Birth date: *4/15/29*
Address: *3401 Elmhurst Ave, Jenkintown, PA*
Hospital I.D. No.: *4227*
Insurer: *Aetna*
Policy No.: *605310P*
Physician: *Joseph Milstein*
Admission date: *1/28/99*
Unit: *3N*

Admitted from:
- ☐ Emergency room
- ☐ Home
- ☑ Doctor's office
- ☐ Transfer from ____

Preoperative teaching according to standard?
☑ Yes ☐ No

Preoperative teaching completed on *1/28/99*

If no, ☐ Surgery not planned
☐ Emergency surgery

Signature *Kate McCauley, RN*

Mode:
- ☐ Ambulatory
- ☑ Wheelchair
- ☐ Stretcher

Accompanied by: *Wife*

T *101° F* **P** *120* **R** *24*

BP (Lying [circled]/sitting) Left: ____
Right: *120 / 68*

Height *5'7"*
Weight *160*

Pulses:
L: *P* Radial *P* DP *P* PT
R: *P* Radial *P* DP *P* PT
Apical pulse *120*
☑ Regular ☐ Irregular

P = Palpable D = Doppler O = Absent

Signature *K. McCauley, RN*

Medical & surgical history

Check (P) if patient or (R) if a blood relative has had any of the following. Check (H) if patient has ever been hospitalized. If it's not appropriate to question patient because of age or sex, cross out option, e.g., ~~infertility.~~

	(H)	(P)	(R)	Interviewer comments
Addictions (e.g., alcohol, drugs)	☐	☐	☐	
Angina	☐	☐	☐	
Arthritis	☐	☐	☐	
Asthma	☐	☑	☑	*lungs clear*
Bleeding problems	☐	☐	☐	
Blood clot	☐	☐	☐	
Cancer	☐	☐	☐	
Counseling	☐	☐	☐	
CVA	☐	☐	☐	
Depression	☐	☐	☐	
Diabetes	☐	☐	☑	
Eating disorders	☐	☐	☐	
Epilepsy	☐	☐	☐	
Eye problems (not glasses)	☐	☐	☐	
Fainting	☐	☐	☐	
Fractures	☐	☐	☐	
Genetic condition	☐	☐	☐	
Glaucoma	☐	☐	☐	
Gout	☐	☐	☐	
Headaches	☐	☐	☐	
Hepatitis	☐	☐	☐	
High cholesterol	☐	☑	☐	
Hypertension	☐	☐	☐	
~~Infertility~~	☐	☐	☐	
Kidney disease/ stones	☐	☐	☐	
Leukemia	☐	☐	☐	
Memory loss	☐	☐	☐	
Mood swings	☐	☐	☐	
Myocardial infarction	☐	☐	☐	
Prostate problems	☐	☐	☐	
Rheumatic fever	☐	☐	☐	
Sexually trans. disease	☐	☐	☐	
Thyroid problems	☐	☐	☐	
TB or positive test	☐	☐	☐	
Other	☐	☐	☐	

List any surgeries the patient has had:

Date	Type of surgery

Has the patient ever had a blood transfusion: ☐ Y ☑ N
Reaction: ☐ Y ☐ N

(continued)

DOCUMENTATION IN ACUTE CARE

Completing the nursing admission assessment *(continued)*

Unit introduction

Patient rights given to patient: ☑ Y ☐ N
Patient verbalizes understanding: ☑ Y ☐ N
☑ Patient ☑ Family oriented to:
Nurse call system/unit policies: ☑ Y ☐ N
Smoking/visiting policy/intercom/ siderails/TV channels: ☑ Y ☐ N

Patient valuables:
☑ Sent home
☐ Placed in safe
☐ None on admission

Patient meds:
☑ Sent home
☐ Placed in pharmacy
☐ None on admission

Allergies or reactions

Medications/dyes ☑ Y ☐ N *PCN*
Anesthesia drugs ☐ Y ☑ N
Foods ☐ Y ☑ N
Environmental (e.g., tape, latex, bee stings, dust, pollen, animals, etc.) ☑ Y ☐ N *Dust, pollen, cats*

Advance directive information

1. Does patient have health care power of attorney? ☐ Y ☑ N
   Name: ______ Phone: ______
   If yes, request copy from patient/family and place in chart. Date done: ______ Init. ______
2. Does patient have a living will? ☑ Y ☐ N
3. Educational booklet given to patient/family? ☑ Y ☐ N
4. Advise attending physician if there is a living will or power of attorney ☑ Y ☐ N

Organ & tissue donation

1. Has patient signed an organ and/or tissue donor card? ☑ Y ☐ N
   If yes, request information and place in chart. Date done: *1/28/99*
   If no, would patient like to know more about the subject of donation? ☐ Y ☐ N
2. Has patient discussed his wishes with family? ☑ Y ☐ N

Medications

Does patient use any over-the-counter medications?
Aspirin ☐ Y ☑ N Laxatives ☑ Y ☐ N
Vitamins ☑ Y ☐ N Weight loss ☐ Y ☑ N

What does the patient usually take for minor pain relief? *Acetaminophen*

Prescribed medication (presently in use)	**Reason**	**Dose**	**Last time taken**
1. *Proventil*	*asthma*	*2 puffs q 4 hr*	*1/27/99*
2.			
3.			
4.			

Signature *Kate McCauley, RN* Date *1/28/99*

tient problem lists, and construct plans of care.

As you complete the form, keep in mind that the Joint Commission on Accreditation of Healthcare Organizations (JCAHO), quality improvement groups, and other parties use admission assessment information to continue accreditation, justify requests for reimbursement, and maintain or improve the standards of quality patient care. The recorded data also serve as a baseline for later comparison with the patient's progress.

Another advantage of this form is its usefulness in describing the patient's living arrangement, caregivers, resources, support groups, and other relevant information needed for discharge planning.

Disadvantages

Sometimes, through no fault of your own, you'll be unable to complete the nursing admission assessment form, especially if the patient is too sick to answer questions or a family member can't answer for him.

Documentation style

Admission assessment forms have typically followed a medical format, emphasizing initial symptoms and a comprehensive review of body systems. Although many facilities still use this format, others have opted for formats that reflect the nursing process. (See Chapter 8, Documentation of the Nursing Process.) Regardless of which format you use, admission assessments are documented in one or a combination of three styles: open-ended, closed-ended, and narrative.

Standard open-ended style

In this style, the assessment form has standard fill-in-the-blank pages with preprinted headings and questions. Information is organized into specific categories so you can easily record and retrieve it. Use phrases and approved abbreviations to complete this form.

Standard closed-ended style

Arranged categorically with preprinted headings, checklists, and questions, a closed-ended admission assessment form requires you simply to check off the appropriate responses. This eliminates the problem of illegible handwriting and makes reviewing documented information easy. The form also clearly establishes the type and amount of information required by the health care facility.

Narrative notes

Handwritten or computer generated, narrative notes summarize information obtained by general observation, the health history interview, and a physical examination. They allow you to list your findings in order of importance. They can be quite time-consuming to write and to read, because they require you to remember and record all significant information in a detailed, logical sequence. (See *Writing a narrative admission assessment,* pages 108 and 109.)

The current trend in hospitals and home care agencies is to avoid writing long narrative note entries. Nursing documentation is no longer judged by quantity but by quality. The narrative note content should be concise, pertinent, and evaluatory. If it is too lengthy, it will interfere with efficient data retrieval.

Documentation guidelines

Acute illness, short hospital stays, and staff shortages sometimes make conducting a thorough and accurate initial interview difficult. In certain circumstances, you can ask the pa-

(Text continues on page 110.)

BETTER CHARTING

Writing a narrative admission assessment

Here's an example of a nursing admission assessment form documented in narrative style. The data begin with the patient's health history.

Patient's name: James McGee
Address: 20 Tomlinson Road, Elgin, IL 60120
Home phone: (555) 203-0704
Work phone: (555) 389-2050
Sex: Male
Age: 48
Birth date: 5/11/50
Social Security no.: 189-30-2415
Place of birth: Waterbury, CT
Race: Caucasian
Nationality: American
Culture: Irish-American
Marital status: Married, Susan, age 45
Dependents: James, age 14; Gretchen, age 12
Contact person: Wife (same address as patient) or Clare Hennigan, sister (1214 Ridge Road, De Kalb, IL 60115; phone (555) 203-1212)
Religion: Roman Catholic
Education: M.S. Degree
Occupation: Chemistry teacher, Park Ridge High School

Chief health complaint

Pt. states, "I've had several episodes of gnawing pain in my stomach, and I feel very tired. My doctor examined me and told me I should have some tests to find out what's wrong."

Health history

Pt. has been feeling unusually tired for about a month. States he lost 12 lb last month and about 5 lb before that without trying. States that he's busier at work than usual. He thinks his fatigue may be caused more by his schedule than by physical problems.

Past health: Had measles, mumps, chickenpox as child. Hospitalized at age 6 for tonsillectomy and adenoidectomy. Had a concussion and a fractured left leg at age 17 from a football accident. Has had no complications from that. Immunizations are up-to-date. Last tetanus shot 5 years ago; received hepatitis B vaccine 1 year ago.

Functional health: Describes himself as having a good sense of humor. Feels good about himself; feels he gets along fairly well with people and has many friends.

Cultural and religious influences: Pt. says he has strong religious background, goes to church regularly — important part of his life.

Family relationships: Because he's enrolled in a doctorate program at night, pt. regrets he doesn't get to spend much time with wife and children. Jimmy and Gretchen get along well together, but sometimes compete for time with him.

Pt. says he's usually easygoing but lately blows up at the kids when stress and deadlines from school have him tied in knots.

Describes relationship with wife, father, and sister as good (mother deceased).

Sexuality: Says he and wife had a "decent [adequate] sex life" before he started work toward PhD. Now he's too tired.

Social support: Has many close friends who live in his neighborhood. Would like to socialize more with friends but schoolwork claims most of his time.

Other:

DOCUMENTATION IN ACUTE CARE

Writing a narrative admission assessment *(continued)*

Personal health perception and behaviors: *Smokes cigarettes — between 1 and 2 packs/day. Never used recreational drugs. Takes vitamin and mineral supplements and occasional nonprescription cold medicines. Diet is eat and run — usually goes to fast-food place for dinner before night class. Drinks 1 or 2 glasses of beer a week when he has time for dinner at home. Drinks 6 to 8 cups black coffee daily.*

Rest and sleep: *Describes himself as a morning person. Gets up at 6:30 a.m., goes to bed between 11:30 p.m. and midnight. Likes to get about 8 hours of sleep, but rarely does. Needs to study at night after kids are asleep.*

Exercise and activity: *Says he'd like to be more active but can't find the time. Occasionally takes a walk in the evening but has no regular exercise regimen.*

Nutrition: *24-hour recall indicates deficiency in iron, protein, and calcium. Takes vitamin and mineral supplements. Skips lunch often. States he's been losing weight without trying.*

Recreation: *Likes swimming, hiking, and camping. Tries to take family camping at least once each summer. Wishes he had more time for recreation.*

Coping: *Describes his way of coping as avoiding problems until they get too big. Feels he copes with day-to-day stresses O.K. Says job is busy and stressful most days. Says he's feeling a lot of pressure trying to juggle family, career, and educational responsibilities.*

Socioeconomic: *Earns around $57,000 a year. Has health insurance and retirement benefits through job. Wife Susan is a secretary earning $25,000.*

Environmental: *No known environmental hazards. Lives in 3-bedroom house in town.*

Occupational: *Works 7 hours a day with 1/2 hr for lunch. Gets along well with coworkers. Feels pressure to attain doctorate to advance his career into educational administration. Has had present position for 12 years.*

Family health history

Maternal and paternal grandfathers are deceased. Both grandmothers are alive and well at ages 87 and 91. Father is alive and well at age 72; mother is deceased (at age 59, of breast cancer). Younger sister is alive and well.

Physical status

General health: *Complains of recent stomach pain and fatigue. Had two head colds last winter. No other illnesses or complaints.*

Skin, hair, and nails: *Pallor, no skin lesions. Hair receding, pale nails*

Head and neck: *Headaches occasionally, relieved by aspirin. No history of seizures. Reports no pain or limited movement*

Nose and sinuses: *No rhinorrhea, has occasional sinus infections, no history of nosebleeds*

Mouth and throat: *Last dental exam and cleaning 6 months ago*

Eyes: *Last eye exam 1 year ago. Reports 20/20 vision.*

Ears: *Reports no hearing problems. No history of ear infections. Last hearing evaluation 2 years ago.*

Respiratory system: *No history of pneumonia, bronchitis, asthma, or dyspnea.*

Cardiovascular system: *No history of murmurs or palpitations. No history of heart disease or hypertension.*

Breasts: *Flat*

GI system: *Frequent episodes of indigestion, sometimes relieved by several doses of an antacid (usually Mylanta). Currently complains of gnawing stomach pain. Regular bowel movements but recently noticed dark, tarry stools.*

Urinary system: *No history of kidney stones or urinary tract infections. Voids clear yellow urine several times a day without difficulty.*

Reproductive system: *No history of sexually transmitted disease. Is currently sexually active, though tired. States that sexual relationship with marriage partner is "fine."*

Nervous system: *Reports no numbness, tingling, or burning in extremities*

Musculoskeletal: *Reports no muscle or joint pains or stiffness*

Immune and hematologic systems: *Pt. says doctor told him his hemoglobin was low. Reports no lymph gland swelling.*

Endocrine system: *No history of thyroid disease*

tient to complete a questionnaire about his past and present health status and use this to document his health history. If he's too ill to be interviewed and family members aren't available, base your initial assessment on your observations and physical examination. Just be sure to document on the admission form why you couldn't obtain complete data.

Conduct an interview and record the complete information on the admission form or progress notes as soon as possible, noting the date and time of the entry. Remember that new information may require you to revise the plan of care accordingly.

Before completing the admission assessment form, consider the patient's ability and readiness to participate. For example, if he's sedated, confused, hostile, angry, or in pain or having breathing problems, ask only the most essential questions. You can perform an in-depth interview later when his condition improves. In the meantime, try to find secondary sources (relatives, for example) to provide needed information. Be sure to document your source.

During your interview, try to alleviate as much of the patient's discomfort and anxiety as possible. Also try to create a quiet, private environment for your talk.

Progress notes

After you've completed your nursing assessment and devised an initial plan of care, use progress notes to record the patient's status and track changes in his condition. Progress notes describe, in chronological order, patient problems and needs, pertinent nursing observations, nursing reassessments and interventions, patient responses to interventions, and progress toward meeting expected outcomes.

These notes promote effective communication among all members of the health care team and continuity of care. Standard progress notes have a column for the date and time and a column for detailed comments. (See *Keeping standard progress notes.*)

Advantages

Because progress notes are written chronologically and usually reflect the patient's problems (the nursing diagnoses), retrieving information can be easy. Also, progress notes contain information that doesn't fit into the space or format of other forms.

Disadvantages

If the notes aren't well organized, you may have to read through the entire form to find what you're looking for. Nurses also may waste time recording information on progress notes that they've already recorded on other forms. In addition, the notes may contain insignificant information because the documenter feels compelled to fill in space.

Documentation guidelines

When writing a progress note, include the date and time of the care given or your observations, what prompts the entry, changes in the patient's condition, and other pertinent data.

Some progress notes are designed to focus on the nursing diagnoses. If your facility uses this type of progress note, be sure to record each nursing diagnosis, problem, goal, or expected outcome that relates to your entry. For example, the nursing diagnosis *Pain* and related problems, such as pain relief and the effectiveness of analgesics, may be the focus of

BETTER CHARTING

Keeping standard progress notes

Use the following example as a guide for completing your progress notes.

PROGRESS NOTES

Date	Time	Comments
2/20/99	0900	Notified Dr. Watts re Ⓛ lower lobe crackles and ineffective cough. R 40 and
		shallow. Skin pale. Nebulizer treatment ordered. ———— Ruth Bullock, RN
2/20/99	1030	Skin slightly pink after nebulizer treatment. Lungs clear. R 24. Showed pt. how to
		do pursed-lip and abdominal breathing. ———— Ruth Bullock, RN
2/20/99	1400	Ⓛ leg wound 3 cm x 1 cm wide x 1 cm deep. Small amount of pink-yellow, non-
		odorous drainage noted on dressing. Surrounding skin reddened and tender.
		Wound irrigated and dressed as ordered. ———— Ruth Bullock, RN
2/20/99	1930	Pt. instructed about upper GI test. Pt. related correct understanding of test
		purpose and procedure. ———— Ann Barrow, RN

a nursing progress note. (See *Using nursing diagnoses to write progress notes,* page 112.)

Chart times

Make sure that every progress note has the specific date and time of the care given or the observation noted. Don't record entries in blocks of time ("1500 to 2330 hours," for example). Years ago, when nurses were required to write progress notes every 2 hours, charting blocks of time was common. Today most nurses use a flow sheet to chart how often they check on a patient. Together, flow sheets and progress notes usually provide adequate evidence of nursing care.

Chart changes in condition

Be sure to document new patient problems ("onset of seizures," for example); resolution of old problems (such as "no complaint of pain in 24 hours"); or deteriorations in the patient's condition (for example, "Pt. has increasing dyspnea, causing him to remain on bed rest. ABG values show PaO_2 of 52. O_2 provided by rebreather mask as ordered.").

Record observations

Document your observations of the patient's response to the plan of care. If the patient's behaviors are similar to agreed-upon objectives, document that the goals are being met. If the reverse is true, document that the goals aren't being met. For example, you might record:

2/9/99	1600	Dyspnea resolving. Pt. can
		perform ADLs and ambulate
		20 feet s̄ SOB. ————
		———— Lois Cahn, RN

BETTER CHARTING

Using nursing diagnoses to write progress notes

Progress notes can be written using a nursing diagnosis, as the example below shows.

Patient identification information
John Adams
111 Oak St.
Centerville, CA
(202) 123-4560

Centerville Hospital, Centerville, CA

PROGRESS NOTES

Date and time	Nursing diagnosis and related problems	Notes
1/9/99 —2300	Pain related to pressure sore on Ⓛ elbow.	Pt. rates pain an 8 on a scale of 1 to 10, with 1 being no pain and 10 being the worst pain ever experienced. Pt. frowning when pointing to wound. BP 130/84; P 96. Pain aggravated by dressing change @ 2200. Percocet ī given P.O. and pt. repositioned on Ⓡ side —— Anne Curry, RN
1/9/99 —2330	Pain related to pressure sore on Ⓛ elbow.	Pt. states that pain is relieved. Will give Percocet 1/2 hour before next dressing change and before future dressing changes. —— Anne Curry, RN

Or you might write:

2/9/99	2000	Dyspnea unrelieved. Pt. continues to have tachypnea and tachycardia 1 hr after receiving O_2 by rebreather mask. Blood drawn for ABG analysis shows Po_2 70; Pco_2 32; pH, 7.40 —— Carol Davis, RN

Don't repeat yourself

Generally, avoid including information that's already on the flow sheet. The exception: a sudden change in the patient's condition, such as a decreased level of consciousness, a change in skin condition, or swelling at an I.V. site.

Be specific

Avoid vague wording when you write a progress note, remember to. For example, using a phrase such as "appears to be" indicates that you're not sure about what you're charting. Phrases such as "no problems" and "had a good day" are also ambiguous and subject to interpretation. Instead, chart specifics, such as the details found in the following example:

1/06/99	1000	Pt. ate 80% of breakfast and 75% of lunch; OOB to bathroom and walked in hallway 3 times for a distance of 10 feet. —— K. Comerford, RN

Respond to needs or complaints

Sometimes, nurses document a problem but fail to describe what they did about it. Outline your interventions clearly—how and when you notified the doctor, what his orders were, when you followed through, and how and when you followed through on a request for nursing orders, information, or services. Here's an example:

1/10/99	400	Pt. wants to know when he'll
		be getting chemotherapy. Dr.
		Milstein notified. Pt. informed
		that Dr. Milstein ordered che-
		motherapy to start this after-
		noon.
		Esther Blake, RN

KARDEX

In use for decades, the patient care Kardex (sometimes called the nursing record or nursing Kardex) gives a quick overview of basic patient care information. A Kardex typically contains boxes for you to check off what applies to each patient as well as current orders for medications, patient care activities, treatments, and tests. (See *Components of a patient care Kardex,* pages 114 and 115.) You'll refer to the Kardex during change-of-shift reports and throughout the day. A Kardex can come in various shapes, sizes, and types. It may also be computer generated.

A Kardex includes the following data:

- the patient's name, age, marital status, and religion (usually on the address stamp)
- allergies
- medical diagnoses, listed by priority
- nursing diagnoses, listed by priority
- current doctors' orders for medication, treatments, diet, I.V. therapy, diagnostic tests, procedures, and other measures
- DNR (do not resuscitate) status
- consultations
- results of diagnostic tests and procedures
- permitted activities, functional limitations, assistance needed, and safety precautions
- emergency contact numbers.

A Kardex can be made more effective by tailoring the information to the needs of a particular setting. For instance, a home health care Kardex should have information on family contacts, doctors, other services, and emergency referrals. Some facilities have eliminated the Kardex and incorporated the information into the patient's plan of care.

Some health care facilities use a Kardex specifically to document medication information or other data, such as test results or nonnursing information, which avoids duplicating what's already written in the nursing plan of care.

MEDICATION KARDEX

If your health care facility uses a separate medication Kardex on acute care units, you'll find this document on the medication cart. The medication Kardex may include the medication administration record (MAR), with medications usually listed at the top of the form. If you don't use a medication cart, the medication sheet needn't be kept separate from the Kardex. (For a sample of a completed medication Kardex, see Chapter 9, Documentation of Everyday Events.)

COMPUTER-GENERATED KARDEX

Typically used to record laboratory or diagnostic test results and X-ray findings, a com-

(Text continues on page 116.)

BETTER CHARTING

Components of a patient care Kardex

Below you'll find the kind of information that might be included on the cover sheet of a patient care Kardex for a medical-surgical unit. Inside the Kardex, which is folded in half horizontally, you'll find additional patient care information.

Keep in mind that the categories, words, and phrases on a Kardex are brief and intended to quickly trigger images of special circumstances, procedures, activities, or patient conditions.

Care status
- Self-care ☐
- Partial care with assistance ☐
- Complete care ☑
- Shower with assistance ☐
- Tub ☐
- Active exercises ☑
- Passive exercises ☑

Special care
- Back care ☑
- Mouth care ☑
- Foot care ☐
- Perineal care ☑
- Catheter care ☑
- Trach care ☐
- Other (specify): ______

Condition
- Satisfactory ☐
- Fair ☑
- Guarded ☐
- Critical ☐
- No code ☑
- Advance directive
  - Yes ☑
  - No ☐
- Date: *1/18/99*

Prosthesis
- Dentures
  - upper ☑
  - lower ☑
- Contact lenses ☐
- Glasses ☑
- Hearing aid ☐
- Other (specify): ______

Isolation
- Strict ☐
- Wound and skin ☐
- Respiratory ☐
- Hepatitis ☐
- Enteric ☐
- Other (specify): ______

Diet
- Type: *2 gm Na*
- Force fluids ☐
- NPO ☐
- Assist with feeding ☑
- Isolation tray ☐
- Calorie count ☐
- Supplements: ______

Tube feedings ☐
- Type: ______
- Rate: ______
- Route: ______
  - NG tube ☐
  - G tube ☐
  - J tube ☐

Admission
- Height: *6' 1"*
- Weight: *161 lb. (73 kg)*
- BP: *118/84*
- Temp: *99.6° F*
- Pulse: *101*
- Resp.: *21*

Frequency
- BP: *q 4 hr.*
- TPR: *q shift*
- Apical pulses: ______
- Peripheral pulses: *q shift*
- Weight: *daily*
- Neuro check: ______
- Monitor: ______
- Strips: ______
- Turn: *q 2 hr.*
- Cough: *q shift*
- Deep breathe: *q shift*
- Central venous pressure: ______
- Other (specify): ______

GI tubes
- Salem sump ☐
- Levin tube ☐
- Feeding tube ☐
- Type (specify): ______
- Other (specify): ______

Activity
- Bed rest ☐
- Chair *t.i.d.* ☑
- Dangle ☐
- Commode ☐
- Commode with assist ☑
- Ambulate ☐
- BRP ☐
- Fall-risk category ☑ (specify): *# 1*
- Other (specify): ______

Mode of transport
- Wheelchair ☑
- Stretcher ☐
- With oxygen ☐

I.V. devices
- Heparin lock ☐
- Peripheral I.V. ☑
- Central line ☐
- Triple-lumen CVP ☐
- Hickman ☐
- Jugular ☐
- Peripherally inserted ☐
- Parenteral nutrition ☐
- Irrigations: ______

Dressings
- Type: ______
- Change: ______

Allergies

______

Emergency contact
- Name: ______
- Telephone no: ______

DOCUMENTATION IN ACUTE CARE

Components of a patient care Kardex *(continued)*

Respiratory therapy
Pulse oximetry
Spo$_2$ level (%) ______
Oxygen ☑
Liters/minute *2 L/min*
Method
Nasal cannula ☑
Face mask ☐
Venturi mask ☐
Partial rebreather mask ☐
Nonrebreather mask ☐
Trach collar ☐
Nebulizer ☐
Chest PT ☑
Incentive spirometry ☑
T-piece ☐
Ventilator ☐
Type: ______
Settings: ______
Other (specify): ______

Drains
Type: ______
Number: ______
Location: ______

Urine output
I & O ☑
Strain urine ☐
Indwelling catheter ☐
Date inserted: ______
Size: ______
Intermittent catheter ☐
Frequency: ______

Side rails
Constant ☐
PRN ☐
Nights ☐

Restraints
Date: ______
Type: ______

Specimens and tests
ACCU check q 6 h
24-hour collection ☐
Other (specify): ______

Stools
Stools negative for occult blood

Special notes
Evaluate pain level q 1 h

Social services
Started 1/18/99

The format and specific information on a Kardex will vary with the needs of the patient population. For instance, the cover sheet of a patient care Kardex on a critical care unit would include the same basic information already shown plus information specific to the unit, including the following:

Monitoring
Hardwire ☐
Telemetry ☐
Arterial line ☐

Pulmonary artery catheter ☐
Pulmonary artery pressure: ______
Pulmonary artery wedge pressure: ______
Other (specify): ______

Mechanical ventilation
Type: ______
Tidal volume: ______
Fio$_2$: ______
Mode: ______
Rate: ______

On an obstetrics unit, you might find the following additional information on the Kardex cover sheet:

Delivery
Date: ______
Time: ______
Type of delivery: ______

Special procedures
Perianal rinse ☐
Sitz bath ☐
Witch hazel compress ☐
Breast binders ☐
Ice ☐
Abdominal binders ☐
Other (specify): ______

Mother
Due date: ______
Gravida: ______
Para: ______
Rh: ______
Blood type: ______
Membranes ruptured: ______
Episiotomy ☐
Lacerations ☐
RhoGAM studies?
Yes ☐ No ☐
Rubella titer?
Yes ☐ No ☐

Infant
Male ☐
Female ☐
Full term ☐
Premature ☐
Weeks: ______
Apgar score ☐
Nursing ☐
Formula ☐
Condition (specify): ______
Other (specify): ______

puterized Kardex usually includes information regarding medical orders, referrals, consultations, specimens (for example, for culture and sensitivity tests or for blood glucose analysis), vital signs, diet, activity restrictions, and so forth. (See *Characteristics of a computer-generated Kardex.*)

Advantages

A patient care Kardex provides quick access to data about task-oriented interventions, such as medication administration and I.V. therapy. Although it duplicates information, the plan of care may be added to the Kardex to provide all the necessary data for patient care.

Disadvantages

Kardexes are only as useful as nurses make them. A Kardex won't be effective if it doesn't have enough space for appropriate data, if it's not updated frequently, if it's not completed, or if the nurse doesn't read it before giving patient care.

Make sure the Kardex doesn't become the working plan of care. Although the Kardex is useful and updated, the plan of care should also be updated. At many facilities, a Kardex is not part of the permanent record and is discarded after the patient is discharged.

Documentation guidelines

The most effective types of Kardex are designed for specific units and reflect the needs of the patients on those units. Keep in mind that you should record information that helps nurses plan daily interventions (for example, the time a particular patient prefers to bathe, his food preferences before and during chemotherapy, and which analgesics or positions are usually required to ease pain).

If you're documenting on a medication Kardex, here are some tips:

- Be sure to include the date; the administration time; the medication dose, route, and frequency; and your initials.
- Indicate whenever you administer a stat dose and, if appropriate, the specific number of doses, as ordered, or the stop date.
- Write legibly, using only standard abbreviations. When in doubt about how to abbreviate a term, spell it out.
- After giving the first dose of a medication, sign your full name, your licensure status, and your initials in the appropriate space.
- After withholding a medication dose, document which dose wasn't given (usually by circling the time it was scheduled or by drawing an asterisk) and the reason it was omitted (for example, withholding oral medications from a patient the morning of scheduled surgery).

If you administer all medications according to the plan of care, you don't need further documentation. However, if your MAR does not have space for information, such as the parenteral administration site, the patient's response to medications given as needed, or deviations from the medication order, you'll need to record this information in the progress notes. Here's an example:

1/12/99	0800	Withheld Procardia per or-
		der of Dr. Patel because pt.'s
		BP: 98/58.
		Dave Bevins, RN

DOCUMENTATION IN ACUTE CARE

BETTER CHARTING

Characteristics of a computer-generated Kardex

In the computer-generated Kardex shown below, you'll find a detailed list of medical orders and other patient care data.

```
3/10/99      539                                          Page 001
= = = = = = = = = = = = = = = = = = = = = = = = = = = = = = = = = = =
Stevens, James                                    M 65
MR#: 000310593                               Acct#: 9400037290
DR: J. Carrio                                     2/W 204-01
DX: Unstable angina                          Date: 3/10/99
= = = = = = = = = = = = = = = = = = = = = = = = = = = = = = = = = = =
SUMMARY: 3/10      0701 to 1501

PATIENT INFORMATION
    3/10     ADVANCE DIRECTIVE: No.
             Advance directive does not exist
    3/10     ORGAN DONOR: Unknown
    3/10     ADMIT DX: Unstable angina
    3/10     MED ALLERGY: None known
    3/10     ISOLATION:

MISC. PATIENT DATA

NURSING PLAN OF CARE PROBLEMS
3/10  Alteration in comfort R/T: anginal pain

ALL CURRENT MEDICAL ORDERS

NURSING ORDERS:
    3/10     Activity, OOB, up as tol.
    3/10     Routine V/S q 8 h
    3/10     Telemetry
    3/10     If 1800 PTT < 50, increase heparin drip to 1200
             units/hr. If 50 to 100, maintain 1000 units/hr. If >100,
             reduce to 900 units/hr.
    3/10     Please contact M. Sweeney to see pt. regarding diabetic
             management and insulin treatment.
DIET:
    3/10     Diabetic: 1600 cal., start with lunch today
I.V.s.:
    3/10     Peripheral line #1. . . . Start D5W 250 ml with heparin
             25,000 units: rate, 1000 units/hr.
```

(continued)

DOCUMENTATION IN ACUTE CARE

Characteristics of a computer-generated Kardex *(continued)*

```
3/10/99        539                                              Page 002
= = = = = = = = = = = = = = = = = = = = = = = = = = = = = = = = = = = = =
Stevens, James                                     M 65
MR#: 000310593                            Acct#:9400037290
DR: J. Carrio                                      2/W 204-01
DX: Unstable angina                       Date: 3/10/99
= = = = = = = = = = = = = = = = = = = = = = = = = = = = = = = = = = = = =
Summary: 3/10      0701 to 1501

SCHEDULED MEDICATIONS:
    3/10     Nitroglycerin oint 2%, 1-1/2 inches, apply to chest wall
             q 8 h, starting on 3/10, 1800 hrs.
    3/10     Diltiazem tab 90 mg, #1, P.O., q 6 h 0800, 1400, 2000,
             0200
    3/10     Furosemide tab 40 mg, #1, P.O., daily 0900
    3/10     Potassium chloride tab 10 mEq, #1, P.O. daily 0900
    3/10     Labetalol tab 100 mg, #1/2, P.O. bid 0900, 1800

STAT/NOW MEDICATIONS:
    3/10     Furosemide tab 40 mg, #1, P.O., today
    3/10     Potassium chloride tab 10 mEq, #1, P.O., today

PRN MEDICATIONS:
    3/10     Procardia nifedipine cap 10 mg, #1, subling. q 6 h, prn
             SBP >170 or DSBP >105
    3/10     Acetaminophen tab 325 mg, #2, P.O., q 4 h, prn for pain
    3/10     Temazepam cap 15 mg, #1, P.O., q HS, prn
    3/10     Alprazolam tab 0.25 mg, #1/2, P.O., q 8 h, prn

LABORATORY:
    3/10     CK & MB 1800 today
    3/10     CK & MB 0200 tomorrow
    3/10     Urinalysis floor to collect
    3/10     PTT 1800 today

ANCILLARY:
    3/10     Stress test persantine, prep H1, Patient handling:
             wheelchair, Schedule: tomorrow

                            Last page
```

Graphic forms

Used for 24-hour assessments, graphic forms usually have a column of data printed on the left side of the page, times and dates printed across the top, and open blocks within the side and top borders. You'll use graphic forms to plot various changes — in the patient's vital signs, weight, intake and output (stools, urine, and vomitus), appetite, and activity level, for instance.

Advantages

Graphic forms present information at a glance, allowing you to trend data. For example, blood pressure that rises, falls, or fluctuates over time can be detected much more readily on a graph than in a narrative accounting of raw numbers. Also, health care personnel such as licensed practical nurses are permitted to document measurements on a graphic form, thereby saving registered nurses valuable time.

Disadvantages

Data placed on the graph must be accurate, legible, and complete. Every vital sign you take should be transcribed onto this form. If these guidelines aren't followed, the form loses its value. For accuracy, double-check the graph after transcribing any information onto it.

Avoid using the information on a graph alone; instead, combine it with narrative documentation to present a complete picture of the patient's clinical condition.

Documentation guidelines

For greater accuracy, try to chart on graphic forms at the same time each day. Document the patient's vital signs on both the graphic form and the progress notes when you administer an analgesic, antihypertensive, or antipyretic drug, for example. This provides a record of the patient's response to a drug that may produce a change in a particular vital sign.

Also document vital signs on both forms for such events as chest pain, chemotherapy, a seizure, or a diagnostic test to indicate the patient's condition at that time.

Be sure to chart legibly, to put data in the appropriate time line, and to make the dots on the graph large enough to be seen easily. Connect the dots if your facility requires you to do so. (See *Using a graphic form,* page 120.)

Flow sheets

Also called abbreviated progress notes, flow sheets have vertical or horizontal columns for recording dates, times, and interventions. You can insert nursing data quickly and concisely, preferably at the time you give care or observe a change in the patient's condition. Because flow sheets provide an easy-to-read record of changes in the patient's condition over time, they allow all members of the health care team to compare data and assess the patient's progress.

Using flow sheets doesn't exempt you from narrative charting to describe your observations, patient teaching, patient responses, detailed interventions, and unusual circumstances. However, flow sheets are handy for charting data related to a patient's ADLs, fluid balance, nutrition, pain management, and skin integrity. They're also useful for recording nursing interventions.

In response to a request by the JCAHO, nurses are using these forms to document basic assessment findings and wound care, hygiene, and routine care interventions. In ad-

BETTER CHARTING

Using a graphic form

Plotting information on a graphic form, such as the sample shown below, helps you visualize changes in your patient's temperature, blood pressure, heart rate, weight, and intake and output.

GRAPHIC FORM

Instructions: Indicate temperature in "O" and pulse in "X"

DATE		4/5/99						4/6/99					
POSTOP. DAY		2											
		4	8	12	4	8	12	4	8	12	4	8	12
PULSE	TEMP.												
150	106°												
140	105°												
130	104°												
120	103°												
110	102°								X				
100	101°		X				X				X		
90	100°						O		O				
80	99°		O								O		
	98.6°												
70	98°												
60	97°												
50	96°												
	95°												
RESPIRATION			18			22			20		18		
BLOOD PRESSURE			120/80				138/80		140/90		132/74		

INTAKE	7-3	3-11	11-7	7-3	3-11	11-7	7-3	3-11	11-7	7-3	3-11	11-7	7-3	3-11	11-7	7-3	3-11	11-7	7-3	3-11	11-7
P.O.	480	800	600	300	250																
I.V.		100	100	50	100																
Blood/Colloid	250	900	0	0	0																
8-hour	730	1800	700	350	350																
24-hour	3230																				
OUTPUT	7-3	3-11	11-7	7-3	3-11	11-7	7-3	3-11	11-7	7-3	3-11	11-7	7-3	3-11	11-7	7-3	3-11	11-7	7-3	3-11	11-7
Urine	800	550	500	450	225																
NG/Emesis	0	50	0	0	0																
Other	0	0	0	0	0																
8-hour	800	600	500	450	225																
24-hour	1900																				
WEIGHT	150 lb																				
STOOL	0	0	÷	0	÷																

DOCUMENTATION IN ACUTE CARE

dition, many facilities document I.V. therapy and patient education on flow sheets. The style and format of flow sheets may be varied to fit the needs of patients on particular units. (See *Using a flow sheet to record routine care,* pages 122 to 124.)

Advantages

Because of their concise format, flow sheets let you evaluate patient trends at a glance, especially if you keep the forms conveniently near the patient's bedside. The format of flow sheets also reinforces nursing standards of care and allows precise nursing documentation.

Disadvantages

Because flow sheets have little space, they're not well suited for recording unusual events. Also, overuse of these forms can lead to incomplete or fragmented documentation that obscures the patient's clinical picture. In addition, flow sheets may cause legal problems if they're not consistent with the progress notes, which may happen if the nurse hurriedly checks off whatever the nurse on the previous shift checked off and then charts the actual care in the progress notes.

In some cases, the flow sheet format fails to reflect the needs of the patients and the documentation needs of the nurses on each unit. If the flow sheet doesn't take these needs into account or isn't revised as needs change, it becomes more of a liability than an asset.

In addition, flow sheets add bulk to the medical record, causing handling and storage problems and duplication of documentation.

Documentation guidelines

Ideally, you'll use flow sheets to document all routine assessment data and nursing interventions, such as repositioning or turning the patient, range-of-motion exercises, patient education, wound care, and medication administration. Then your progress notes need only include the patient's progress toward achieving desired outcomes and any unplanned assessments.

Make sure data on the flow sheet are consistent with data in your progress notes. Of course, all entries should accurately reflect the care given. Discrepancies can damage your credibility and increase your chance of liability.

Sometimes, recording only the information requested isn't sufficient to give a complete picture of the patient's status. In such cases, record additional information in the space provided on the flow sheet. If additional information isn't necessary, draw a line through this space to indicate that further information isn't required. If your flow sheet doesn't have additional space and you need to record more information, use the progress notes.

Fill out flow sheets completely, using the key symbols provided, such as a check mark, an "X," initials, circles, or the time to indicate that a parameter was observed or an intervention was carried out. When necessary, use the abbreviation "N/A" (not applicable) or another abbreviation recognized by your facility.

Don't leave blank spaces — they imply that an intervention wasn't completed, wasn't attempted, or wasn't recognized. If you have to omit something, document the reason.

Clinical pathways

A clinical pathway (also known as a critical pathway) integrates the principles of case management into nursing documentation. It

(Text continues on page 125.)

BETTER CHARTING

Using a flow sheet to record routine care

As this sample shows, a patient care flow sheet lets you quickly document your routine interventions.

PATIENT CARE FLOW SHEET

Date 1/22/99	**2300–0700**	**0700–1500**	**1500–2300**
Respiratory			
Breath sounds	Clear 2330 PW	Crackles ⓁLL 0800 SR	Clear 1600 MLF
Treatments/results	———	Nebulizer 0830 SR	———
Cough/results	÷ PW	Mod. amt. tenacious yellow mucus, 0900 SR	÷
O_2 therapy	Nasal cannula @ 2 L/min PW	Nasal cannula @ 2 L/min SR	Nasal cannula @ 2 L/min MLF
Cardiac			
Chest pain	÷ PW	÷ SR	÷ MLF
Heart sounds	Normal S_1 and S_2 PW	Normal S_1 and S_2 SR	Normal S_1 and S_2 MLF
Telemetry	N/A	N/A	N/A
Pain			
Type and location	Ⓛ flank 0400 PW	Ⓛ flank 1000 SR	Ⓛ flank 1600 MLF
Intervention	Meperidine 0415 PW	Repositioned and meperidine 1010 SR	Meperidine 1615 MLF
Pt. response	Improved from #9 to #3 in 1/2 hr PW	Improved from #8 to #2 in 45 min. SR	Complete relief in 1 hr MLF
Nutrition			
Type	———	Regular SR	Regular MLF
Toleration %	———	90% SR	80% MLF
Supplement	———	1 can Ensure SR	———
Elimination			
Stool appearance	÷ PW	÷ SR	÷ soft dark brown MLF
Enema	N/A	N/A	N/A
Results	———	———	———
Bowel sounds	Present all quadrants 2330 PW	Present all quadrants 0800 SR	Hyperactive all quadrants 1600 MLF
Urine appearance	Clear, amber 0400 PW	Clear, amber 1000 SR	Dark yellow 1500 MLF
Indwelling urinary catheter	N/A	N/A	N/A
Catheter irrigations	———	———	———

Using a flow sheet to record routine care *(continued)*

PATIENT CARE FLOW SHEET

Date 1/22/99	2300–0700	0700–1500	1500–2300
I.V. therapy			
Tubing change	———	1100 SR	———
Dressing change	———	1100 SR	———
Site appearance	No edema, no redness 2330 PW	No redness, no edema, no drainage 0800 SR	No redness, no edema 1600 MLF
Wound			
Type	Ⓛ flank incision 2330 PW	Ⓛ flank incision 1200 SR	Ⓛ flank incision 2000 MLF
Dressing change	Dressing dry and intact 2330 PW	1200 SR	2000 MLF
Appearance	Wound not observed PW	See progress note. SR	See progress note. MLF
Tubes			
Type	N/A	N/A	N/A
Irrigation	———	———	———
Drainage appearance	———	———	———
Hygiene			
Self/partial/complete	———	Partial 1000 SR	Partial 2100 MLF
Oral care	———	1000 SR	2100 MLF
Back care	0400 PW	1000 SR	2100 MLF
Foot care	———	1000 SR	———
Remove/reapply elastic stockings	0400 PW	1000 SR	2100 MLF
Activity			
Type	Bed rest PW	OOB to chair X 20 min. 1000 SR	OOB to chair X 20 min. 1800 MLF
Toleration	Turns self PW	Tol. well SR	Tol. well MLF
Repositioned	2330 Supine PW 0400 Ⓛ side PW	Ⓛ side 0800 SR Ⓡ side 1400 SR	Self MLF
ROM	———	1000 (active) SR 1400 (active) SR	1800 (active) MLF 2200 (active) MLF

(continued)

Using a flow sheet to record routine care *(continued)*

PATIENT CARE FLOW SHEET

Date 1/22/99	2300–0700	0700–1500	1500–2300
Sleep			
Sleeps well	0400 PW 0600 PW	N/A	N/A
Awake at intervals	2330 PW 0400 PW	———	———
Awake most of the time	———	———	———
Safety			
Side rails up	2330 PW 0200 PW 0400 PW	1500 SR	1800 MLF
Call button in reach	2330 PW 0200 PW 0400 PW	0800 SR	1600 MLF
Equipment			
Type IVAC pump	Continuous 2300 PW	Continuous 0800 SR	Continuous 1600 MLF
Teaching			
Wound splinting	0400 PW	1000 SR	———
Deep breathing	0400 PW	1000 SR	1600 MLF
Initials/Signature/Title	PW / Pam Watts, RN	SR / Susan Reynolds, RN	MLF / Mary La Farge, RN

PROGRESS SHEET

Date	Time	Comments
1/22/99	1/22/99	Ⓛ flank dressing saturated with serosang. drng. Dressing removed. Wound edges well-approximated except for 2-cm opening noted at lower edge of incision. Small amount serosang. drng noted oozing from this area. No redness noted along incision line. Sutures intact. Incision line painted with povidone-iodine. Five 4" x 4" gauze pads applied and taped in place. Dr. Wong notified of increased amt. of drng. ——— Susan Reynolds, RN
1200	2000	Dr. Wong to see pt. Ⓛ flank drsg. removed. 2-cm opening noted at lower edges of incision. Otherwise, wound edges well-approximated. Dr. Wong sutured opening with one 3-0 silk suture. No redness or drng. noted along incision line. Painted incision line with povidone-iodine and applied two 4" x 4" gauze pads. Taped drsg. in place. ——— Mary La Farge, RN.

outlines the standard of care for a specific diagnosis-related group (DRG). It incorporates multidisciplinary diagnoses and interventions, such as nursing-related problems, combined nursing and medical interventions, and key events that must occur for the patient to be discharged by a target date.

These events include consultations, diagnostic tests, treatments, medications, procedures, activities, diet, patient teaching, discharge planning, and anticipated outcomes. Other events or interventions may be added and the pathway's categories may be presented in various formats and combinations.

Within the managed care system, clinical pathways set the standard for patient progress and track it as well. They provide the nursing staff with necessary written criteria to guide and monitor patient care. In some health care facilities, the nursing diagnosis forms the clinical pathway's basis for patient care, although critics believe that structuring the pathway in this way interferes with communication and coordination of care among non-nursing members of the health care team.

A clinical pathway is usually organized by categories according to the patient's diagnosis, which dictates his expected length of stay, daily care guidelines, and expected outcomes. The care guidelines specified for each day may be organized into such categories as activity, diet or nutrition, treatments, medications, patient teaching, discharge planning, and so forth.

The structure and categories may vary from one facility to the next and depend on which are appropriate for the specific DRG. (For an example of a completed clinical pathway, see *Following a clinical pathway,* pages 126 and 127.)

Advantages

Using a clinical pathway form as a permanent documentation tool can eliminate duplicate charting. Narrative notes need only be written when a standard on the pathway remains unmet or when the patient's condition warrants a deviation in care as planned on the pathway. Like the traditional plan of care — and unlike the Kardex — the clinical pathway becomes part of the patient's permanent record.

As long as standardized orders or standing protocols have been determined and accepted, nurses can advance the patient's activity level, diet, and treatment regimens without waiting for a doctor's order. Also, doctors receive fewer phone calls because nurses have the freedom to make nursing decisions.

Clinical pathways improve communication among all members of the health care team because everyone works from the same plan. Proponents of clinical pathways believe that shared accountability for patient outcomes also improves the overall quality of care.

Some health care facilities adapt certain clinical pathways for distribution to patients, finding that many patients feel less anxiety and cooperate more with therapy because they know what to expect. What's more, some patients seem to recover more quickly and go home sooner than anticipated. A secondary benefit of clinical pathways seems to be improved patient teaching and discharge planning.

Disadvantages

Clinical pathways prove most effective for a patient who has only one diagnosis; they're less effective for a patient with several diagnoses or one who experiences complications

(Text continues on page 128.)

BETTER CHARTING

Following a clinical pathway

At any point in a treatment course, a glance at the clinical pathway allows you to compare the patient's progress and your performance as a caregiver with care standards. Below is a sample pathway.

CLINICAL PATHWAY: COLON RESECTION WITHOUT COLOSTOMY

	Patient visit	Presurgery Day 1	O.R. Day	Postop Day 1
Assessments	History and physical with breast, rectal, and pelvic exam Nursing assessment	Nursing admission assessment	Nursing admission assessment on TBA patients in holding area Review of systems assessment*	Review of systems assessment*
Consults	Social service consult Physical therapy consult	Notify referring physician of impending admission		
Labs and diagnostics	Complete blood count (CBC) Coagulation profile ECG Chest X-ray (CXR) Chem profile CT ABD w/wo contrast CT pelvis Urinalysis Barium enema & flex sigmoidoscopy/colonoscopy Biopsy report	Type and screen for patients with hemoglobin (Hgb) <10	Type and screen for patients in holding area with Hgb <10	CBC
Interventions	Many or all of the above labs/diagnostics will have already been done. Check all results and fax to the surgeon's office.	Admit by 8 a.m. Check for bowel prep orders Bowel prep* Antiembolism stockings Incentive spirometry Ankle exercises* I.V. access* Routine vital signs (VS)* Pneumatic inflation boots	Shave and prep in O.R. Nasogastric (NG) tube maint.* Intake and output (I/O) VS per routine* Catheter care* Incentive spirometry* Ankle exercises* I.V. site care* Head of bed (HOB) 30°* Safety measures* Wound care* Mouth care*	NG tube maintenance* I/O* VS per routine* Catheter care* Incentive spirometry* Ankle exercises* I.V. site care* HOB 30°* Safety measures* Wound care* Mouth care* Antiembolism stockings
I.V.s		I.V. fluids, D_5½ NSS	I.V. fluids, D_5LR	I.V. fluids, D_5LR
Medication	Prescribe GoLYTELY/Nulytely 10a—2p Neomycin @ 2p, 3p, and 10p Erythromycin @2p, 3p, and 10p	GoLYTELY/Nulytely 10a—2p Erythromycin @ 2p, 3p, and 10p Neomycin @ 2p, 3p and 10p	Preop antibiotics (ABX) in holding area Postop ABX × 2 doses PCA (basal rate 0.5 mg) S.C. heparin	PCA (basal rate 0.5 mg) S.C. heparin
Diet/GI	Clears presurgery day NPO after midnight	Clears presurgery day NPO after midnight	NPO/NG tube	NPO/NG tube
Activity			4 hours after surgery, ambulate with abdominal binder* D/C pneumatic inflation boots once patient ambulates	Ambulate t.i.d. with abdominal binder* May shower Physical therapy b.i.d.
KEY: *NSG activities V = Variance N = No var.	1. V (N) 2. V N 3. V N	1. V (N) 2. V (N) 3. V (N)	1. V (N) 2. V (N) 3. V (N)	1. V (N) 2. V (N) 3. V (N)
Signatures:	1. *C. Molloy, RN* 2. 3.	1. *M. Connel, RN* 2. *C. Roy, RN* 3. *J. Kane, RN*	1. *L. Singer, RN* 2. *J. Smith, RN* 3. *P. Joseph, RN*	1. *L. Singer, RN* 2. *J. Smith, RN* 3. *P. Joseph, RN*

Following a clinical pathway *(continued)*

CLINICAL PATHWAY: COLON RESECTION WITHOUT COLOSTOMY

	Postop Day 2	Postop Day 3	Postop Day 4	Postop Day 5
Assessments	Review of systems assessment*	Review of systems assessment*	Review of systems assessment*	Review of systems assessment*
Consults		Dietary consult		Oncology consult if indicated (or to be done as outpatient)
Labs and diagnostics	Electrolyte 7 (EL-7) CXR	CBC EL-7	Pathology results on chart	CBC EL-7
Interventions	D/C NG tube if possible* (per guidelines) I/O* VS per routine* D/C catheter* Ambulating* Incentive spirometry* Ankle exercises* I.V. site care* HOB 30°* Safety measures* Wound care* Mouth care* Antiembolism stockings	I/O* VS per routine* Incentive spirometry* Ankle exercises* I.V. site care* Safety measures* Wound care* Antiembolism stockings	I/O* VS per routine* Incentive spirometry* Ankle exercises* I.V. site care* Safety measures* Wound care* Antiembolism stockings	Consider staple removal Replace with Steri-Strips Assess that patient has met d/c criteria*
I.V.s	I.V. fluids D_5½ NSS+ MVI	I.V.-Heplock	Heplock	D/C Heplock
Medication	PCA (5 mg basal rate)	D/C PCA P.O. analgesia Resume routine home meds	P.O. analgesia	P.O. analgesia
Diet/GI	D/C NG tube per guidelines: (Clamp tube at 8 a.m. if no N/V and residual <200 ml, D/C tube @ 12 noon)* (Check with doctor first)	Clears if pt. has BM/flatus Advance to postop diet if tolerating clears (at least one tray of clears)*	House	House
Activity	Ambulate q.i.d. with abdominal binder* May shower Physical therapy b.i.d.	Ambulate at least q.i.d. with abdominal binder* May shower Physical therapy b.i.d.	Ambulate at least q.i.d. with abdominal binder* May shower Physical therapy b.i.d.	
Teaching	Reinforce preop teaching* Patient and family education p.r.n.* re: family screening	Reinforce preop teaching* Patient and family education p.r.n.* re: family screening Begin D/C teaching	Reinforce preop teaching* Patient and family education p.r.n.* D/C teaching re: reportable s/s, F/U and wound care*	Review all D/C instructions and Rx including* follow-up appointments: with surgeon within 3 weeks, with oncologist within 1 month if indicated
KEY: *NSG activities **V = Variance** **N = No var.**	1. 2. 3. V V V (N) (N) (N)	1. 2. 3. V V V (N) (N) (N)	1. 2. 3. V V V (N) (N) (N)	1. 2. 3. V V V (N) (N) (N)
Signatures:	1. A. McCarthy, RN 2. R. Moyer, RN 3. P. Drake, RN	1. A. McCarthy, RN 2. R. Moyer, RN 3. P. Drake, RN	1. L. Singer, RN 2. J. Smith, RN 3. P. Joseph, RN	1. L. Singer, RN 2. J. Smith, RN 3. P. Joseph, RN

DOCUMENTATION IN ACUTE CARE

(because of the difficulty establishing a time line for such a patient). For example, treatment progress is usually predictable for a patient who undergoes a cholecystectomy and is otherwise healthy. However, if the same patient has diabetes and coronary artery disease, the expected treatment course is fairly unpredictable. What's more, the plan of care is likely to change. The result? Lengthy and fragmented documentation.

Documentation guidelines

When developing a clinical pathway to distribute to patients, use simple vocabulary and keep your instructions short. Avoid unapproved abbreviations and complex medical terminology. Ideally, this version of the pathway should explain the diagnosis, review any tests and care the patient can expect, and inform him about activity restrictions, diet, medications, and home health care services.

When writing a clinical pathway, you'll need to collaborate with the doctor and other members of the health care team. Keep in mind that the standardized orders for the clinical pathway require the doctor's signature on admission of the patient.

To ensure consistent documentation from shift to shift, review the clinical pathway during the change-of-shift report with the nurse who's taking over. Point out any critical events, note any changes in the patient's expected length of stay, and discuss any variances that may have occurred during your shift.

If an objective for a particular day remains unmet, document this fact on the appropriate form. Variances from the plan may result for several reasons: the plan itself, patient complications, or unforeseeable events.

Document variances as justifiable or unjustifiable. For instance, you may have a patient who doesn't walk in the hall as scheduled. If he has a secondary infection that prevents him from walking, the variance is justifiable. If he prefers to stay in bed to read or watch TV, the variance is unjustifiable. You'll need to take steps to correct the problem and then document your interventions.

Patient-teaching documents

A preprinted patient-teaching form lets you clearly and completely document the dates, times, and results of your patient-teaching sessions. The form provides evidence that you implemented a teaching plan and that you're evaluating its effectiveness. Completed, the form also documents the patient's progress toward an acceptable level of self-care or assisted care.

Of course, you'll need to construct a patient-teaching plan before you can perform patient-teaching services, complete patient-teaching forms, or distribute educational materials.

Patient-teaching plans

Because standard-setting and reimbursing agencies require the health care facility to instruct patients about their condition and treatment regimen, you'll need to draw up teaching plans to meet your patient's particular needs.

Beginning with your assessment findings, compile a list of topics and strategies that the patient needs to know or perform to attain his maximum level of health and self-care.

These are called *learning outcomes* or *objectives.* Next, devise teaching activities, methods, and tools (such as brochures, one-on-one discussions, and videotapes) to convey and reinforce the information. Then design a way to evaluate your teaching effectiveness, such as a written quiz or an oral question-and-answer session. (See *Filing a teaching plan,* pages 130 and 131.)

Identifying what needs to be learned and how you will teach it constitutes the patient-teaching plan. Translated into reality, the instructive elements and activities should:

- define the patient's condition. If the patient has hypertension, the plan will probably begin with a working definition of normal blood pressure — both systolic and diastolic — and the roles played by the heart and blood vessels. Then the lesson will continue with an explanation of what happens in abnormal blood pressure.
- identify risk factors associated with the patient's condition. General risk factors usually have something to do with family history, age, race, diet, activity patterns, personal habits (such as smoking cigarettes or drinking alcohol), and so forth.
- explain what causes the patient's condition. For example, a patient-teaching plan for hypertension would include a simplified lesson on the dynamics of cardiac output and peripheral vascular resistance. (The teacher might use a model blood vessel for illustration.) If appropriate, the teaching plan should include an explanation of variations of the patient's condition (such as essential or secondary hypertension).
- point out the importance of therapy, emphasizing, if necessary, the consequences of untreated disease. (In untreated hypertension, for example, consequences include cardiovascular disease, stroke, and kidney damage.)
- explain the goals of treatment and identify the components of the treatment plan. In hypertension, for example, the goal of treatment would be stable, normal blood pressure; the components of the treatment plan might include dietary modifications, weight reduction, medications, exercise, stress management, self-monitoring, and regular health care follow-up.
- define the patient's anticipated learning outcomes and provide a time frame. Again using hypertension as an example, some timed learning outcomes might include:
  - By discharge, the patient will be able to plan three well-balanced, low-sodium meals from the food list supplied by the nutritionist.
  - Within 48 hours, the patient will be able to name his medications, explain their purposes, state how and when to take them, and list related adverse reactions that he should report to the doctor or nurse.
  - By discharge, the patient will develop a doctor-approved exercise program.

Advantages

Though the patient-teaching plan doesn't stand alone as a document in the medical record, it is part of the patient's plan of care, which is part of the medical record. The teaching plan tells health care team members at a glance what the patient learned and what he still needs to learn and do about his health condition. It also shows quality-improvement measures in progress and meets professional and accrediting requirements as well.

(Text continues on page 132.)

BETTER CHARTING

Filing a teaching plan

Your teaching plan should include your assessment findings; projected learning outcomes, along with the activities, methods, and tools needed to accomplish the outcomes; and the techniques you'll use to evaluate the effectiveness of teaching.

The teaching plan below was structured for Harold Harmon, a patient who has heart failure.

Assessment findings	Learning outcomes	Activities
Mr. Harmon needs to understand the action of his medication.	Mr. Harmon will: —explain the action of digoxin. —state when to take the drug.	—Present written brochures. —Discuss content. —Check Mr. Harmon's knowledge.
Mr. Harmon needs to learn how to take his pulse.	Mr. Harmon will take his pulse and come within two beats of his doctor's or nurse's results.	—Show Mr. Harmon a videotape that includes instruction on how to take a pulse. —Instruct him to study printed materials. —Demonstrate the procedure. —Provide feedback and practice time. —Ask Mr. Harmon to demonstrate the procedure.
Mr. Harmon reports feeling increased anxiety. He needs to learn how to cope with this anxiety and to control stress in his life.	Mr. Harmon will explain two techniques that he'll use to help him relax.	—Invite Mr. Harmon to watch a videotape on how to control stress. —Encourage him to read printed materials (booklets, pamphlets) on techniques to reduce stress. —Demonstrate deep-breathing and progressive muscle relaxation techniques. —Role-play a guided imagery scene. —Present a case study on how other people cope with stress.

Teaching methods	Teaching tools	Evaluation methods
— One-on-one discussion	— Printed materials describing digoxin's action — Patient-teaching aid on digoxin — Illustration of a medication clock	— Question and answer — Written test
— Demonstration — Supervised practice sessions — One-on-one discussion	— Videotape — Printed materials — Photographs or illustrations of key steps in the procedure	— Question and answer — Return demonstration
— One-on-one discussion — Group discussion (with family) — Role-playing — Case study — Self-monitoring	— Printed materials — Videotape	— Question and answer — Interview — Observation — Return demonstration of relaxation techniques

Disadvantages

Constructing individual teaching plans requires time and thought. Fortunately, some health care facilities have patient education departments that focus on developing and implementing standard teaching plans for many common disorders.

Documentation guidelines

Check your facility's policies and procedures to learn where you're expected to file the patient-teaching plan — for example, within the plan of care, on charts, in progress notes, in the patient education office, or elsewhere.

When writing the teaching plan, be sure to follow the nursing process. Assess the patient's learning needs first, formulate a list of learning diagnoses (or learning outcomes), plan ways to meet the patient's learning needs, implement the plan, and periodically evaluate the results of your teaching by assessing your patient's responses.

Be sure to keep the plan succinct and precise. Most important of all, be sure to talk with the patient about the patient-teaching plan and agree on realistic learning outcomes.

Encourage and expect the patient's participation in the plan. Doing so usually increases his cooperation and your effectiveness.

Patient-teaching forms

Despite their similar content, patient-teaching forms vary according to the health care facility. For the most part, they contain general information about the patient's learning abilities, goals to be met, and skills to be acquired by the time of discharge. They may also focus on teaching aspects as they relate to a patient's particular disease. You can document information by filling in blanks, checking boxes, or writing brief narrative notes. (See *Documenting your teaching.*)

Additional documentation materials include patient-teaching aids, such as preprinted instructional materials, illustrations, models, games, dolls, audiocassettes, and videotapes.

Advantages

Patient-teaching forms make documenting your patient education quicker and easier by creating a record of a patient's outcomes, responses, and level of learning. Correct use of these forms may be your legal defense for many years against charges of inadequate patient care. These forms also prevent duplication of patient-teaching efforts by other staff members. There are no disadvantages of using patient-teaching forms.

Documentation guidelines

Aim to have your completed patient-teaching forms include the patient's learning ability, his response to teaching, and the outcomes. If your facility doesn't have a preprinted form, talk to your supervisor about developing one. In the meantime, document your patient teaching in accurate, detailed progress notes. (See Chapter 8, Documentation of the Nursing Process, for more information on patient-teaching forms.)

Whether you chart on a preprinted form or on progress notes, remember these tips:

- Check your facility's policies and procedures regarding when, where, and how to document your teaching.
- Each shift, ask yourself these questions: What part of the teaching plan did I complete? What other instruction did I give the

(Text continues on page 136.)

BETTER CHARTING

Documenting your teaching

Use the model patient-teaching form below — for a patient with diabetes mellitus — as a guideline for documenting your teaching sessions clearly and completely.

PATIENT TEACHING
Instructions for Diabetic Patients

County Hospital, Waltham, MA

Bernard Miller
7 Main St.
Waltham, MA 04872

Admission date: 1/3/99 **Anticipated discharge:** 1/8/99 **Diagnosis:** TIA/NIDDM

Educational assessment

Comprehension level
Ability to grasp concepts
- [x] High
- [ ] Average
- [ ] Needs improvement

Comments: ______

Motivational level
- [x] Asks questions
- [ ] Eager to learn
- [ ] Anxious
- [ ] Uncooperative
- [ ] Disinterested
- [ ] Denies need to learn

Comments: ______

Knowledge and skill levels
Understanding of health condition and how to manage it
- [ ] High (>75% working knowledge)
- [ ] Adequate (50% to 75% working knowledge)
- [x] Needs improvement (25% to 50% working knowledge)
- [ ] Low (<25% working knowledge)

Comments: ______

Learning barriers
- [ ] Language (specify: foreign, impairment, laryngectomy, other): ______
- [ ] Vision (specify: blind, legally blind, other): ______
- [ ] Hearing (impaired, deaf)
- [ ] Memory
  - [ ] Change in long-term memory (specify): ______
  - [ ] Change in short-term memory (specify): ______
- [ ] Other (specify): ______

Instructor's initials: CW

Anticipated outcomes
Patient will be prepared to perform self-care at the following level:
- [x] High (total self-care)
- [ ] Moderate (self-care with minor assistance)
- [ ] Minimal (self-care with more than 50% assistance)

(continued)

Documenting your teaching *(continued)*

Key

P = patient taught
F = caregiver or family taught
R = reinforced
N/A = not applicable
A = asked questions
B = nonattentive, poor concentration
C = expressed denial, resistance
D = verbalized recall
E = demonstrated ability

Date	1/4/99	1/5/99	1/5/99	1/5/99	1/6/99	1/7/99	1/7/99	1/8/99	
Time	1900	0800	1330	1830	1000	0800	1830	0800	
Assessed educational needs Assessment of patient's (or caregiver's) current knowledge of disease (include medical, family, and social histories)	A/CW								
Assessment of learner's reaction to diagnosis (verbal and nonverbal responses)	A/CW								
General diabetic education goals The patient (or caregiver) will:									
■ define diabetes mellitus.	P/A/CW	R/EG	D/ME					D/EG	
■ state hormone produced in the pancreas.	P/A/CW	R/EG	D/ME					D/EG	
■ identify three signs and symptoms of diabetes.	P/CW	R/EG	D/ME					D/EG	
■ discuss risk factors associated with the disease.	P/CW	R/EG	D/ME					D/EG	
■ differentiate between type 1 and type 2 diabetes.	P/A/CW	R/EG	D/ME					D/EG	
Survival skill goals The patient (or caregiver) will:									
■ identify the name, purpose, dose, and time of administration of medication ordered.		P/EG	R/ME	D/LT				D/EG	
■ properly administer insulin.	N/A								
– draw up insulin properly.	N/A								
– discuss and demonstrate site selection and rotation.	N/A								
– demonstrate proper injection technique with needle angled appropriately.	N/A								
– explain correct way to store insulin.	N/A								
– demonstrate correct disposal of syringes.	N/A								
■ distinguish among types of insulin.	N/A								
– species (pork, beef, recombinant DNA)	N/A								
– regular	N/A								
– NPH/Ultralente (longer acting)	N/A								
■ Properly administer mixed insulins.	N/A								
– demonstrate injecting air into vials.	N/A								

Documenting your teaching *(continued)*

Date	1/4/99	1/5/99	1/5/99	1/5/99	1/6/99	1/7/99	1/7/99	1/8/99	
Time	1900	0800	1330	1830	1000	0800	1830	0800	
– draw up mixed insulin properly (regular before NPH).	N/A								
■ demonstrate knowledge of oral antidiabetic agents.									
– identify name of medication, dose, and time of administration.		P/EG	A/ME		D/EG	F/EG	R/LT	D/EG	
– identify purpose of medication.		P/EG	A/ME		D/EG	F/EG	R/LT	D/EG	
– state possible adverse effects.		P/EG	A/ME		D/EG	F/EG	R/LT	D/EG	
■ list signs and symptoms, causes, implications, and treatments of hyperglycemia and hypoglycemia.		P/EG	A/ME			F/EG		D/EG	
■ monitor blood glucose levels satisfactorily.									
– demonstrate proper use of blood glucose monitoring device.				P/LT	E/EG	E/EG	R/LT	E/EG	
– perform fingerstick.				P/LT	E/EG	E/EG	R/LT	E/EG	
– obtain accurate blood glucose reading.				P/LT	E/EG	E/EG	R/LT	E/EG	
Healthful living goals The patient (or caregiver) will:									
■ consult with the nutritionist about meal planning.			P/ME	R/LT	A/EG			D/EG	
■ follow the diet recommended by the American Diabetes Association.			P/ME	R/LT	A/EG			D/EG	
■ state importance of adhering to diet.			P/ME	R/LT	A/EG			D/EG	
■ give verbal feedback on 1-day meal plan.			P/ME	D/LT	A/EG			D/EG	
■ state the effects of stress, illness, and exercise on blood glucose levels.			P/ME	D/LT	A/EG			D/EG	
■ state when to test urine for ketones and how to address results.			P/ME	D/LT	A/EG			D/EG	
■ identify self-care measures for periods when illness occurs.			P/ME	D/LT	A/EG			D/EG	
■ list precautions to take while exercising.			P/ME	D/LT	A/EG			D/EG	
■ explain what steps to take when patient doesn't want to eat or drink on proper schedule.			P/ME	D/LT	A/EG			D/EG	
■ agree to wear medical identification (for example, a Medic Alert bracelet).			P/ME	A/LT				D/EG	

(continued)

Documenting your teaching *(continued)*

Date	1/4/99	1/5/99	1/5/99	1/5/99	1/6/99	1/7/99	1/7/99	1/8/99	
Time	1900	0800	1330	1830	1000	0800	1830	0800	
Safety goals The patient (or caregiver) will:									
■ state the possible complications of diabetes.	P/CW	R/EG		D/LT		F/EG		D/EG	
■ explain the importance of careful, regular skin care.	P/CW	R/EG		D/LT		F/EG		D/EG	
■ demonstrate healthful foot care.	P/CW	R/EG		D/LT		F/EG		D/EG	
■ discuss the importance of regular eye care and examinations.	P/CW	R/EG		D/LT					
■ state the importance of oral hygiene	P/CW	R/EG		D/LT					
Individual goals									
Initial Signature									
CW Carol Witt, RN, BSN									
EG Ellie Grimes, RN, MSN									
ME Marianne Evans, RN									
LT Lynn Tata, RN, BSN									

patient or his family? Then document your answers.

- Be sure to document that the patient's ongoing educational needs are being met.
- Before discharge, document the patient's remaining learning needs and note whether you provided him with printed or other patient-teaching aids.
- Be sure to evaluate your teaching. One way is by using a checklist. (See *Evaluating your teaching: The checklist method.*)

Discharge summary–patient instruction forms

To comply with JCAHO requirements related to discharge planning, you must document your assessment of a patient's continuing care needs as well as any referrals for such care. To facilitate this kind of documentation, many health care facilities combine discharge summaries and patient instructions in one form. This form contains sections for recording discharge documentation, patient assessment, patient education, and detailed special instructions. On such forms, a narrative style coexists with open- and closed-ended styles.

Another form summarizes the discharge plans made by the different services on one

CHARTING GUIDELINES

Evaluating your teaching: The checklist method

A checklist is a simple, quick way of obtaining information, evaluating your teaching, and gauging your patient's progress at various learning stages. It clearly shows you and the patient which goals he's achieved and which goals remain. To devise a useful checklist, follow these tips:

- Make the list concise but wide-ranging enough to cover all aspects of the skill or activity being evaluated.
- Limit the items on the checklist to a group of related activities, such as the steps in tracheostomy care or the segments of a cardiac rehabilitation plan.
- Arrange items in a logical order — sequentially, chronologically, or in order of importance.
- Identify the essential steps of the activities or behavior you're evaluating.
- Relate items on the list to the patient's learning goals and to your teaching methods.
- Use only one idea or concept for each item.
- Phrase each item succinctly and accurately.
- Test your checklist on at least two patients before adopting it permanently.
- Use the checklist along with other evaluation tools to promote balance and avoid giving it undue importance.

The sample checklist below might be used for evaluating how well a diabetic patient has learned to draw up insulin.

DRAWING UP INSULIN

Yes	No	
☐	☐	Disinfects top of vial thoroughly
☐	☐	Inserts needle into vial without contamination
☐	☐	Withdraws proper amount of insulin
☐	☐	Expels air from syringe
☐	☐	Retains exact dose of insulin in syringe
☐	☐	Replaces cap on needle without contamination

page, emphasizing and documenting a team approach to discharge planning. This form is started at admission, updated during the hospital stay, and completed as discharge arrangements are finalized. (See *Using a multidisciplinary discharge document,* pages 138 and 139.)

Advantages

The combination discharge summary–patient instruction form provides useful information about additional teaching needs and points out whether the patient has the information he needs to care for himself or get further help. It establishes compliance with JCAHO requirements and helps to safeguard you from malpractice accusations.

A multidisciplinary discharge document allows all members of the health care team to reinforce information that may be discipline-specific. For example, the nutritionist may reinforce a special diet or a social worker may provide information regarding assistance in the home. This type of form eliminates second-guessing. There are no disadvantages

BETTER CHARTING

Using a multidisciplinary discharge document

Many health care facilities use a multidisciplinary discharge form. The sample form below has spaces that can be filled in by the nurse, doctor, and other health care providers.

ADMISSION/DISCHARGE DOCUMENT

Patient name: Mary Mayer
Address: 312 Woodlake Drive, Philadelphia, PA
Birth date: 4/12/38
Date of admission: 2/1/99

Patient no.: 34719284
HMO no.: 43217575
Doctor: Dr. Michael Bloom
Discharge date: 2/9/99 Unit: 5N

Discharged to:
☑ Home
☐ Transfer to: ______

Discharged by:
☐ Ambulatory
☑ Wheelchair
☐ Stretcher

Accompanied by: husband

Valuables w/patient ☑ Y ☐ N
Meds w/patient ☑ Y ☐ N
I.V. access DC'd ☑ Y ☐ N

Discharge planning **Family/Friend contacts**

	Name	Relationship	Phone (H)	(W)
1.	Frank Mayer	Husband	492-7342	
2.	Rose Hayes	Sister	492-1965	
3.				
4.				
5.				

Health team referrals

Date	Discipline contacted	Reason	Signature
2/1/99	Nutritional services	Dietary compliance	C. Weir, RN
2/5/99	Respiratory therapy	Treatments	P. Cummins, RT
2/7/99	Physical therapy	Weight bearing	L. Doyle, RN

Supplies/Equipment needed at home

Date	Item	Provider	Signature
2/8/99	Walker	DME R US	B. Frank, MSW
2/8/99	O_2 supplies	DME R US	B. Frank, MSW

Community resources — Resource information provided (list resources)

Date		Signature	Date		Signature
2/9/99	1. Meals On Wheels	B. Frank, MSW		3.	
	2.			4.	

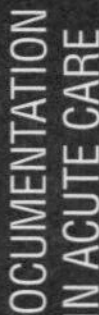

Using a multidisciplinary discharge document *(continued)*

Education needs — Teaching topic completed (refer from 24-hour document)

Date		Signature	Date		Signature
2/1/99	1. Cardiac medications	C. Weir, RN		6.	
2/2/99	2. Low-salt diet restrictions	P. Brown, NT		7.	
	3.			8.	
	4.			9.	
	5.			10.	

Learning ability — Knowledge assessment of discharge needs

Date		Patient		Caregiver (Indicate relationship)			Signature
2/9/99	States diagnosis/disease	☑ Y	☐ N	☑ Y	☐ N	husband	C. Weir, RN
2/9/99	States prognosis	☑ Y	☐ N	☑ Y	☐ N		C. Weir, RN
2/9/99	States medication regimen	☑ Y	☐ N	☑ Y	☐ N		C. Weir, RN
2/9/99	States complications	☑ Y	☐ N	☑ Y	☐ N		C. Weir, RN
2/9/99	Asks pertinent questions	☑ Y	☐ N	☑ Y	☐ N		C. Weir, RN
	Other	☐ Y	☑ N	☐ Y	☑ N		C. Weir, RN

Adapted with permission from Carol Weir. *Core Charting.* Thornberry Ltd., 1-800-775-0878. Doc. #654

of using a discharge summary–patient instruction form or a multidisciplinary discharge document.

Documentation guidelines

Upon discharge, give your patient a copy of his discharge instructions. Document a final physical assessment, including vital signs. Enter a final note in the narrative section or another predetermined location summarizing the patient's condition from admission to discharge with interventions. This summary should include the date, time, location, and mode of discharge.

Make sure that your discharge summary outlines the patient's care, provides useful information for further teaching and evaluation, and documents that the patient has the information he needs to care for himself or to get further help.

Dictated documentation

In some situations, nurses dictate from a nursing unit or clinical setting, and clerical personnel transcribe the information for the written clinical record. This occurs commonly among visiting nurses who may dictate into a recorder or a car phone between patient visits.

Advantages

Convenient and fast, dictated documentation can be performed without the distractions and interruptions encountered in a clinical setting. Using this documentation technique allows the nurse more time for patient care. Dictation can be done at any time of day or night, and studies show that this kind of documentation is highly accurate. What's more, it complies with JCAHO standards and may actually improve the quality of documentation.

Disadvantages

Delays in transcription time can prevent necessary documentation from being made readily available to doctors and other health care team members. Also, supplies for recorded documentation may be more costly than for handwritten charting. In addition, the nurse may need time to adjust to this type of documentation.

Documentation guidelines

Before dictating a report, familiarize yourself with the recording equipment. Then review the existing records and the notations you made during contact with your patient. Here are some tips for more effective dictation:

- Refer to your health care facility's policy and procedures manual for dictation guidelines, and consult the transcriptionist if you have related questions.
- Prepare a brief outline of your report so that it illustrates the nursing process.
- At the beginning of your dictation, name the patient and give his identification number, if necessary.
- Tell the transcriptionist when the report begins and ends. Be sure to provide the date of the report and the date of the visit with the patient. Instruct the transcriptionist to provide the date of transcription. At the end of the report, include a summary, evaluation, and recommendations. Discuss your plans for the next time you'll see the patient.
- Use a checklist as you dictate to be sure that you include all the necessary information. For example, state the purpose of your time with the patient, list assessments performed and findings, discuss any new or changing patient problems, list interventions and patient responses, identify future care needs, explain patient teaching provided, and describe the patient's response.
- Try to dictate the information as near to the time that you provided care as possible so that your activities and observations are fresh in your mind.
- Speak clearly and slowly, avoiding unnecessary medical terminology or uncommon abbreviations.
- If you need to add information or change something you've said, give clear and specific directions to the transcriptionist.

Patient self-documentation

Although self-documentation obviously isn't feasible or desirable for every patient, it can be effective for patients who must perform considerable self-care (diabetic patients, for example) or for patients trying to discover what precipitates a problem (such as those with chronic headaches).

In using self-documentation, a diabetic patient may record information on his diet, insulin dose, self-tested blood glucose levels, and activity level. The accumulated information can help him avoid insulin reactions and delay, prevent, or even reverse complications from hyperglycemia or hypoglycemia. Self-documentation may also provide valuable information for the doctor as well.

A patient with chronic headaches may be asked to chart, among other things, when a headache occurred, what warning signs he noticed, and what pain relief measures he tried. Analyzing this information may help ward off future headaches. (See *Teaching self-documentation skills,* page 142.)

The patient can document entries on preprinted forms or in journal style. Such records can be used in both inpatient and outpatient care settings. Depending on health care facility policies, they may or may not become a permanent part of the medical record. (See *Keeping a record of monitored activity,* page 143.)

Advantages

Having the patient document data and events related to his own condition teaches him about his problem and its causes, symptoms, and treatment. It also may provide needed clues to the problem's precipitators and suggest solutions to the problem.

Data recorded by the patient may actually be more accurate than data interpreted by someone else. For example, a nurse or doctor may better understand the character of a patient's problem if he describes it in his own words.

Self-documentation also improves therapeutic compliance by making the patient an active participant in his treatment and providing him with some control.

Disadvantages

Self-documentation isn't difficult, but it takes time, patience, planning, motivation, and perseverance — on the part of both the nurse and the patient. The patient needs to understand how to keep careful records, what's important to document, and when to document. Otherwise, the records won't be useful and may even adversely affect his treatment and recovery.

Documentation guidelines

The patient must fully understand what needs to be documented and why it's important. If he will use preprinted forms, take the time to review each aspect of a form with him. If he will use a chart or a graph, show him how to use the form. If possible, show him examples of self-documentation.

Identify the person that the patient can contact if he has questions.

Emphasize the benefits of self-documentation to the patient (increased knowledge about his condition and increased control of his treatment, for example). By doing so, you may help boost his interest in keeping his records updated.

Finally, show him the results of his self-documentation, pointing out how or what the data contribute to his treatment.

Adapted or new forms

You may find that one or several documentation forms you've been using no longer suit your needs. This may occur because of changes in therapies, patient populations, or reimbursement criteria. Duplicated and fragmented documentation data are among the first signs that the forms in use aren't filling

BETTER CHARTING

Teaching self-documentation skills

For some patients, self-documentation has wide-ranging benefits. By learning to keep a log or a journal, for example, a patient may find out what triggers certain health problems (such as headaches, asthma attacks, or hypoglycemic episodes). Once the trigger emerges, the patient and caregiver can implement preventive strategies.

To help a patient learn self-documentation skills, some health care facilities use individual self-documentation forms such as the sample headache log shown at right.

Reviewing instructions

Give the patient instructions and review them with him. Tell him to complete the headache log daily. Inform him that doing so may help him to identify what triggers his headaches (for example, environmental factors, foods, or stress). Explain that information collected in the log may also help him discover effective ways to relieve a headache once it starts.

Instruct the patient to describe the details of each headache in a diary, log, or small notebook.

Checking the boxes

Review these steps with the patient:

- Using the log page at right as a guide, note the date and time of the headache and any warning signs.
- Put a check mark in the appropriate box to indicate the headache's intensity.
- Next, check the box to mark how long you've had the headache.
- Check the appropriate box for any other signs or symptoms that accompany your headache, such as nausea, vomiting, or sensitivity to light.
- Continue by checking the steps you took to relieve the headache (for example, medication, biofeedback, rest) as well as the effectiveness of these measures.

Completing the log

Urge the patient to think carefully about the events that occurred before the headache. For instance, was his headache triggered by emotional stress, by drinking a cup of coffee, or by something else? Tell him to write down the details of such potential triggers in his log.

HEADACHE LOG

Date and time headache began

2/25/99 – 5:00 p.m.

Warning signs

- ☑ Flashing lights
- ☐ Blind spots
- ☐ Colors
- ☐ Zigzag patterns
- ☐ None
- ☐ Other

Intensity

- ☐ Mild
- ☑ Moderate
- ☐ Severe
- ☐ Disabling

Duration

- ☑ Less than 4 hours
- ☐ 4 to 7.5 hours
- ☐ 8 to 11.5 hours
- ☐ 12 to 24 hours
- ☐ More than 1 day
- ☐ More than 2 days

Associated signs and symptoms

- ☐ Upset stomach
- ☑ Nausea or vomiting
- ☐ Dizziness
- ☑ Sensitivity to light
- ☐ Sensory, motor, or speech disturbances
- ☐ Other

Measures for relief

- ☑ Medication
- ☐ Rest
- ☑ Sleep
- ☐ Biofeedback
- ☐ Ice pack
- ☐ Relaxation exercises

Extent of relief

- ☐ None
- ☑ Mild
- ☐ Moderate
- ☐ Marked
- ☐ Complete

Possible triggers

Caffeine and sugar

BETTER CHARTING

Keeping a record of monitored activity

In many situations, your patient can provide more information more accurately than can a member of the health care team. A case in point: a patient who wears a Holter monitor to evaluate the effect of medication on his heart and his daily activities.

Keeping this in mind, some health care facilities prepare patient instructional materials in conjunction with a diary-like chart (such as the example below), which the patient refers to and completes for the medical record.

Date	Time	Activity	Feelings
1/15/99	10:30 a.m.	Rode home from hospital in cab	Legs tired, felt short of
			breath
	11:30 a.m.	Watched TV in living room	Comfortable
	12:15 p.m.	Ate lunch, took propranolol	Indigestion
	1:30 p.m.	Walked next door to see neighbor	Felt short of breath
	2:45 p.m.	Walked home	Very tired, legs hurt
	3:00 to 4:00 p.m.	Urinated, took nap	Comfortable
	5:30 p.m.	Ate dinner slowly	Comfortable
	7:20 p.m.	Had bowel movement	Felt short of breath
	9:00 p.m.	Watched TV, drank one beer	Heart beating fast for about
			1 minute, no pain
	11:00 p.m.	Took propranolol, urinated,	Tired
		and went to bed	
1/16/99	8:15 a.m.	Woke up, urinated, washed	Very tired, rapid heartbeat
		face and arms	for about 30 seconds
	10:30 a.m.	Returned to hospital	Felt better

first signs that the forms in use aren't filling current needs.

When developing a new form or adapting an old one, remember to ask yourself these questions:

- What problems exist with the old forms?
- What information is really needed?
- What changes would correct these problems?
- Which parts of the old forms remain valuable and need to be retained?

Even if your health care facility uses a computerized documentation system, ask staff members to help design the new form or reprogram the system. To develop an effective form, follow these guidelines:

- If your facility uses a specific nursing theory or framework for delivering nursing care, make sure that the nursing assessment form reflects it.
- If the old nursing assessment form reflects a medical format, change it to highlight the nursing process. For example, reorganize the form according to human response patterns or functional health care designs.
- Ask staff members who'll be using the form to evaluate possible formats and indicate which they prefer. Ask for their ideas about how best to organize and document their data.
- List all information the form must include. Be sure to document this information to comply with professional practice standards published by such organizations as the American Nurses Association (ANA) and the JCAHO.
- Consider combining documentation styles in one form. Decide which style is most appropriate for each type of information included in the form. For instance, a narrative note may best suit one part of the form, whereas an open-ended style may best convey information on another part.
- After developing the form, write procedural guidelines for its use. Provide clear explanations and completed examples for each section.
- Ask staff members not involved in developing the form to analyze both the form and the guidelines. This helps identify potentially confusing sections that require more detailed explanation or revision.
- Before adopting the form, have staff members test it to make sure they can use it easily for entering information and retrieving it as well.
- If you expect the form will become a permanent part of the medical record, check the section devoted to form adoptions in your policy and procedures manual. Some health care facilities require a form to be approved by the medical records committee or certain departments before official use.

Selected references

Coyne, M.L., et al. "Describing Pain Management Documentation," *MEDSURG Nursing* 7(1):45-51, February 1998.

Goodstein, S. "Documentation by Dictation," *Nursing Spectrum* 94(5):12, March 10, 1997.

"Hospital Boosts Documentation with Wireless Laptop Links," *Report on Healthcare Information Management* 6(2):1-2, February 1998.

"Materials Help Hospitals Meet JCAHO Standards," *Patient Education Management* 3(11): 124-26, November 1996.

Rode, D. "Medicare Audits and the Importantance of Ducmentation," *Healthcare Financial Management* 51(10):82-84, October 1997.

"Successful Forms for Outpatient Documentation," *Patient Education Management* 5(2):23-24, February 1998.

Using Performance Improvement Tools in Home Care. Oakbrook Terrace, Ill.: Joint Commission on Accreditation of Healthcare Organizations, 1996.

6

Documentation in Long-term Care

A long-term care facility provides continuing care for chronically ill or disabled patients in an effort to promote the highest level of functioning possible. Long-term care is an increasingly important form of health care delivery because the elderly segment of the population is rapidly growing and people are living longer with chronic illnesses.

Maintaining accurate, complete documentation in long-term care is vital for the following reasons:

- Documentation of assessment findings, therapeutic interventions, and patient outcomes helps maintain communication among the many disciplines involved in caring for patients in a long-term care facility.
- Because long-term care facilities are highly regulated by state and federal agencies, strict documentation standards are required.
- Documentation may be used to defend the health care facility and its personnel in court.
- Good documentation ensures certification, licensure, reimbursement, and accreditation.

Documenting the status, care, and events affecting patients in a long-term care facility is every bit as important as it is in acute care and home health care settings. (See Chapters 5 and 7, respectively.) Although forms and requirements of documentation in these settings share many similarities, long-term care documentation differs in two important ways:

- Because patients stay at long-term care facilities for weeks or months, documentation isn't done as often. This shifts the emphasis from charting to helping patients reach the goals set out in their care plans.
- Some of the government forms required for long-term care facilities are lengthy and complex. But when used appropriately, they can provide the health care team with a comprehensive assessment tool to help determine the needs and plan of care for each patient.

Whether you're an independent practitioner or a staff member in a rehabilitation center or nursing home, accurate and complete records provide your employer with evidence of standard, quality nursing care. In long-term patient care settings, documentation requirements are based on professional standards, state and federal regulations, and the health care facility's policies.

Skilled vs. intermediate care

The type of care provided in long-term care facilities is usually categorized as either skilled or intermediate. Patients in a skilled care facility require more extensive care and more specialized nursing skills (such as I.V. therapy, parenteral nutrition, respiratory care, mechanical ventilation, and physical, occupational, and speech therapy).

An intermediate care facility focuses on patients who have chronic illnesses but who need less complex care. For example, these patients may simply need assistance with activities of daily living (ADLs), such as bathing and dressing.

Many facilities offer both skilled and intermediate care. Residents from either group may need care on a short- or long-term basis and may move from one level to another according to their progress or decline. You should consider care level a primary factor when documenting patient information.

Requirements of regulatory bodies

Among the government programs, laws, and agencies that influence the kind of documentation required in long-term care facilities are the Medicare and Medicaid programs, the Omnibus Budget Reconciliation Act (OBRA) of 1987, and the Health Care Financing Administration (HCFA).

Medicare

The Medicare administration provides little reimbursement for services provided in long-term care facilities except for services requiring skilled care, such as chemotherapy and tube feeding. For such services, Medicare guidelines require that charting clearly show that the patient needed care by a professional or technical staff member.

To justify the need for skilled rehabilitative care, you must document a reasonable expectation of improvement or services needed to establish a maintenance program. The amount, duration, and frequency of services must be reasonable and necessary.

If the patient doesn't improve or isn't expected to improve according to the plan of care, he becomes ineligible for Medicare coverage. When a patient is improving, you must document his progress. If the patient's status changes, you'll need to supply a revised plan of care within 7 days. Of course, you must document the need for any new or continuing skilled services provided. Medicare also requires documentation of your evaluations for expected outcomes.

Medicaid

Patients in long-term care facilities who are under age 65 and are receiving skilled care are usually paying for the service themselves or, if they have coverage and qualify, are receiving reimbursement through the Medicaid program. To secure Medicaid reimbursement, you must document skilled care daily.

Intermediate care must be documented weekly unless a change in the patient's status necessitates a change in services. In such cases, you'll need to chart the change and document the patient's status more frequently. Medications and treatments must still be documented daily for reimbursement.

Additionally, you'll need to perform a monthly reevaluation. Like Medicare, Medicaid also requires an evaluation of expected outcomes on the plan of care.

OBRA

This law requires that a comprehensive assessment be performed within 4 days of a patient's admission to a long-term care facility. The lengthy form that's required is known as the *Minimum Data Set for Resident Assessment and Care Screening*— or MDS for short. The assessment and care screening process must be reviewed every 3 months and repeated annually— sooner if the patient's condition progresses or declines in two or more assessment areas of the MDS.

OBRA also requires that a plan of care be completed within 7 days of admission.

HCFA

This branch of the Department of Health and Human Services was developed to ensure compliance (especially by the states) with federal Medicare and Medicaid standards. Accordingly, to comply with regulations for residential long-term care patients, the facility's staff must complete the MDS within 14 days of a patient's admission, review the patient's status every 3 months, and perform a comprehensive reassessment annually.

Standard and required documents

As you would in any other setting, you'll use the nursing process as the basis for documenting care in a long-term facility. Required documents consist of the MDS (including the Resident Assessment Protocol summary), the Preadmission Screening Annual Resident Review, the initial nursing assessment form, and nursing summaries.

Minimum Data Set

Mandated by OBRA, this federal regulatory form must be filled out for every resident admitted to a long-term care facility. The MDS provides the health care team with a comprehensive assessment tool. It's used to comply with quality improvement and reimbursement requirements, to standardize information, and to facilitate communication among agencies and among members of the health care team.

Different sections of this form must be completed and signed by staff members from various professions, including nurses; physical, occupational, and speech therapists; social workers; and medical records personnel. (See *Minimum Data Set.*)

Resident Assessment Protocol

The Resident Assessment Protocol (RAP), another form mandated by federal regulations, has now been incorporated in the MDS as section V. The RAP section provides a summary of the assessment that lists the patient's problems and helps develop the plan of care. For example, if the patient has a stage 2 pressure ulcer documented in section M of the MDS, the RAP summary (section V) will indicate the need for a plan of care for a pressure ulcer.

Preadmission Screening Annual Resident Review

Just as a patient's physical status must be documented to qualify for Medicare or Medicaid reimbursement, so must his mental status. Federal regulations require long-term care facilities to perform a complete mental status assessment and to document the findings on a form known as the Preadmission Screening Annual Resident Review (PASARR). In most long-term care facilities, the PASARR is completed by a social worker. (See *Preadmission Screening Annual Resident Review,* pages 170 to 175.)

Initial nursing assessment form

The initial nursing assessment must be performed and documented for all patients in a long-term care facility. In this setting, you'll place special emphasis on the patient's functional status, as reflected by his ability to perform ADLs. Among the areas you'll assess are hearing and vision, bowel and bladder control, communication, safety, need for adaptive

(Text continues on page 176.)

BETTER CHARTING

Minimum Data Set

The Omnibus Budget Reconciliation Act of 1987 mandated that all patients admitted to a long-term care facility that receives federal funds must undergo a comprehensive assessment within 4 days of their admission. A completed sample of the required form, known as the Minimum Data Set (MDS), appears below.

Minimum Data Set (MDS)—Version 2.0
For Nursing Home Resident Assessment and Care Screening
Basic Assessment Tracking Form

General instructions: Complete this information for submission with all full and quarterly assessments (Admission, Annual, Significant Change, State or Medicare required assessments, or Quarterly Reviews, etc.)

Section AA. Identification information

1. Resident's name	John (a.) First; D. b.(Middle initial); Walker c. (Last); Jr. d.(Jr./Sr.)	
2. Gender	1. Male 2. Female	1
3. Birth date	03 — 10 — 1920 (Month, Day, Year)	
4. Race/Ethnicity	1. American Indian/Alaskan Native 2. Asian/Pacific Islander 3. Black, not of Hispanic origin 4. Hispanic 5. White, not of Hispanic origin	3
5. Social Security and Medicare numbers *(C in 1st box if non med. no.)*	a. Social Security number 123 — 43 — 6789 b. Medicare number (or comparable railroad insurance number) 123456789A	
6. Facility provider no.	a. State No. 7455103 b. Federal No. 6126555482	
7. Medicaid no. *("+" if pending, "N" if not a Medicaid recipient)*	N	
8. Reasons for assessment	*(Note – Other codes do not apply to this form)* a. Primary reason for assessment **02** 1. Admission assessment (required by day 14) 2. Annual assessment 3. Significant change in status assessment 4. Significant correction of prior full assessment 5. Quarterly review assessment 10. Significant correction of prior quarterly assessment 0. NONE OF ABOVE b. Codes for assessments required for Medicare PPS or the State **00** 1. Medicare 5-day assessment 2. Medicare 30-day assessment 3. Medicare 60-day assessment 4. Medicare 90-day assessment 5. Medicare readmission/return assessment 6. Other state required assessment 7. Medicare 14-day assessment 8. Other Medicare-required assessment	
9. Signatures of persons completing these items:	a. Signatures Tina D'Agostino Title RN Date 2/10/99 b. Date	

(continued)

BETTER CHARTING

Minimum Data Set *(continued)*

Minimum Data Set (MDS) –Version 2.0
For Nursing Home Resident Assessment and Care Screening
Full Assessment Form
(Status in last 7 days, unless other time frame indicated)

Section A. Identification and background information

1. Resident's name	John (a.) First · D. b.(Middle initial) · Walker c. (Last) · Jr. d.(Jr./Sr.)	
2. Room no.	3 2 2	
3. Assessment reference date	Last day of MDS observation period 0 2 — 1 0 — 1 9 9 9 Month Day Year Original (0) or corrected copy of form (enter number of correction)	0
4a. Date of reentry	Date of reentry from most recent temporary discharge to a hospital in last 90 days (or since last assessment or admission if less than 90 days) — — Month Day Year	
5. Marital status	1. Never married 2. Married 3. Widowed 4. Separated 5. Divorced	3
6. Medical record no.	6 9 2 4 0 5	
7. Current payment sources for N.H. stay	*(Billing Office to indicate; check all that apply in last 30 days)* Medicaid per diem a. Medicare per diem b. X Medicare ancillary Part A c. X Medicare ancillary Part B d. CHAMPUS per diem e. VA per diem f. Self or family pays for full per diem g. Medicaid resident liability or Medicare co-payment h. Private insurance per diem (including co-payment) i. Other per diem j.	
8. Reasons for assessment *(Note—if this is a discharge summary or reentry assessment, only a limited subset of MDS items need to be completed.)*	a. Primary reason for assessment 1. Admission assessment (required by day 14) 2. Annual assessment 3. Significant change in status assessment 4. Significant correction of prior full assessment 5. Quarterly review assessment 6. Discharged—return not anticipated 7. Discharged—return anticipated 8. Discharge prior to completing initial assessment 9. Reentry 10. Significant correction of prior quarterly assessment 0. *None of above*	0 2

Minimum Data Set *(continued)*

Section A. Identification and background information *(continued)*

8. Reasons for assessment *(continued)*	b. Codes for assessments required for Medicare PPS or the State 1. Medicare 5-day assessment 2. Medicare 30-day assessment 3. Medicare 60-day assessment 4. Medicare 90-day assessment 5. Medicare readmission/return assessment 6. Other state required assessment 7. Medicare 14-day assessment 8. Other Medicare required assessment	0 0
9. Responsibility/Legal guardian	*(Check all that apply)* Legal guardian — a. X Other legal oversight — b. Durable power of attorney/ health care — c. Durable power of attorney/financial — d. Family member responsible — e. Patient responsible for self — f. *None of above* — g.	
10. Advance directives	*(For those items with supporting documentation in the medical record, check all that apply.)* Living will — a. X Do not resuscitate. — b. Do not hospitalize. — c. Organ donation — d. Autopsy request — e. Feeding restrictions — f. Medication restrictions — g. Other treatment restrictions — h. *None of above* — i.	

Section B. Cognitive patterns

1. Comatose	*(Persistent vegetative state/no discernible consciousness)* 0. No 1. Yes (If yes, skip to Section G)	0
2. Memory	*(Recall of what was learned or known)* a. Short-term memory OK—seems/appears to recall after 5 minutes 0. Memory OK 1. Memory problem	0
	b. Long-term memory OK—seems/appears to recall long past 0. Memory OK 1. Memory problem	0
3. Memory/Recall ability	*(Check all that resident was normally able to recall during last 7 days)* Current season — a. X Location of own room — b. X Staff names/faces — c. X That he/she is in a nursing home — d. X *None of the above* are recalled — e.	
4. Cognitive skills for daily decision making	*(Made decisions regarding tasks of daily life)* 0. Independent—decisions consistent/reasonable 1. Modified independence—some difficulty in new situations only 2. Moderately impaired—decisions poor; cues/supervision required 3. Severely impaired—never/rarely made decisions	0

(continued)

BETTER CHARTING

Minimum Data Set *(continued)*

Section B. Cognitive patterns *(continued)*

5. Indicators of delirium; periodic disordered thinking/awareness	*(Code for behavior in the last 7 days.) (Note: Accurate assessment requires conversations with staff and family who have direct knowledge of resident's behavior over this time.)* 0. Behavior not present 1. Behavior present, not of recent onset 2. Behavior present over last 7 days appears different from resident's usual functioning (e.g., new onset or worsening)	
	a. Easily distracted (e.g., difficulty paying attention; gets sidetracked)	0
	b. Periods of altered perception or awareness of surroundings (e.g., moves lips or talks to someone not present; believes he/she is somewhere else; confuses night and day)	0
	c. Episodes of disorganized speech (e.g., speech is incoherent, nonsensical, irrelevant, or rambling from subject to subject; loses train of thought)	0
	d. Periods of restlessness (e.g., fidgeting or picking at skin, clothing, etc.; frequent position changes; repetitive physical movements or calling out)	0
	e. Periods of lethargy (e.g., sluggishness, staring into space, difficult to arouse, little body movement)	0
	f. Mental function varies over the course of the day (e.g., sometimes better, sometimes worse; behaviors sometimes present, sometimes not)	0
6. Change in cognitive status	Resident's cognitive status, skills, or abilities have changed as compared to status of 90 days ago (or since last assessment if less than 90 days) 0. No change 1. Improved 2. Deteriorated	0

Section C. Communication/Hearing patterns

1. Hearing	*(With hearing appliance, if used)* 0. Hears adequately — normal talk, TV, phone 1. Minimal difficulty when not in quiet setting 2. Hears in special situations only — speaker has to adjust tonal quality and speak distinctly 3. Highly impaired — absence of useful hearing	1
2. Communication devices/techniques	*(Check all that apply during last 7 days)*	
	Hearing aid present and used	a.
	Hearing aid present and not used regularly	b. X
	Other receptive comm. techniques used (e.g., lip reading)	c.
	None of above	d.

3. Modes of expression	*(Check all used by resident to make needs known)*			
	Speech	a. X	Communication board	e.
	Writing messages to express or clarify needs	b.	Other	f.
	American sign language or Braille	c.	*None of above*	g.
	Signs/gestures/sounds	d.		

Minimum Data Set *(continued)*

Section C. Communication/Hearing patterns *(continued)*

Item	Codes	Entry
4. Making self understood	*(Expressing information content — however able)* 0. Understood 1. Usually understood — difficulty finding words or finishing thoughts 2. Sometimes understood — ability is limited to making concrete requests 3. Rarely/Never understood	0
5. Speech clarity	*(Code for speech in the last 7 days)* 0. Clear speech — distinct, intelligible words 1. Unclear speech — slurred, mumbled words 2. No speech — absence of spoken words	0
6. Ability to understand others	*(Understanding verbal information content — however able)* 0. Understands 1. Usually understands — may miss some part/intent of message 2. Sometimes understands — responds adequately to simple, direct communication 3. Rarely/Never understands	0
7. Change in communication/hearing	Resident's ability to express, understand, or hear information has changed as compared to status of 90 days ago (or since last assessment if less than 90 days) 0. No change 1. Improved 2. Deteriorated	0

Section D. Vision patterns

Item	Codes	Entry
1. Vision	*(Ability to see in adequate light and with glasses if used)* 0. Adequate — sees fine detail, including regular print in newspapers/books 1. Impaired — sees large print, but not regular print in newspapers/books 2. Moderately impaired — limited vision; not able to see newspaper headlines, but can identify objects 3. Highly impaired — object identification in question, but eyes appear to follow objects 4. Severely impaired — no vision or sees only light, colors, or shapes; eyes do not appear to follow objects	1
2. Visual limitations/ difficulties	Side vision problems — decreased peripheral vision (e.g., leaves food on one side of tray, difficulty traveling, bumps into people and objects, misjudges placement of chair while seating self)	a.
	Experiences any of the following: sees halos or rings around lights, sees flashes of light, sees "curtain" over eyes	b.
	None of above	c. X
3. Visual appliances	Glasses; contact lenses; magnifying glass 0. No 1. Yes	1

Section E. Mood and behavior patterns

1. Indicators of depression, anxiety, sad mood	*(Code for indicators observed in last 30 days, irrespective of the assumed cause)* 0. Indicator not exhibited in last 30 days 1. Indicator of this type exhibited up to 5 days a week 2. Indicator of this type exhibited daily or almost daily (6, 7 days a week)

(continued)

DOCUMENTATION IN LONG-TERM CARE

BETTER CHARTING

Minimum Data Set *(continued)*

Section E. Mood and behavior patterns *(continued)*

1. Indicators of depression, anxiety, sad mood *(continued)*	***Verbal expressions of distress***		i. Repetitive anxious complaints/concerns (non-health related), e.g., persistently seeks attention/reassurance regarding schedules, meals, laundry, clothing, relationship issues	0
	a. Resident made negative statements — e.g., "Nothing matters; would rather be dead; what's the use; regrets having lived so long; Let me die"	1	***Sleep cycle issues***	
	b. Repetitive questions — e.g., "Where do I go; What do I do?"	0	j. Unpleasant mood in morning	0
	c. Repetitive verbalizations — e.g., calling out for help ("God help me")	0	k. Insomnia/change in usual sleep pattern	1
	d. Persistent anger with self or others — e.g., easily annoyed, anger at placement in nursing home, anger at care received.	0	***Sad, apathetic, anxious appearance***	
	e. Self deprecation — e.g., "I am nothing; I am of no use to anyone"	1	l. Sad, pained, worried facial expressions — e.g., furrowed brows	1
	f. Expressions of what appear to be unrealistic fears — e.g., fear of being abandoned, left alone, being with others	0	m. Crying, tearfulness	0
	g. Recurrent statements that something terrible is about to happen — e.g., believes he or she is about to die, have a heart attack	0	n. Repetitive, physical movements — e.g., pacing, hand-wringing, restlessness, fidgeting, picking	0
	h. Repetitive health complaints — e.g., persistently seeks medical attention, obsessive concern with body functions	0	***Loss of interest***	
			o. Withdrawal from activities of interest — e.g., no interest in long-standing activities or being with family/friends	1
			p. Reduced social interaction	1
2. Mood persistence	One or more indicators of depressed, sad, or anxious mood were not easily altered by attempts to "cheer up," console, or reassure the resident over last 7 days. 0. No mood indicators 1. Indicators present, easily altered 2. Indicators present, not easily altered			1
3. Change in mood	Resident's mood status has changed as compared to status of 90 days ago (or since last assessment if less than 90 days) 0. No change 1. Improved 2. Deteriorated			2

		A.	B.
4. Behavioral symptoms	(A) Behaviorial symptom frequency in last 7 days 0. Behavior not exhibited in last 7 days 1. Behavior of this type occurred 1 to 3 days in last 7 days 2. Behavior of this type occurred 4 to 6 days, but less than daily 3. Behavior of this type occurred daily (B) Behavioral symptom alterability in last 7 days 0. Behavior not present or behavior was easily altered 1. Behavior was not easily altered		
	a. Wandering (moving with no rational purpose, seemingly oblivious to needs or safety)	0	0
	b. Verbally abusive behavioral symptoms (others were threatened, screamed at, cursed at)	0	0

Minimum Data Set *(continued)*

Section E. Mood and behavior patterns *(continued)*

4. Behavioral symptoms *(continued)*	c. Physically abusive behavioral symptoms (others were hit, shoved, scratched, sexually abused)	0	0
	d. Socially inappropriate/disruptive behavioral symptoms (made disruptive sounds, noisiness, screaming, self-abusive acts, sexual behavior or disrobing in public, smeared/threw food/feces, hoarding, rummaged through others' belongings)	0	0
	e. Resists care (resisted taking medications/injections, ADL assistance, or eating)	0	0
5. Change in behavioral symptoms	Resident's behavior status has changed as compared to status of 90 days ago (or since last assessment if less than 90 days) 0. No change 1. Improved 2. Deteriorated		0

Section F. Psychosocial well-being

1. Sense of initiative/involvement	At ease with others	a.
	At ease doing planned or structured activities	b.
	At ease doing self-initiated goals	c.
	Establishes own goals	d.
	Pursues involvement in life of facility (e.g., makes/keeps friends, involved in group activities, responds positively to new activities, assists at religious services)	e.
	Accepts invitations into most group activities	f.
	None of above	g. X
2. Unsettled relationships	Covert/open conflict with or repeated criticism of staff	a.
	Unhappy with roommate	b.
	Unhappy with residents other than roommate	c.
	Openly expresses conflict/anger with family/friends	d.
	Absence of personal contact with family/friends	e. X
	Recent loss of close family member/friend	f.
	Does not adjust easily to change in routines	g.
	None of above	h.
3. Past roles	Strong identification with past roles and life status	a.
	Expresses sadness/anger/empty feeling over lost roles/status	b. X
	Resident perceives that daily routine (customary routine, activities) is very different from prior pattern in the community	c.
	None of above	d.

(continued)

BETTER CHARTING

Minimum Data Set *(continued)*

Section G. Physical functioning and structural problems

1. (A) ADL self-performance — (Code for resident's performance over all shifts during last 7 days — not including setup)
   0. Independent — No help or oversight — OR — Help/oversight provided only 1 or 2 times during last 7 days
   1. Supervision — Oversight, encouragement, or cueing provided 3 or more times during last 7 days — OR — Supervision (3 or more times) plus physical assistance provided only 1 or 2 times during last 7 days
   2. Limited assistance—Resident highly involved in activity; received physical help in guided maneuvering of limbs or other nonweight-bearing assistance 3 or more times — OR — More help provided only 1 or 2 times during last 7 days
   3. Extensive assistance —While resident performed part of activity over last 7-day period, help of following type(s) provided 3 or more times:
      - Weight-bearing support
      - Full staff performance during part (but not all) of last 7 days
   4. Total dependence — Full staff performance of activity during entire 7 days
   8. Activity did not occur during entire 7 days

   (B) ADL support provided — (Code for most support provided over all shifts during last 7 days; code regardless of resident's self-performance classification)
   0. No setup or physical help from staff
   1. Setup help only
   2. One person physical assist
   3. Two+ person physical assist
   8. ADL activity itself does not occur during entire 7 days

		(A) Self-perf	(B) Support
a. **Bed mobility**	How resident moves to and from lying position, turns side to side, and positions body while in bed	0	0
b. **Transfer**	How resident moves between surfaces — to/from bed, chair, wheelchair, standing position (EXCLUDE to/from bath/toilet)	0	0
c. **Walk in room**	How resident walks between locations in his/her room	0	0
d. **Walk in corridor**	How resident walks in corridor on unit	0	0
e. **Locomotion on unit**	How resident moves between locations in his/her room and adjacent corridor on same floor. If in wheelchair, self-sufficiency once in chair.	0	0
f. **Locomotion off unit**	How resident moves to and returns from off-unit locations (e.g., areas set aside for dining, activities, or treatments). If facility has only one floor, how resident moves to and from distant areas on the floor. If in wheelchair, self-sufficiency once in chair.	0	0
g. **Dressing**	How resident puts on, fastens, and takes off all items of street clothing, including donning/removing prosthesis	1	1
h. **Eating**	How resident eats and drinks (regardless of skill), including intake of nourishment by other means (e.g., tube feeding, total parenteral nutrition)	0	0
i. **Toilet use**	How resident uses the toilet room (or commode, bedpan, urinal); transfer on/off toilet, cleanses, changes pad, manages ostomy or catheter, adjusts clothes	0	0
j. **Personal hygiene**	How resident maintains personal hygiene, including combing hair, brushing teeth, shaving, applying makeup, washing/drying face, hands, and perineum (EXCLUDE baths and showers)	0	0

Minimum Data Set *(continued)*

Section G. Physical functioning and structural problems *(continued)*

2. Bathing	How resident takes full-body bath/shower, sponge bath, and transfers in/out of tub/shower. (EXCLUDE washing of back and hair.) Code for most dependent in self-performance and support. (A) Bathing self-performance codes appear below 0. Independent — No help provided 1. Supervision — Oversight help only 2. Physical help limited to transfer only 3. Physical help in part of bathing activity 4. Total dependence 8. Activity itself did not occur during entire 7 days *(Bathing support codes are as defined in item 1, code B above)*	(A) /	(B) /
3. Test for balance (see training manual)	*(Code for ability during test in the last 7 days)* 0. Maintained position as required in test 1. Unsteady, but able to rebalance self without physical support 2. Partial physical support during test; or stands (sits) but does not follow directions for test 3. Not able to attempt test without physical help		
	a. Balance while standing		O
	b. Balance while sitting — position, trunk control		O
4. Functional limitation in range of motion (see training manual)	*(Code for limitations during last 7 days that interfered with daily functions or placed resident at risk of injury)* (A) Range of motion 0. No limitation 1. Limitation on one side 2. Limitation on both sides (B) Voluntary movement 0. No loss 1. Partial loss 2. Full loss	(A)	(B)
	a. Neck	O	O
	b. Arm — including shoulder or elbow	O	O
	c. Hand — including wrist or fingers	O	O
	d. Leg — including hip or knee	O	O
	e. Foot — including ankle or toes	O	O
	f. Other limitation or loss	O	O
5. Modes of locomotion	*(Check all that apply during last 7 days)* Cane/walker/crutch — a. Wheeled self — b. Lifted manually — c. Wheelchair primary mode of locomotion — d. *None of above* — e. X		
6. Modes of transfer	*(Check all that apply during last 7 days)* Bedfast all or most of time — a. Bed rails used for bed mobility or transfer — b. Lifted manually — c. Lifted mechanically — d. Transfer aid (e.g., slide board, trapeze, cane, walker, brace) — e. *None of above* — f. X		

(continued)

BETTER CHARTING

Minimum Data Set *(continued)*

Section G. Physical functioning and structural problems *(continued)*

7. Task segmentation	Some or all of ADL activities were broken into subtasks during last 7 days so that resident could perform them. 0. No 1. Yes	O
8. ADL functional rehabilitation potential	Resident believes he/she is capable of increased independence in at least some ADLS	a.
	Direct care staff believe resident is of capable of increased independence in at least some ADLS	b.
	Resident able to perform tasks/activity but is very slow	c.
	Difference in ADL self-performance or ADL support, comparing morning to evenings	d.
	None of above	e. X
9. Change in ADL function	Resident's ADL self-performance status has changed as compared to status of 90 days ago (or since last assessment if less than 90 days) 0. No change 1. Improved 2. Deteriorated	O

Section H. Continence in last 14 days

1. Continence self-control categories
(Code for resident's performance over all shifts)

0. Continent — Complete control (includes use of indwelling urinary catheter or ostomy device that does not leak urine or stool)
1. Usually continent — BLADDER, incontinent episodes once a week or less; BOWEL, less than weekly
2. Occasionally incontinent — BLADDER, 2 or more times a week but not daily; BOWEL, once a week
3. Frequently incontinent — BLADDER, tended to be incontinent daily, but some control present (e.g, on day shift); BOWEL, 2 to 3 times a week
4. Incontinent — Had inadequate control BLADDER, multiple daily episodes; BOWEL, all (or almost all) of the time

a. Bowel continence	Control of bowel movement, with appliance or bowel incontinence programs, if employed	O
b. Bladder continence	Control of urinary bladder function (if dribbles, volume insufficient to soak through underpants), with appliances (e.g., Foley) or continence programs, if employed	/

2. Bowel elimination pattern	Bowel elimination pattern regular — at least one movement every three days	a.	Diarrhea	c.
			Fecal impaction	d.
	Constipation	b. X	*None of above*	e.
3. Appliances and programs	Any scheduled toileting plan	a.	Did not use toilet room/commode/urinal	f.
	Bladder retraining program	b.	Pads/briefs used	g.
	External (condom) catheter	c.	Enemas/irrigation	h. X
	Indwelling catheter	d.	Ostomy present	i.
	Intermittent catheter	e.	*None of above*	j.

4. Change in urinary continence	Resident's urinary continence has changed as compared to status of 90 days ago (or since last assessment if less than 90 days) 0. No change 1. Improved 2. Deteriorated	2

Minimum Data Set *(continued)*

Section I. Disease diagnoses

Check only those diseases that have a relationship to current ADL status, cognitve status, mood and behavior status, medical treatments, nursing monitoring, or risk of death. (Do not list inactive diagnoses.)

1. Diseases	*(If none apply, check the "None of above" box)*			
	Endocrine/Metabolic/Nutritional		Multiple sclerosis	w.
	Diabetes mellitus	a. X	Paraplegia	x.
	Hyperthyroidism	b.	Parkinson's disease	y.
	Hypothyroidism	c.	Quadriplegia	z.
	Heart/Circulation		Seizure disorder	aa.
	Arteriosclerotic heart disease (ASHD)	d. X	Transient ischemic attack (TIA)	bb.
	Cardiac dysrhythmias	e.	Traumatic brain injury	cc.
	Congestive heart failure	f. X	***Psychiatric/Mood***	
	Deep vein thrombosis	g.	Anxiety disorder	dd.
	Hypertension	h. X	Depression	ee.
	Hypotension	i.	Manic depression (bipolar disease)	ff.
	Peripheral vascular disease	j.	Schizophrenia	gg.
	Other cardiovascular disease	k.	***Pulmonary***	
	Musculoskeletal		Asthma	hh.
	Arthritis	l.	Emphysema/COPD	ii.
	Hip fracture	m.	***Sensory***	
	Missing limb (e.g., amputation)	n.	Cataracts	jj.
	Osteoporosis	o.	Diabetic retinopathy	kk.
	Pathological bone fracture	p.	Glaucoma	ll.
	Neurological		Macular degeneration	mm.
	Alzheimer's disease	q.	***Other***	
	Aphasia	r.	Allergies	nn.
	Cerebral palsy	s.	Anemia	oo.
	Cerebrovascular accident (stroke)	t.	Cancer	pp.
	Dementia other than Alzheimer's disease	u.	Renal failure	qq.
	Hemiplegia/hemiparesis	v.	*None of above*	rr.
2. Infections	*(If none apply, check the "None of above" box)*			
	Antibiotic-resistant infection (e.g., methicillin-resistant staph)	a.	Septicemia	g.
	Clostridium difficile (c. diff.)	b.	Sexually transmitted diseases	h.
	Conjunctivitis	c.	Tuberculosis	i.
	HIV infection	d.	Urinary tract infection in last 30 days	j.
	Pneumonia	e.	Viral hepatitis	k.
	Respiratory infection	f.	Wound infection	l.
			None of above	m. X

(continued)

BETTER CHARTING

Minimum Data Set *(continued)*

Section I. Disease diagnoses *(continued)*

3. Other current or more detailed diagnoses and ICD-9 codes	a. Cerebral arteriosclerosis	437-0
	b.	
	c.	
	d.	
	e.	

Section J. Health conditions

1. Problem conditions	*(Check all problems present in last 7 days unless other time frame is indicated)*			
	Indicators of fluid status		Edema	g. X
	Weight gain or loss of 3 or more pounds within a 7-day period	a.	Fever	h.
	Inability to lie flat due to shortness of breath	b.	Hallucinations	i.
	Dehydrated; output exceeds input	c.	Internal bleeding	j.
	Insufficient fluid; did NOT consume all/almost all liquids provided during last 3 days	d.	Recurrent lung aspirations in last 90 days	k.
	Other		Shortness of breath	l.
	Delusions	e.	Syncope (fainting)	m.
	Dizziness/Vertigo	f.	Unsteady gait	n.
			Vomiting	o.
			None of above	p.
2. Pain symptoms	*(Code the highest level of pain present in the last 7 days)*			
	a. FREQUENCY with which resident complains or shows evidence of pain 0. No pain (skip to J4) 1. Pain less than daily 2. Pain daily	0	b. INTENSITY of pain 1. Mild pain 2. Moderate pain 3. Times when pain is horrible or excruciating	
3. Pain site	*(If pain present, check all sites that apply in last 7 days)*			
	Back pain	a.	Incisional pain	f.
	Bone pain	b.	Joint pain (other than hip)	g.
	Chest pain while doing activities	c.	Soft tissue pain (e.g., lesion, muscle)	h.
	Headache	d.	Stomach pain	i.
	Hip pain	e.	Other	j.
4. Accidents	*(Check all that apply)*			
	Fell in past 30 days	a.	Other fracture in last 180 days	d.
	Fell in past 31-180 days	b.	*None of above*	e. X
	Hip fracture in last 180 days	c.		

Minimum Data Set *(continued)*

Section J. Health conditions *(continued)*

5. Stability of conditions	Conditions/diseases make resident's cognitive, ADL, mood or behavior patterns unstable (fluctuating, precarious, or deteriorating)	a. X
	Resident experiencing an acute episode or flare-up of a recurrent or chronic problem	b.
	End-stage disease, 6 or fewer months to live	c.
	None of above	d.

Section K. Oral/Nutritional status

1. Oral problems	Chewing problem	a.
	Swallowing problem	b.
	Mouth pain	c.
	None of above	d. X
2. Height and weight	*Record (a.) height in inches and (b.) weight in pounds. Base weight on most recent measure in last 30 days; measure weight consistently in accord with standard facility practice — e.g., in a.m. after voiding, before meal, with shoes off, and in night-clothes.* a. HT (in.) 7 0 b. WT (lb.) 1 8 5	
3. Weight change	a. Weight loss—5% or more in last 30 days; or 10% or more in last 180 days. 0. No 1. Yes	0
	b. Weight gain —5% or more in last 30 days; or 10% or more in last 180 days 0. No 1. Yes	0

4. Nutritional problems	Complains about the taste of many foods	a. X	Leaves 25% or more of food uneaten at most meals	c.
	Regular or repetitive complaints of hunger	b.	*None of above*	d.
5. Nutritional approaches	*(Check all that apply in last 7 days)*		Dietary supplement between meals	f.
	Parenteral/I.V.	a.	Plate guard, stabilized built-up utensil, etc.	g.
	Feeding tube	b.	On a planned weight change program	h.
	Mechanically altered diet	c.	*None of above*	i.
	Syringe (oral feeding)	d.		
	Therapeutic diet	e. X		

6. Parenteral or enternal intake	*(Skip to section L if neither 5a nor 5b is checked)*	
	a. Code the proportion of total calories the resident received through parenteral or tube feedings in the last 7 days. 0. None 1. 1% to 25% 2. 26% to 50% 3. 51% to 75% 4. 76% to 100%	
	b. Code the average fluid intake per day by I.V. or tube in last 7 days 0. None 1. 1 to 500 cc/day 2. 501 to 1000 cc/day 3. 1001 to 1500 cc/day 4. 1501 to 2000 cc/day 5. 2001 or more cc/day	

(continued)

BETTER CHARTING

Minimum Data Set *(continued)*

Section L. Oral/Dental status

1. Oral status and disease prevention	Debris (soft, easily movable substances) present in mouth prior to going to bed at night	a.
	Has dentures or removable bridge	b.
	Some/all natural teeth lost — does not have or does not use dentures (or partial plates)	c.
	Broken, loose or carious teeth	d.
	Inflamed gums (gingiva); swollen or bleeding gums; oral abscesses; ulcers or rashes	e.
	Daily cleaning of teeth/dentures or daily mouth care by resident or staff	f. X
	None of above	g.

Section M. Skin condition

1. Ulcers (due to any cause)	*(Record the number of ulcers at each ulcer stage — regardless of cause. If none present at a stage, record "0" (zero). Code all that apply during last 7 days. Code 9 = 9 or more.) (Requires full body exam.)*	
	a. Stage 1. A persistent area of skin redness (without a break in the skin) that does not disappear when pressure is relieved.	0
	b. Stage 2. A partial-thickness loss of skin layers that presents clinically as an abrasion, blister, or shallow crater	0
	c. Stage 3. A full thickness of skin is lost, exposing the subcutaneous tissues — presents as a deep crater with or without undermining adjacent tissue	0
	d. Stage 4. A full thickness of skin and subcutaneous tissue is lost, exposing muscle or bone	0
2. Type of ulcer	*(For each type of ulcer, code for the highest stage in the last 7 days using scale in item M1 — i.e., 0 = none; stages 1, 2, 3, 4)*	
	a. Pressure ulcer — any lesion caused by pressure resulting in damage of underlying tissue	0
	b. Stasis ulcer — open lesion caused by poor circulation in the lower extremities	0
3. History of resolved ulcers	Resident had an ulcer that was resolved or cured in last 90 days. 0. No 1. Yes	0
4. Other skin problems or lesions present	*(Check all that apply during last 7 days)*	
	Abrasions, bruises	a.
	Burns (second or third degree)	b.
	Open lesions other than ulcers, rashes, cuts (e.g., cancer lesions)	c.
	Rashes — e.g., intertrigo, eczema, drug rash, heat rash, herpes zoster	d.
	Skin desensitized to pain or pressure	e. X
	Skin tears or cuts (other than surgery)	f.
	Surgical wounds	g.
	None of above	h.

Minimum Data Set *(continued)*

Section M. Skin condition *(continued)*

5. Skin treatments	*(Check all that apply during last 7 days)*	
	Pressure-relieving device(s) for chair	a.
	Pressure-relieving device(s) for bed	b.
	Turning/repositioning program	c.
	Nutrition or hydration intervention to manage skin problems	d.
	Ulcer care	e.
	Surgical wound care	f.
	Application of dressings (with or without topical medications) other than to feet	g.
	Application of ointments/medications (other than to feet)	h.
	Other preventative or protective skin care (other than to feet)	i.
	None of above	j. X
6. Foot problems and care	*(Check all that apply during last 7 days)*	
	Resident has one or more foot problems — e.g., corns, calluses, bunions, hammer toes, overlapping toes, pain, structural problems	a.
	Infection of the foot — e.g., cellulitis, purulent drainage	b.
	Open lesions of the foot	c.
	Nails/calluses trimmed during last 90 days	d.
	Received preventive or protective foot care (e.g., used special shoes, inserts, pads, toe separators)	e. X
	Application of dressings (with or without topical medications)	f.
	None of above	g.

Section N. Activity pursuit patterns

1. Time awake (If resident is comatose, skip to Section O)	*(Check appropriate time periods over last 7 days)*	
	Resident awake all or most of time (i.e., naps no more than one hour per time period) in the:	
	Morning	a. X
	Afternoon	b. X
	Evening	c. X
	None of above	d.
2. Average time involved in activities	(When awake and not receving treatments or ADL care) 0. Most — more than ⅔ of time 2. Little — less than ⅓ of time 1. Some — from ⅓ to ⅔ of time 3. None	2
3. Preferred activity settings	*(Check all settings in which activities are preferred)*	
	Own room	a. X
	Day/activity room	b.
	Inside NH/off unit	c.
	Outside facility	d. X
	None of above	e.

(continued)

BETTER CHARTING

Minimum Data Set *(continued)*

Section N. Activity pursuit patterns *(continued)*

4. General activity preferences (adapted to resident's current abilities)	*(Check all preferences whether or not activity is currently available to resident)*			
	Cards/other games	a. X	Walking/wheeling outdoors	h.
	Crafts/arts	b.	Watching TV	i. X
	Exercise/sports	c.	Gardening or plants	j.
	Music	d. X	Talking or conversing	k.
	Reading/writing	e. X	Helping others	l.
	Spiritual/religious activities	f.	*None of above*	m.
	Trips/shopping	g.		
5. Prefers change in daily routine	*Code for resident preferences in daily routines* 0. No change 1. Slight change 2. Major change			
	Type of activities in which resident is currently involved			0
	Extent of resident involvement in activities			1

Section O. Medications

1. Number of medications	*(Record the number of different medications used in the last 7 days; enter "0" if none used)*			0 5
2. New medications	*(Resident currently receiving medications that were initiated during the last 90 days)* 0. No 1. Yes			0
3. Injections	*(Record the number of days injections of any type were received during the last 7 days; enter "0" if none used)*			7
4. Days received the following medications	*(Record the number of days during the last 7 days; enter "0" if not used. Note—enter "1" for long-acting meds used less than weekly)*			
	a. Antipsychotic	0	d. Hypnotic	0
	b. Antianxiety	0	e. Diuretic	7
	c. Antidepressant	0		

Section P. Special treatments and procedures

1. Special treatments, procedures, and programs	a. SPECIAL CARE — *Check treatments or programs received during the last 14 days*			
	Treatments		Ventilator or respirator	l.
	Chemotherapy	a.	***Programs***	
	Dialysis	b.	Alcohol/drug treatment program	m.
	I.V. medication	c.	Alzheimer's/dementia special care unit	n.
	Intake/output	d.	Hospice care	o.
	Monitoring acute medical condition	e. X	Pediatric unit	p.
	Ostomy care	f.	Respite care	q.
	Oxygen therapy	g.	Training in skills required to return to the community (e.g., taking medications, housework, shopping, transportation, ADLs)	r.
	Radiation	h.	None of above	s.
	Suctioning	i.		
	Tracheostomy care	j.		
	Transfusions	k.		

Minimum Data Set *(continued)*

Section P. Special treatments and procedures *(continued)*

1. Special treatments, procedures, and programs *(continued)*	b.THERAPIES – *Record the number of days and total minutes each of the following therapies was administered (for at least 15 minutes a day) in the last 7 calendar days; enter "0" if none or less than 15 min daily (Note — count only post-admission therapies)*					
	(A) = # of days administered for 15 minutes or more	DAYS	MIN			
	(B) = total # of minutes provided in last 7 days	(A)	(B)			
	a. Speech – language pathology and audiology services	0	0	0	0	0
	b. Occupational therapy	0	0	0	0	0
	c. Physical therapy	0	0	0	0	0
	d. Respiratory therapy	0	0	0	0	0
	e. Psychological therapy (by any licensed mental health professional)	0	0	0	0	0

2. Intervention programs for mood, behavior, cognitive loss	*(Check all interventions or strategies used in last 7 days—no matter where received)*	
	Special behavior symptom evaluation program	a.
	Evaluation by a licensed mental health specialist in the last 90 days	b.
	Group therapy	c.
	Resident-specific deliberate changes in the environment to address mood/behavior patterns — e.g., providing bureau in which to rummage	d.
	Reorientation — e.g., cueing	e.
	None of above	f. X

3. Nursing rehabilitation/restorative care	*Record the number of days each of the following rehabilitation or restorative techniques or practices was provided to the resident for more than or equal to 15 minutes per day in the last 7 days. (Enter "0" if none or less than 15 minutes daily)*			
	a. Range of motion (passive)	0	f. Walking	0
	b. Range of motion (active)	0	g. Dressing or grooming	0
	c. Splint or brace assistance	0	h. Eating or swallowing	0
	Training and skill practice in:		i. Amputation/prosthesis care	0
	d. Bed mobility	0	j. Communication	0
	e. Transfer	0	k. Other	0

4. Devices and restraints	*(Use the following codes for last 7 days)* 0. Not used 1. Used less than daily 2. Used daily	
	Bed rails	
	a. Full bed rails on all open sides of bed	0
	b. Other types of side rails used (e.g., half rail, one side)	0
	c. Trunk restraint	0
	d. Limb restraint	0
	e. Chair prevents rising	0

(continued)

DOCUMENTATION IN LONG-TERM CARE

BETTER CHARTING

Minimum Data Set *(continued)*

Section P. Special treatments and procedures *(continued)*

5. Hospital stays	Record number of times resident was admitted to hospital with an overnight stay in last 90 days (or since last assessment if less than 90 days). (Enter "0" if no hospital admissions)	0 0
6. Emergency room (ER) visits	Record number of times resident visited ER without an overnight stay in last 90 days (or since last assessment if less than 90 days. (Enter "0" if no ER visits)	0 0
7. Physician visits	In the LAST 14 DAYS (or since admission if less than 14 days in facility), how many days has the physician (or authorized assistant or practitioner) examined the resident? (Enter "0" if none)	0 1
8. Physician orders	In the LAST 14 DAYS (or since admission if less than 14 days in facility), how many days has the physician (or authorized assistant or practitioner) changed the resident's orders? Do not include order renewals without change. (Enter "0" if none)	0 0
9. Abnormal lab values	Has the resident had any abnormal lab values during the last 90 days (or since admission)? 0. No 1. Yes	1

Section Q. Discharge potential and overall status

1. Discharge potential	a. Resident expresses/indicates preference to return to the community 0. No 1. Yes	1
	b. Resident has a support person who is positive towards discharge 0. No 1. Yes	0
	c. Stay projected to be of a short duration — discharge projected within 90 days (do not include expected discharge due to death) 0. No 2. Within 31-90 days 1. Within 30 days 3. Discharge status uncertain	0
2. Overall change in care needs	Resident's overall self-sufficiency has changed significantly as compared to status of 90 days ago (or since last assessment if less than 90 days) 0. No change 1. Improved — receives fewer supports, needs less restrictive level of care 2. Deteriorated — receives more support	0

Section R. Assessment information

1. Participation in assessment	a. Resident:	0. No	1. Yes		1
	b. Family	0. No	1. Yes	2. No family	0
	c. Significant other	0. No	1. Yes	2. None	0

2. Signatures of persons completing the assessment

Tina D'Agostino, RN

a. Signature of RN Assessment Coordinator (sign on above line)

b. Date RN Assessment Coordinator signed as complete: 0 2 – 1 2 – 1 9 9 9 (Month – Day – Year)

c. Other signatures	Title	Sections	Date
Brian Devlin	*RN*	*S*	*2/12/99*

d. ______

e. ______

f. ______

Minimum Data Set *(continued)*

Section S. State-specific information

1. MA resident determination (admission, reentry, MA change)	a. Recipient number from PA ACCESS card (if applicable)	
	b. MA NF Effective date from PA/FS 162 (if applicable) — Month – Day – Year	
	c. Is the resident funded through a long-term care capitated assistance program? 0. No 1. Yes	0
	d. Is the resident Medical Assistance for MA CASE-MIX? (see instructions) 0. No 1. Yes	0
2. Date of change to/from MA (MA change)	Date of change to/from Medical Assistance for MA CASE-MIX — Month – Day – Year	
3. Resident admission information (admission)	a. Is the resident DAY ONE MA eligble? 0. No 1. Yes	
	b. Has the resident been assisted by an OPTIONS Level II site? 0. No 1. Yes	
	c. Is the resident funded through a managed care organization? 0. No 1. Yes	
4. Schedule II drugs (full, quarterly)	During the last 7 days, did the resident receive any Schedule II (controlled substances) drugs? 0. No 1. Yes	0

Section T. Therapy supplement for Medicare PPS

1. Special treatments and procedures	a. Recreation therapy — *Enter number of days and total minutes of recreation therapy administered (for at least 15 minutes a day) in the last 7 days (Enter "0" if none)* (A) = # of days administered for 15 minutes or more (B) = total # of minutes provided in last 7 days	DAYS (A): 0; MIN (B): 0 0 0 0
	Skip unless this is a Medicare 5 day or Medicare readmission/return assessment. b. Ordered therapies — Has physician ordered any of the following therapies to begin in first 14 days of stay — physical therapy, occupational therapy, or speech pathology service? 0. No 1. Yes *If not ordered, skip to item 2.*	
	c. Through day 15, provide an estimate of the number of days when at least 1 therapy service can be expected to have been delivered.	
	d. Through day 15, provide an estimate of the number of therapy minutes (across the therapies) that can be expected to be delivered.	

(continued)

BETTER CHARTING

Minimum Data Set *(continued)*

Section T. Therapy supplement for Medicare PPS *(continued)*

2. Walking when most self-sufficient	*Complete item 2 if ADL self-performance score for TRANSFER (G1.b.a.) is 0, 1, 2, or 3 AND at least one of the following is present:* • Resident received physical therapy involving gait training (P.1.b.c.) • Physical therapy was ordered for the resident involving gait training (T.1.b) • Resident received nursing rehabilitation by walking (P.3.f) • Physical therapy involving walking has been discontinued within the past 180 days *Skip to item 3 if resident did not walk in last 7 days.* *(For following five items, base coding on the episode when the resident walked the farthest without sitting down. Include walking during rehabilitation sessions.)*
	a. Furthest distance walked without sitting down during this episode: 0. 150+ feet 1. 51-149 feet 2. 26-50 feet 3. 10-25 feet 4. Less than 10 feet b. Time walked without sitting down during this episode: 0. 1-2 minutes 1. 3-4 minutes 2. 5-10 minutes 3. 11-15 minutes 4. 16-30 minutes 5. 31+ minutes c. Self-performance in walking during this episode: 0. INDEPENDENT — No help or oversight 1. SUPERVISION — Oversight, encouragement, or cueing provided 2. LIMITED ASSISTANCE — Resident highly involved in walking; received physical help in guided maneuvering of limbs or other nonweight-bearing assistance 3. EXTENSIVE ASSISTANCE — Resident received weight-bearing assistance while walking d. Walking support provided associated with this episode (code regardless of resident's self-performance classification): 0. No setup or physical help from staff 1. Setup help only 2. One person physical assist 3. Two + persons physical assist e. Parallel bars used by resident in association with this episode 0. No 1. Yes
3. Case mix group	Medicare ☐☐☐☐☐ State ☐☐☐☐☐

Minimum Data Set *(continued)*

Section V. Resident assessment protocol summary

Resident's name: John D. Walker, Jr. **Medical record no.:** 692405

1. Check if RAP is triggered.
2. For each triggered RAP, use the RAP guidelines to identify areas needing further assessment. Document relevant assessment information regarding the resident's status.
   - Describe:
     - Nature of the condition (may include presence or lack of objective data and subjective complaints)
     - Complications and risk factors that affect your decision to proceed to care planning
     - Factors that must be considered in developing individualized care plan interventions
     - Need for referrals/further evaluation by appropriate health professionals.
   - Documentation should support your decision-making regarding whether to proceed with a care plan for a triggered RAP and the type(s) of care plan interventions that are appropriate for a particular resident.
   - Documentation may appear anywhere in the clinical record (e.g., progress notes, consults, flowsheets, etc.)
3. Indicate under the "Location and Date of RAP" column where information related to the RAP assessment can be found.
4. For each triggered RAP, indicate whether a new care plan, care plan revision, or continuation of current care plan is necessary to address the problem(s) identified in your assessment. The "Care Planning Decision" column must be completed within 7 days of completing the RAI (MDS and RAPs).

A. RAP problem area	(a) Check if triggered	Location and date of RAP assessment documentation	(b) Care planning decision — Check if addressed in care plan
Delirium			
Cognitive loss			
Visual function			
Communication			
ADL functional/ rehabilitation potential			
Urinary incontinence and indwelling catheter			
Psychosocial well-being	✓		
Mood state	✓		
Behavioral symptoms			
Activities			
Falls			
Nutritional status			
Feeding tubes			
Dehydration/fluid maintenance			
Dental care			
Pressure ulcers			
Psychotropic drug use			
Physical restraints			

B. Susan Weiss RN — 02 12 1999
Signature of RN Coordinator for RAP Assessment Process — Month Day Year

Signature of Person Completing Care Planning Decision — Month Day Year

BETTER CHARTING

Preadmission Screening Annual Resident Review

Before a patient covered by Medicare or Medicaid can be admitted to a long-term care facility, he must undergo an evaluation of his mental status, known as the Preadmission Screening Annual Resident Review (PASARR). A completed sample of this form appears below.

IDENTIFICATION FORM PA-PASARR-ID

Applicant's/resident's name (last, first)	Social security number	Date
Perrone, Marie	127-30-1228	2/10/99

I. What are the appllcant's/resident's current diagnoses? The individual named above is being considered for nursing facility services on the basis of the following medical diagnoses (Dx).

Primary Dx:	Fractured Ⓛ hip—Total Ⓛ hip replacement
Secondary Dx:	NIDDM
Target Dx:	Depression

II. An individual is considered to have a serious mental illness if he/she meets all of the following requirements regarding diagnosis, level of impairment, and duration of illness.

A. **Diagnosis:** The individual has a serious mental disorder diagnosable under the *Diagnostic and Statistical Manual of Mental Disorders*, 4th edition, revised in 1994.

This mental disorder is:

schizophrenia, delusional (paranoid) disorder, mood disorder, or psychotic disorder not otherwise specified; panic or other severe anxiety disorder; somatoform disorder; personality disorder; or another mental disorder that may lead to a chronic disability. Specify: Depression

NOTE: For this purpose, individuals whose primary diagnosis is not considered a serious mental illness and who have a diagnosis of dementia (including Alzheimer's disease and other organic brain diseases) are to be excluded from PASARR evaluation and continue with regular admission.

☑ Yes ☐ No

B. **Level of impairment:** The mental disorder resulted in functional limitations in major life activities within the past 3 to 6 months that were not appropriate for the individual's developmental stage. An individual typically has at least one of the following characteristics on a continuing or intermittent basis. Check the appropriate box(es):

☑ 1. *Interpersonal functioning.* The individual has serious difficulty interacting appropriately and communicating effectively with other individuals; has a possible history of altercations, evictions, firing, fear of strangers, avoidance of interpersonal relationships, and social isolation.

☑ 2. *Concentration, persistence, and pace.* The individual has serious difficulty in sustaining focused attention for a long enough period to permit the completion of tasks commonly found in work settings or in worklike structured activities occurring in school or home settings. This manifests as difficulty in concentration, inability to complete simple tasks within an established time period, making frequent errors, or requiring assistance in the completion of these tasks.

☑ 3. *Adaptation to change.* The individual has serious difficulty in adapting to typical changes in circumstances associated with work, school, family, or social interaction. This manifests in agitation, exacerbated signs and symptoms associated with the illness, or withdrawal from the situation, or requires intervention by the mental health or judicial system.

Preadmission Screening Annual Resident Review *(continued)*

C. **Recent treatment:** The treatment history indicates that the individual has experienced at least one of the following (check the appropriate boxes):

☑ 1. Psychiatric treatment more intensive than outpatient psychiatric care more than once in the past 2 years (such as partial hospitalization or inpatient hospitalization). Name of inpatient facility partial program or other mental health treatment: *Westover Hospital*

☑ 2. Within the last 2 years, due to his mental disorder, the individual experienced an episode of significant disruption to the normal living situation, for which supportive services were required to maintain functioning at home or in a residential treatment environment, or which resulted in intervention by housing or law enforcement officials.

D. Does the applicant/resident meet all of the requirements of having a serious mental illness listed in Section II A-C?

☑ Yes ☐ No

III. An applicant/resident is considered to be mentally retarded if all of the criteria listed below in A through C are met. If evidence is not present to at least suspect that the individual meets each of the three criteria, the individual should not be identified within the mental retardation target population. Documentation is not necessary to support each criterion as long as the individual is suspected to meet each criterion based on observations and knowledge about the individual. The individual completing this form is responsible for reporting the documentation used in making the identification and should complete the entire section, including "Related questions."

A. The individual has significantly subaverage intellectual functioning (i.e., two standard deviations below the norm, an I.Q. of around 70 or below).

☐ Yes ☑ No

Related questions:

Is intellectual functioning documented on a standardized general intelligence test?

☐ Yes ☑ No

If yes, what is the name and date of the test and the tester's professional qualifications?

If no, what is the basis of the reviewer's finding?
General response of patient to questions

B. The individual has impairments in adaptive behavior that show (check all that apply):

☐ 1. Significant limitation in meeting the standards of maturation, learning, personal independence, and/or social responsibility of his/her age and cultural group.

(continued)

BETTER CHARTING

Preadmission Screening Annual Resident Review *(continued)*

☐ 2. Substantial functional limitation in three or more of the following areas of major life activity that is not related to the normal aging process (check all that apply):

☐ a. Self-care ☐ b. Receptive and expressive language ☐ c. Learning

☐ d. Mobility ☐ e. Self-direction ☐ f. Capacity for independent living

☐ g. Economic self-sufficiency

Related questions:

Are impairments in adaptive behavior documented by a standardized test?

☐ Yes ☐ No

If yes, what is the name and date of the test and the tester's professional qualifications?

____

____

If no, what is the basis for the reviewer's finding?

____

____

C. Is there documentation to substantiate that these conditions occurred between the individual's birth and 22nd birthday?

☐ Yes ☐ No

Related questions:

What documentation substantiates that these conditions occurred between the individual's birth and 22nd birthday?

____

____

D. Does the applicant/resident have presenting evidence to indicate mental retardation based on the criteria listed in A through C above?

☐ Yes ☑ No

E. Has the applicant/resident received mental retardation services from an MR agency in the past?

☐ Yes Identify agency: ______________________________

☑ No

IV. **"Other related condition"** (ORC) includes physical, sensory, or neurologic disabilities that manifested before age 22, are likely to continue indefinitely, and result in substantial functional limitations in three or more of the following areas of major life activity: economic self-sufficiency, capacity for independent living, mobility, self-direction, learning, understanding and use of language, and self-care. Examples of individuals with other related conditions include those with paraplegia or quadriplegia (due to spinal cord injuries), spina bifida, cerebral palsy, blindness or deafness, epilepsy, and head injuries or other injuries (such as gunshot wounds) so long as the injuries were sustained before age 22. It is important to note that an individual can have an ORC regardless of whether the ORC impairs his intellectual abilities.

Preadmission Screening Annual Resident Review *(continued)*

The key to determining whether an individual has an ORC is the age of onset of the disability. It's the obligation of the nursing facility to determine age of onset. If the clinical record does not clearly eliminate the possibility that the individual's physical disability occurred before the age of 22, the nursing facility must ask the individual (or the individual's family, if necessary), document the response, and target the individual accordingly. This information must be available upon request to representatives of the Department, which include the Community Services Program for Persons with Physical Disabilities (CSPPPD) contractors who serve individuals with other related conditions.

A. An individual is considered to have an ORC, which is a severe chronic developmental disability, if he meets all of the conditions in 1 through 4 below.

1. The ORC is attributable to:

   a. Cerebral palsy, autism, epilepsy, Tourette syndrome, meningitis, encephalitis, hydrocephalus, multiple sclerosis, polio, anoxic brain damage, paraplegia or quadriplegia (due to spinal cord injuries), spina bifida, blindness or deafness, head injuries or other injuries (such as gunshot wounds) so long as the injuries were sustained before age 22. Circle applicable condition(s).

   b. Any other condition, other than a serious mental illness, found to be closely related to mental retardation because this condition has resulted in impairment of general intellectual functioning or adaptive behavior similar to that of individuals with mental retardation, and requires treatment or services similar to those required for individuals with mental retardation.

2. The ORC is manifested before the individual reaches age 22.

3. The ORC is likely to continue indefinitely.

4. The ORC results in substantial functional limitations in three or more of the following areas of major life activity. Check all areas of substantial functional limitation that were present prior to age 22 and were directly the result of the ORC:

   ☐ a. Self-care ☐ b. Understanding and use of language ☐ c. Learning

   ☐ d. Mobility ☐ e. Self-direction ☐ f. Capacity for independent living

   ☐ g. Economic self-sufficiency

B. Does the applicant/resident meet the criteria of an ORC as defined in IV-A?

☐ Yes ☑ No

C. Is there documentation that indicates the presence of an ORC as defined in IV-A?

☐ Yes ☑ No

D. Was the individual referred for care by an agency that serves individuals with developmental disabilities, or is the applicant/resident eligible for that agency's services?

☐ Yes ☑ No

IF YOU ANSWER "YES" IN SECTIONS II-D (MH), III-D (MR), OR *IV-B (ORC), GO TO SECTION V.*

IF YOU ANSWER "NO" IN SECTIONS II-D (MH), III-D (MR), AND *IV-B (ORC), GO TO SECTION VI-A-B.*

(continued)

BETTER CHARTING

Preadmission Screening Annual Resident Review *(continued)*

V. Does the applicant/resident meet the criteria for exceptional admission to a facility without PAS evaluation? Criteria defined in A, B, and C of this section apply to applicants/residents who answered "Yes" in Sections II-D, III-D, or IV-B.

A. Is the person an exempted hospital discharge?

☑ Yes ☐ No

Although identified as an individual with a serious mental illness, mental retardation, or an ORC, an applicant/resident who is not dangerous to himself and/or others may be directly admitted for nursing facility services from an acute care hospital for a period up to 30 days without further evaluation if such admission is based on a written, medically prescribed period of recovery for the conditions requiring hospitalization.

If the individual is admitted under this criterion and continues in residence for more than 30 days, a new PA-PASARR-ID form must be completed. The department must be notified on the MA 408, and an evaluation must be completed within 40 calendar days of admission to the nursing facility. Failure to report these changes in condition in a timely manner may result in financial sanctions against the nursing facility.

B. Does the person require respite care?

☐ Yes ☑ No

Although identified as an individual with a serious* mental illness, mental retardatlon, or ORC, an applicant/resident who is not dangerous to himself or others may be admitted for respite care for a period up to 14 days without further evaluation if he/she is certified by a referring or attending physician to require 24-hour nursing facility services and supervision.

If the individual's condition changes from respite to long-term and he/she is going to stay in the nursing facility, the department must be notified on the MA 408, and an evaluatlon must be completed within 24 days of admission to the nursing facility. Failure to report these changes in condition in a timely manner may result in financial sanctions against the nursing facility.

C. Is the person in a coma or functioning at brain stem level?

☐ Yes ☑ No

Although identified as an individual with a serious* mental illness, mental retardation, or ORC, an applicant/resident who is not dangerous to himself and/or others may receive nursing facility services without further evaluation if certified by the referring or attending physician to be in a coma or functioning at brain stem level. The condition must require intense 24-hour nursing facility services and supervision and be so extreme that the individual cannot focus upon, participate in, or benefit from specialized services.

If there is a "No" response in Sections II-D, III-D, and IV-B, complete Sections VI A-B.

If there is a "Yes" response in Sections II-D (MH), III-D (MR), or IV-B (ORC), and if all answers to Section V (Exceptional Criteria) are "No," complete Sections VI-A and VI-C.

If there is a "Yes" response to any question in Section V (Exceptional Criteria), complete Sections VI-A and VI-D.

* *Serious* applies only to mental illness.

VI. Certifications

A. Individual completing form:

Jean Krenshaw, MSW	(615) 222-8100	2/11/99
SIGNATURE	TELEPHONE NUMBER	DATE

Preadmission Screening Annual Resident Review *(continued)*

GO TO APPROPRIATE BLOCK: B, C, OR D.

B. Regular Admission — No further PASARR evaluation is needed. (Answers in Sections II-D, III-D, and IV-B are all "No.") This is to certify that the applicant does not need to have a PASARR evaluation completed.

SIGNATURE	TELEPHONE NUMBER	DATE

GO TO SECTION VII.

C. Target Group — PASARR evaluation is required. (Answers in Sections II-D, III-D, or IV-B are "Yes" and answers to Section V are "No.") This is to certify that the applicant meets criteria for referral to the designated Area Agency on Aging for PAS evaluation or will be referred to the Department's Utilization Management Review Team for PASARR evaluation.

SIGNATURE	TELEPHONE NUMBER	DATE

GO TO SECTION VII.

D. Exceptional Admission (when answers in Sections II-D, III-D, or IV-B are "Yes" and one or more answers in Section V are "Yes"). This is to certify that the applicant/resident was targeted for evaluation but has a condition that meets the criteria for exceptional admission indicated in Section V.

Dr. Jorge Marcos	(615) 222-8839
PRINT PHYSICIAN'S NAME	TELEPHONE NUMBER
Jorge Marcos, MD	2/11/99
PHYSICIAN'S SIGNATURE	DATE

Medical Director Confirmation (must be completed for all exceptional admissions).
This is to confirm that I have reviewed the diagnosis and medical need of the applicant for the level of nursing services and medical services to be provided by the facility.

Dr. Molly VandenHeuvel	(615) 222-7177
PRINT MEDICAL DIRECTOR'S NAME	TELEPHONE NUMBER
M. VandenHeuvel, MD	2/12/99
MEDICAL DIRECTOR'S SIGNATURE	DATE

GO TO SECTION VII.

VII. Does the applicant/resident need an interpreter or other assistance to participate in or understand the PASARR evaluation process?

- ☐ Yes Describe ____________________
- ☑ No

GO TO SECTION VIII.

VIII. Type of admission

☐ Target group	☑ Exceptional admission	☐ Regular
1. Report on MA 408	1. Report on MA 408 admission	
2. Refer to OPTIONS/UMR team		

devices to assist dexterity and mobility, family relationships, and the patient's transition from home or hospital to the long-term care facility.

Some facilities are decreasing the nurse's role in this initial assessment, relying on the history and physical examination findings obtained from the doctor.

Nursing summaries

Care and status updates in long-term care facilities must be completed regularly. The nurse usually completes a nursing care summary at least once a week for patients requiring skilled care and every 2 weeks for patients requiring intermediate care.

The summary should address such topics as ADLs, nutrition and hydration, needed safety measures (such as adaptive devices), medications and other treatments, and adjustment problems related to the transition from home or hospital to the facility.

Medicare and Medicaid standards require that you complete a nursing assessment summary at least monthly.

ADL checklists or flow sheets

Commonly filled out by the nurses' assistants on each shift, ADL checklists and flow sheets must be reviewed and signed by the nurse. These forms include data related to such categories as diet, personal and oral hygiene, bowel and bladder function, skin care, and ambulation. Commonly used ADL forms include the Katz index, the Barthel index, and the Lawton scale.

The Katz index, the most commonly used checklist, describes the patient's functional level at a specific time and rates his performance on three levels: without help, some help needed, and having complete disability. (See *Katz index.*) Other scales closely assess the patient's performance of basic ADLs, such as using the telephone and preparing meals. (See *Lawton scale,* page 178.)

Documents that satisfy internal policies and procedures

Like government agencies, long-term care facilities have their own strict and comprehensive protocols (for bowel and bladder monitoring, physical and chemical restraints, safety, and infection control, for example). Documentation related to these care categories should reflect the nursing process, especially in the areas of assessment and intervention.

Plans of care

Usual standards for plans of care developed for residents of long-term care facilities require that they be completed by the nurse within 7 days of the patient's admission. Usual standards also require that a review of the plan of care be completed and documented every 3 months or whenever the patient's status progresses or deteriorates in two or more areas.

In long-term care facilities, the plan of care is typically developed using an interdisciplinary approach. Ideally, the patient, his family, and all involved departments — nursing, dietary, physical therapy, and social services, for example — contribute to the plan.

BETTER CHARTING

Katz index

Below you'll find a sample of the Katz index, which is used to assess six basic activities of daily living (ADLs).

Evaluation Form

Name *Henry Dancer* Date *3/2/99*

For each area of functioning listed below, check the description that applies.

Indicates independence	Indicates assistance needed	Indicates dependence
Bathing: Sponge bath, tub bath, or shower. ☑ Receives no assistance; gets into and out of tub, if tub is usual means of bathing.	☐ Receives assistance in bathing only one part of the body, such as the back or leg.	❍ Receives assistance in bathing more than one part of the body, or can't bathe.
Dressing: Gets outer garments and underwear from closets and drawers and uses fasteners, including suspenders, if worn. ☑ Gets clothes and gets completely dressed without assistance.	☐ Gets clothes and gets dressed without assistance except for tying shoes.	❍ Receives assistance in getting clothes or in getting dresses, or stays partly or completely undressed.
Toileting: Goes to the room termed "toilet" for bowel movement and urination, cleans self afterward, and arranges clothes. ☑ Goes to toilet room, cleans self, and arranges clothes without assistance. May use object for support, such as cane, walker, or wheelchair and may manage night bedpan or commode, emptying it in the morning.	❍ Receives assistance in going to toilet room or in cleaning self or arranging clothes after elimination or in use of night bedpan or commode.	❍ Doesn't go to toilet room for the elimination process.
Transfer ☑ Moves into and out of bed and chair without assistance. May use object, such as cane or walker for support.	❍ Moves into or out of bed or chair with assistance.	❍ Doesn't get out of bed.
Continence ☑ Controls urination and bowel movement completely by self.	❍ Has occasional accidents.	❍ Supervision helps keep control of urination or bowel movement, or catheter is used, or is incontinent.
Feeding ☐ Feeds self without assistance.	☑ Feeds self except for assistance in cutting meat or buttering bread.	❍ Receives assistance in feeding or is fed partly or completely through tubes or by I.V. fluids.

Evaluator: *Germaine Fried, RN*

Overall evaluation: *B*

A: Independent in all six functions.
B: Independent in all but one of these functions.
C: Independent in all but bathing and one additional function.
D: Independent in all but bathing, dressing, and one additional function.
E: Independent in all but bathing, dressing, toileting, and one additional function.
F: Independent in all but bathing, dressing, toileting, transferring, and one additional function.
G: Dependent in all six functions.
Other: Dependent in at least two functions but not classifiable as C, D, E, or F.

Adapted with permission from Katz, S. et al. "Studies of Illness in the Aged: The Index of ADL-A Standardized Measure of Biological and Psychosocial Function," *JAMA* 185:914-19, ©1963.

BETTER CHARTING

Lawton scale

The Lawton scale evaluates more sophisticated functions — known as instrumental activities of daily living — than the Katz index. Patients or caregivers can complete the form in a few minutes. The first answer in each case — except for 8a — indicates independence; the second indicates capability with assistance; and the third, dependence. In this version, the maximum score is 29, although scores have meaning only for a particular patient, as when declining scores over time reveal deterioration. Question 4 to 7 tend to be gender specific; modify them as necessary.

Name *Julia Lippey* **Rated by** *Katherine Mitchell, RN* **Date** *January 18, 1999*

1. Can you use the telephone?
   Without help . . . . (3) [circled]
   With some help 2
   Completely unable 1

2. Can you get to places beyond walking distance?
   Without help . . . . (3) [circled]
   With some help 2
   Completely unable 1

3. Can you go shopping for groceries?
   Without help . . . . (3) [circled]
   With some help 2
   Completely unable 1

4. Can you prepare your own meals?
   Without help . . . . (3) [circled]
   With some help 2
   Completely unable 1

5. Can you do your own housework?
   Without help 3
   With some help . . . . (2) [circled]
   Completely unable 1

6. Can you do your own handyman work?
   Without help 3
   With some help . . . . (2) [circled]
   Completely unable 1

7. Can you do your own laundry?
   Without help . . . . (3) [circled]
   With some help 2
   Completely unable 1

8a. Do you take medicines or use any medications?
   Yes (If yes, answer Question 8b.) . . . . (1) [circled]
   No (If no, answer Question 8c.) 2

8b. Do you take your own medicine?
   Without help (in the right doses at the right times) . . . . (3) [circled]
   With some help (if someone prepares it for you and/or reminds you to take it) 2
   Completely unable 1

8c. If you had to take medicine, could you do it?
   Without help (in the right doses at the right times) 3
   With some help (if someone prepares it for you and/or reminds you to take it) 2
   Completely unable 1

9. Can you manage your own money?
   Without help . . . . (3) [circled]
   With some help 2
   Completely unable 1

Adapted with permission from Lawton, M.P., and Brody, E.M. "Assessment of Older People: Self-Maintaining and Instrumental Activites of Daily Living," *The Gerontologist* 9(3):179-186, Autumn 1969.

DOCUMENTATION GUIDELINES

Consider the following points when updating your records:

- When writing nursing summaries, be sure to address all specific patient problems noted in the plan of care.
- When writing progress notes, confirm that the patient's progress is being evaluated and reevaluated continually in relation to the goals or outcomes defined in the plan of care. If goals aren't met, this also needs to be addressed. Any additional actions should be described and documented.
- Record transfers and discharges according to your facility's protocol.
- Be sure to report and document any change in the patient's condition (for example, a change resulting from an accident or a treatment) to the doctor and the patient's family.
- Document any follow-up interventions or other measures implemented in response to a reported change in the patient's condition.
- Keep a record in your notes of all visits to and phone calls about the patient from family or friends. An institution may be fined by state or federal regulators if omissions such as these occur.
- If an incident involving the patient occurs, such as a fall or a treatment error, be sure to maintain follow-up documentation for at least 48 hours after the event.
- Ensure that records for newly admitted patients are maintained in a thorough and detailed manner by the nursing staff on each shift during the patient's first week of residence.
- Like patients who experience an incident and those who need special monitoring, new patients should become well known to all staff members. Some long-term care facilities use a flagging system (such as a red dot on the patient's chart, bed, or door) to identify new patients.
- When documenting, never lose sight of funding. To qualify for reimbursement, the records must reflect the level of care given to the patient. If you're providing care for your patient's pressure ulcer, for example, Medicare requires documentation that describes daily activity; skin condition; turning and positioning measures; the ulcer's location, size, and degree of healing; the patient's nutritional status and dietary intake; and so forth.
- Be certain that your records accurately reflect any skilled service that the patient receives.
- Always record a doctor's verbal and telephone orders, and make sure that the doctor countersigns these orders within 48 hours.
- If appropriate, record when the doctor sees the patient because standards require that the doctor see each patient in a long-term care facility at least once every 60 days.

Selected references

Blaum, C.S., et al. "Validity of the Minimum Data Set for Assessing Nutritional Status in Nursing Home Residents," *American Journal of Clinical Nutrition* 66(4):787-94, October 1997.

Fitzgerald, R.P., et al. "Applying Performance Measures to Long-Term Care," *Joint Commission Journal on Quality Improvement* 22(7):505-17, July 1996.

Ganser, T. "Quality Variable for Documentation in Long-Term Care," *Topics in Health Information Management* 18(1):32-37, August 1997.

Heiker, D.M. "A Narrative Approach to Quality Care in Long-Term Care Facilities," *Journal of Holistic Nursing* 15(1):68-81, March 1997.

Jaffe, M.S. *The OBRA Guidelines for Quality Improvement.* Aurora, Colo.: Skidmore-Roth Pub., 1996.

Kleyman, P. "HCFA Proposes First System of Integrated Long-Term Care," *Aging Today* 18(3):1-2, May-June 1997.

Lyons, E. "Documenting in Skilled Nursing Facilities," *Topics in Geriatric Rehabilitation* 13(1):44-60, September 1997.

Marek, K.D., et al. "OBRA '87: Has It Resulted in Positive Change in Nursing Homes?" *Journal of Gerontological Nursing* 22(12):32-40, December 1996.

"Medicare/Medicaid: Resident Assessment in Long-term Care Facilities — HCFA's Final Rule," *Legal Eagle Eye Newsletter for the Nursing Profession* 6(2):2-3, 6, February 1998.

Pepe, M.C., et al. "Evaluating the Effectiveness of Nursing Home Pre-Admission Review: A State Example," *Journal of Long-Term Home Health Care* 16(3):15-23, Summer 1997.

Wiener, J.M. "Managed Care and Long-Term Care: The Integration of Financing and Services," *Generations* 20(2):47-52, Summer 1996.

7

Documentation in Home Care

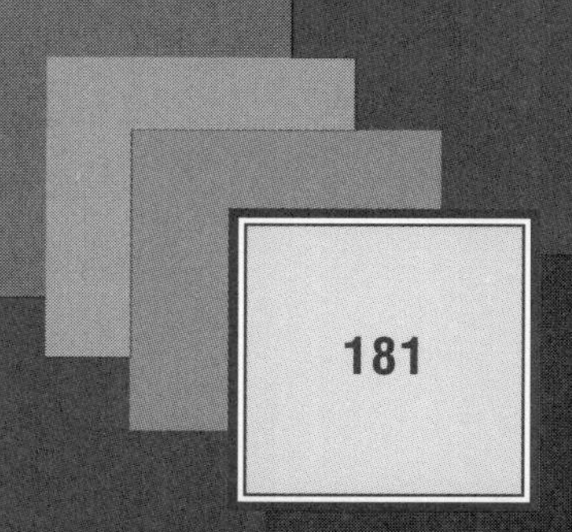

Like hospitals, rehabilitation centers, and nursing homes, home health care agencies are regulated by state and federal laws and bodies. These standard bearers require accurate and complete documentation as well as the standard of care from home health care agencies. Without these features, a home health care agency may fail to earn licensure, accreditation, and reimbursement—or may have current licensure, accreditation, and reimbursement revoked.

Accreditation and quality improvement programs are available through the Foundation for Hospice and Homecare, the Joint Commission on Accreditation of Healthcare Organizations (JCAHO), and the American Nurses Association (ANA), which has instituted the ANA Standards of Home Care Nursing Practice. The nursing process forms the basis of these standards.

The newest credentialing body for home health care agencies is the National Committee for Quality Assurance (NCQA). This private, nonprofit organization evaluates and provides information about the quality of managed health care. It has two purposes: accrediting managed care companies and measuring patient care outcomes. In the future, the NCQA may be used to compare home health care agencies within specified regions.

NCQA standards originated with the Health Plan Employer Data and Information Set (HEDIS), which was developed by a coalition of health maintenance organizations (HMOs). Some states use HEDIS to compare hospitals within regions. The Health Care Financing Administration (HCFA), the watchdog agency for Medicare and Medicaid disbursements, is aggressively urging states to use HEDIS to compare the performance of Medicaid HMOs, to make purchasing decisions, and to hold plans accountable.

Home health care growth

In light of the speedy discharge of patients from hospitals, the increasing number of elderly people, and the availability of safe, easily operated health care equipment, home health care has a bright future. Services provided range from caretaking and assistance with activities of daily living (ADLs) to such highly complex and advanced interventions as I.V. therapy delivered by central and peripheral lines, mechanical ventilation, and chemotherapy.

Providing nursing care to patients in their home requires you to assume many roles, including those of skilled-care provider, educator, and communicator. The skilled home care practitioner must be highly competent and well organized—especially in the area of documentation.

In no other health care setting are you as responsible for ensuring reimbursement payments as you are in the home health care setting. Your success or failure virtually depends on your documentation skills. For this reason, home health care organizations have a tightly structured documentation system.

STANDARDIZED AND REQUIRED DOCUMENTS

Home health care nurses are bound by all the controls imposed by the professional standards and nurse practice acts that govern nurses in all other settings. In addition, every home health agency has its own standards, requirements, and forms to be used when documenting a patient's care. Naturally, you'll want to be familiar with your agency's requirements and follow them to the best of your ability. For the most part, however, you'll find that all agencies and payers require certain types of documentation, even if they use different forms to report the information.

The areas in which you'll need to ensure documentation typically include the referral for home care, Medicare and Medicaid, assessment (including the Outcome and Assessment Information Set B [OASIS-B]), plan of care, medical update, progress notes, nursing summaries, patient or caregiver teaching, recertification, discharge summary, and referral to community resources.

Referral forms

Before you begin caring for a patient in his home, your agency will receive information about that patient on a referral, or intake, form. This form is used to make sure that the patient is eligible for home care and that the agency can provide the services he needs before it agrees to take the new case. (See *Using a referral form for home care,* pages 184 and 185.)

Medicare and Medicaid forms

By mandate in 1985, HCFA required home health care agencies to standardize and update their record keeping and documentation methods. For each qualified Medicare or Medicaid recipient, the agency must complete a Home Health Certification and Plan of Care form (Form 485) and submit it for approval every 60 days. (See *Certifying home health care needs,* page 186.) A medical update and patient information form is completed when Medicare requests it or to obtain recertification for additional home care.

These data allow Medicare reviewers to evaluate each claim in accordance with the criteria for coverage. Medicare will provide no payment unless the required forms are properly completed, signed, and submitted. These forms are usually completed by the nurse assigned to the patient, although the nursing supervisor can also complete them. The data are usually filed after completing a comprehensive nursing assessment and devising a suitable plan of care. Forms must be signed by the nurse and the attending doctor.

To meet Medicare's criteria for home care reimbursement, the patient needs to meet all of the following conditions:

- He must be confined to his home.
- He must need skilled services.
- He must need those skilled services on an intermittent basis.
- The care he needs must be reasonable and medically necessary.
- He must be under a doctor's care.

Agency assessment forms

When a patient is referred to a home health care agency, the agency must complete a thorough and specific assessment of the patient's:

- physical status
- nutritional status
- mental and emotional status
- home environment in relation to safety and supportive services and groups, such as family, neighbors, and community
- knowledge of his disease or current condition, prognosis, and treatment plan
- potential for complying with the treatment plan.

HCFA's proposed "Conditions of Participation for Home Health Agencies" requires that Medicare-certified agencies complete a

(Text continues on page 187.)

BETTER CHARTING

Using a referral form for home care

Also called an intake form, a referral form is used to document a new patient's needs when you begin your evaluation. Use the sample below as a guide.

Date of referral: 1/17/99 Branch: North Chart #: 97-413 H ✓
Info taken by: Beth Isham, RN Admit date: 1/18/99
Patient's name: Geraldine Rush
Address: 66 Newton St.
City: Burlington State: VT Zip: 05402
Phone: (802) 123-4567 Date of birth: 4/3/20
Primary caregiver name & phone number: husband (Dennis) (802) 123-4567
Insurance name: Medicare Ins. #: 123-45-6789
Is this a managed care policy (HMO)? no
Primary Dx: (Code 162.5) lung cancer Date: 12/11/96
(Code 877) decubitus ulcer (coccyx) Date: 3/13/97
(Code 714.0) rheumatoid arthritis Date: 1980s
Procedures: (Code 86.28) decubitus care Date: 3/14/97
Referral source: J. Silva, hospital SW Phone: 765-2813
Doctor name & phone #: Frank Crabbe Phone: 765-4321
Doctor address: 9073 Parkway Drive, Burlington
Hospital: University Hospital Admit: 1/1/99 Discharge: 1/16/99
Functional limitations: Pain management, nonambulatory, poor fine motor skills 2° rheumatoid arthritis
ORDERS/SERVICES: (specify amount, frequency and duration)
(SN:) SN visits 3x/week & p.r.n. x 2 months
(AL:) CNA visits daily 5 days/week x 2 months
(PT, OT), ST: PT & OT evaluations and visits 2-3 x/week & p.r.n. x 2 months
(MSW:) MSW evaluation & weekly visits x 2 months
Spiritual coordinator: Rev. Carlson, St. Paul's Lutheran Church
Counselor: JoAnne Knowton, MSW
Volunteer: Rosalie Marshall (niece) will provide care on weekends
Other services provided: shopping, laundry, meal prep
Goals: wound care, pain management, terminal care @ home
Equipment: Needs commode, hospital bed, bedpan, Hoyer lift, side rail w/c
Company & phone number: Scott Medical Equipment 765-9931
Safety measures: side rails up X 4 Nutritional req diet as tolerated

FUNCTIONAL LIMITATIONS: (Circle applicable)			ACTIVITIES PERMITTED: (Circle applicable)		
1. Amputation	5. Paralysis	9. Legally blind	1. Complete bed rest	6. Partial wgt bearing	(A) Wheelchair
2. Bowel/Bladder	(6.) Endurance	A. Dyspnea with minimal exer	2. Bed rest BRP	7. Independent at home	B. Walker
3. Contracture	(7.) Ambulation		3. Up as tolerated	8. Crutches	C. No restriction
4. Hearing	8. Speech	(B.) Other RA	(4.) Transfer bed/chair	9. Cane	D. Other -specify

Accessibility to bath: Y - (N) Shower Y - (N) Bathroom Y - (N) Exit (Y) - N
Mental status: (Circle) Oriented Comatose Forgetful (Depressed) Disoriented Lethargic Agitated Other

Using a referral form for home care *(continued)*

Allergies: *none known*

• Hospice appropriate meds • Med company: *Walker Pharmacy*

MEDICATIONS:

morphine sulfate liq. 20 mg/ml 40 mg P.O. q6h p.r.n. pain
Compazine 10 mg P.O. or P.R. q4–6h p.r.n. n/v
Colace 200 mg P.O. q.d. p.r.n. constipation
Benadryl 25 – 50 mg P.O. @ h.s. p.r.n. sleeplessness

Living will Yes ✓ No ____ Obtained ____ Family to mail to office ____
Guardian, POA, or responsible person: *husband*
Address & phone number: *same*
Other family members: ____
ETOH: *0* Drug use: *0* Smoker: *2 ppd x 40 years; quit 2 yrs ago*
History: *Other than problems associated with arthritis, was in general good health until 12/96, Dx: lung CA – husband cared for @ home until 1/1/99.*

Social history (place of birth, education, jobs, retirement, etc.): *Born & raised in Toronto, became U.S. citizen when married in 1951. 2 yrs. college – majored in music. Retired church organist.*

ADMISSION NOTES: VS: T *98.4° P.O.* AP *86* RR *18* BP *140/72*
Lungs: *breath sounds LLL* Extremities: *cool to touch; pedal pulses present*
Wgt: *118* Recent wgt (loss)/gain of *40 lb over 6 months*
Admission narrative: *Visit made to pt/husband in hospital before discharge. Both have been told that she is failing rapidly, and would like her to return home with Hospice services. Niece willing to help 2 days/week. Pt apprehensive; husband blames himself for the coccygeal decubitus ulcer which developed under his care.*
Psychosocial issues: *Pt has always cared for husband. Describes self as depressed that she is no longer able to do so; worries who will care for him after she dies.*
Environmental concerns: *Need smoke detectors*

Are there any cultural or spiritual customs or beliefs of which we should be aware before providing Hospice services? *Pt would like Holy Communion just before death (& weekly)*
Funeral home: *not yet chosen* Contact made: Yes *X* No ____

DIRECTIONS: *Corner Newton & Elm; duplex, white with green trim. Door on Ⓛ says 66. Bell broken – knock loudly.*

Agency representative signature: *Beth Isham, RN* Date: *1/18/99*
Home Care Supervisor

BETTER CHARTING

Certifying home health care needs

The Home Health Certification and Plan of Care form (also known as Form 485) is the official form required by Medicare to authorize coverage for home care. To maintain Medicare coverage, this form must be updated and resubmitted every 62 days.

Department of Health and Human Services
Health Care Financing Administration

Form Approved
OMB No. 0938-0357

HOME HEALTH CERTIFICATION AND PLAN OF CARE

1. Patient's HI Claim No.	2. Start Of Care Date	3. Certification Period	4. Medical Record No.	5. Provider No.
111-111	03/08/99	From 07/08/99 To: 09/08/00	78-9101	11-1213

6. Patient's Name and Address
Mary Long
2218 Central Ave.
Wichita, Kansas

7. Provider's Name, Address and Telephone Number
Home Health Agency
301 Main Street
Wichita, Kansas

8. Date of Birth 06/04/29 9. Sex ☐ M ☑ F

10. Medications: Dose/Frequency/Route (N)ew (C)hanged
digoxin 0.125 mg P.O. q.d.; Lasix 20 mg P.O. q.d.; warfarin 5 mg P.O. q.d.; Capoten 12.5 mg b.i.d.; Proventil 2 puffs q.i.d./p.r.n.; MVI one P.O. q.d.; $FeSO_4$ 325 mg q.d.; Ex-Strength Tylenol 500 mg q4h p.r.n.; albuterol 0.5 cc with 3 cc NSS via nebulizer b.i.d.; aspirin 325 mg 1 P.O. qd

		Date
11. ICD-9-CM 4-27-31	Principal Diagnosis: atrial fibrillation	01/20/99
12. ICD-9-CM 0000	Surgical Procedure: gastrostomy tube insertion	03/3/99
13. ICD-9-CM 4280	Other Pertinent Diagnoses: heart failure	03/1/99
496	chronic airway obstruction	11/29/97

14. DME and Supplies: Gastrostomy tube supplies, cane

15. Safety Measures: Prevent falls

16. Nutritional Req.: Magnacal 80 ml/hr

17. Allergies: NKA

18.A. Functional Limitations
1 ☐ Amputation
2 ☐ Bowel/Bladder (Incontinence)
3 ☐ Contracture
4 ☐ Hearing
5 ☐ Paralysis
6 ☑ Endurance
7 ☐ Ambulation
8 ☐ Speech
9 ☐ Legally Blind
A ☐ Dyspnea With Minimal Exertion
B ☐ Other (Specify)

18.B. Activities Permitted
1 ☐ Complete Bedrest
2 ☐ Bedrest BRP
3 ☑ Up As Tolerated
4 ☐ Transfer Bed/Chair
5 ☐ Exercises Prescribed
6 ☐ Partial Weight Bearing
7 ☐ Independent At Home
8 ☐ Crutches
9 ☑ Cane
A ☐ Wheelchair
B ☐ Walker
C ☐ No Restrictions
D ☐ Other (Specify)

19. Mental Status: 1 ☑ Oriented 2 ☐ Comatose 3 ☐ Forgetful 4 ☐ Depressed 5 ☐ Disoriented 6 ☐ Lethargic 7 ☐ Agitated 8 ☐ Other

20. Prognosis: 1 ☐ Poor 2 ☐ Guarded 3 ☐ Fair 4 ☑ Good 5 ☐ Excellent

21. Orders for Discipline and Treatments (Specify Amount/Frequency/Duration)
RN: Assess heart failure, effects of digoxin, monitor complaints of arthritis pain control; monitor gastrostomy tube site, help with gastrostomy feedings and tube care. Draw blood as ordered by MD.
AID 2-3wk; assist with personal care and ADLs.

22. Goals/Rehabilitation Potential/Discharge Plans
Pt needs teaching reinforcement and emotional support for colostomy.
Rehab potential is good. Skilled nursing facility.

23. Nurse's Signature and Date of Verbal SOC Where Applicable: N. Smith, RN 03/08/99

25. Date HHA Received Signed POT: 03/08/99

24. Physician's Name and Address
M. Raser, MD
555 Main St.
Wichita, Kansas

26. I certify/recertify that this patient is confined to his/her home and needs intermittent skilled nursing care, physical therapy and/or speech therapy or continues to need occupational therapy. The patient is under my care, and I have authorized the services on this plan of care and will periodically review the plan.

27. Attending Physician's Signature and Date Signed
M. Raser, MD 03/8/99

28. Anyone who misrepresents, falsifies, or conceals essential information required for payment of Federal funds may be subject to fine, imprisonment, or civil penalty under applicable Federal laws.

Form HCFA-485 (C-4) (02-94) (Print Aligned)

PROVIDER

comprehensive assessment of home care patients using a standardized form called the Outcome and Assessment Information Set (OASIS). The revised version of the OASIS form is now known as OASIS-B. HCFA is preparing to mandate the use of OASIS-B by the end of 1998. However, many home health agencies already use this form in their documentation. (See *Using the OASIS-B form,* pages 188 to 203.)

The OASIS form was developed specifically to measure outcomes for adults who receive home care. Using this instrument, you'll collect data to measure changes in your patient's health status over time. Typically, you'll collect OASIS data when a patient starts home care, at the 60-day recertification point, and when the patient is discharged or transferred to another facility, such as a hospital or a subacute care facility.

Plan of care

As in any health care setting, the nursing process forms the basis for developing the plan of care. However, because the patient's care occurs in the home — usually with family participation — you have less control than you would in an institutional setting. The patient and his family become the decision makers in many aspects and have greater control of the situation. You should address these factors realistically when developing the plan of care. Remember that you are a guest in the patient's home; you may need to adjust your interventions, patient goals, and teaching accordingly.

Many agencies use the Home Health Certification and Plan of Care form as the patient's official plan of care. Other agencies require a separate plan of care, whereas still others see the two plans as redundant and time-consuming.

Medical update

Whenever you update your plan of care, you must do so on a form accepted by your agency. To continue providing skilled nursing care to a patient at home, you must submit the information that the insurer requests on an approved agency form. You are not required to submit the Medical Update and Patient Information form (Form 486) unless Medicare requests it. (See *Providing updated medical and patient information,* page 204.)

If you must complete Form 486 for Medicare patients, use the following treatment codes to describe the skilled nursing care delivered to the patient:

A1: Skilled observation and assessment (including vital signs, response to medications, etc.)
A2: Indwelling urinary catheter insertion
A3: Bladder instillation
A4: Open wound care and dressing
A5: Decubitus care (partial tissue loss with signs of infection or full tissue loss, etc.)
A6: Venipuncture
A7: Restorative nursing
A8: Postcataract care
A9: Bowel and bladder training
A10: Chest physiotherapy (percussion and postural drainage)
A11: Administration of vitamin B_{12}
A12: Administration of insulin
A13: Administration of other I.M. or S.C. medications
A14: Administration of I.V. clysis
A15: Teaching ostomy or ileostomy conduit care
A16: Teaching nasogastric feeding
A17: Reinsertion of nasogastric feeding tube
A18: Teaching gastrostomy feeding
A19: Teaching parenteral nutrition

(Text continues on page 203.)

BETTER CHARTING

Using the OASIS-B form

The OASIS-B form includes more than 80 topics, including sociodemographic, physiologic, and functional data; service utilization information; and mental, behavioral, and emotional data. Keep in mind that this form is not a comprehensive assessment tool, nor is it suitable for use with pediatric or Ob/Gyn patients.

OUTCOME AND ASSESSMENT INFORMATION SET (OASIS-B)

Items to be Used at Specific Time Points

Start of Care (or Resumption of Care Following Inpatient Facility Stay): 1-79
Follow-Up: 1-11, 14, 19-21, 23, 26-36, 39-81
Discharge (not to inpatient facility): 1-11, 14, 19-21, 23, 26-36, 39-84, 88-89
Transfer to Inpatient Facility (with or without agency discharge): 1-11, 80-82, 85-89
Death at Home: 1-11, 89
Note: For items 61-77, please note special instructions at the beginning of the section.

DEMOGRAPHICS AND PATIENT HISTORY

1. (M0010) Agency ID: 2 7 3 9 6 4 2 8
2. (M0020) Patient ID number: QCB/811757
3. (M0030) Start of care date: 0 2 / 0 8 / 1 9 9 9 (month day year)
4. (M0040) Patient's last name: P E R E Z
5. (M0050) Patient state of residence: P A
6. (M0060) Patient ZIP code: 1 9 1 4 7
7. (M0063) Medicare number: 1 3 4 7 6 5 4 8 2 A (including suffix if any)
   ☐ NA- No Medicare
8. (M0066) Birth date: 0 7 / 0 7 / 1 9 1 2 (month day year)
9. (M0080) Discipline of person completing assessment:
   ☒ 1-RN ☐ 2-LPN ☐ 3-PT
   ☐ 4-SLP/ST ☐ 5-OT ☐ 6-MSW
10. (M0090) Date assessment information recorded: 0 2 / 0 8 / 1 9 9 9 (month day year)
11. (M0100) This assessment is currently being completed for the following reason:
    - ☒ 1 - Start of care
    - ☐ 2 - Resumption of care (after inpatient stay)
    - ☐ 3 - Discharge from agency — not to an inpatient facility [Go to M0150]
    - ☐ 4 - Transferred to an inpatient facility — discharged from agency [Go to M0830]
    - ☐ 5 - Transferred to an inpatient facility — not discharged from agency [Go to M0830]
    - ☐ 6 - Died at home [Go to M0906]
    - ☐ 7 - Recertification reassessment (follow-up) [Go to M0150]
    - ☐ 8 - Other follow-up [Go to M0150]
12. (M0130) Gender:
    ☐ 1-Male ☒ 2-Female
13. (M0140) Race/Ethnicity (as identified by patient):
    - ☐ 1 - White, non-Hispanic
    - ☐ 2 - Black, African-American
    - ☒ 3 - Hispanic
    - ☐ 4 - Asian, Pacific Islander
    - ☐ 5 - American Indian, Eskimo, Aleut
    - ☐ 6 - Other
    - ☐ UK - Unknown

Using the OASIS-B form *(continued)*

14. (M0150) Current payment sources for home care: (Mark all that apply.)
    - ☐ 0 - None: no charge for current services
    - ☒ 1 - Medicare (traditional fee-for-service)
    - ☐ 2 - Medicare (HMO/managed care)
    - ☐ 3 - Medicaid (traditional fee-for-service)
    - ☐ 4 - Medicaid (HMO/managed care)
    - ☐ 5 - Workers' compensation
    - ☐ 6 - Title programs (e.g., Title III, V, or XX)
    - ☐ 7 - Other government (e.g., CHAMPUS, VA, etc.)
    - ☐ 8 - Private insurance
    - ☐ 9 - Private HMO/managed care
    - ☐ 10 - Self-pay
    - ☐ 11 - Other (specify) ____________
    - ☐ UK - Unknown

15. (M0160) Financial factors limiting the ability of the patient/family to meet basic health needs: (Mark all that apply.)
    - ☐ 0 - None
    - ☐ 1 - Unable to afford medicine or medical supplies
    - ☒ 2 - Unable to afford medical expenses that are not covered by insurance/Medicare (e.g., copayments)
    - ☐ 3 - Unable to afford rent/utility bills
    - ☐ 4 - Unable to afford food
    - ☐ 5 - Other (specify) ____________

16. (M0170) From which of the following inpatient facilities was the patient discharged <u>during the past 14 days</u>? (Mark all that apply.)
    - ☒ 1 - Hospital
    - ☐ 2 - Rehabilitation facility
    - ☐ 3 - Nursing home
    - ☐ 4 - Other (specify) ____________
    - ☐ NA - Patient was not discharged from an inpatient facility [If NA, go to M0200]

17. (M0180) Inpatient discharge date (most recent):
    02/01/1999
    month day year
    - ☐ UK - Unknown

18. (M0190) Inpatient diagnoses and three-digit ICD code categories <u>for only those conditions treated during an inpatient facility stay within the last 14 days</u> (no surgical or V-codes):

	<u>Inpatient facility diagnosis</u>	<u>ICD</u>
a.	Heart failure	(4 2 8)
b.	Sacral decubitus	(7 0 7)

19. (M0200) Medical or treatment regimen change within past 14 days: Has this patient experienced a change in medical or treatment regimen (e.g., medication, treatment, or service change due to new or additional diagnosis, etc.) within the last 14 days?
    - ☐ 0 - No [If no, go to M0220]
    - ☒ 1 - Yes

20. (M0210) List the patient's medical diagnoses and three-digit ICD code categories <u>for those conditions requiring changed medical or treatment regimen</u> (no surgical or V-codes):

	<u>Changed medical regimen diagnosis</u>	<u>ICD</u>
a.	Urinary Retention	(7 8 8)
b.	____________	(_ _ _)
c.	____________	(_ _ _)
d.	____________	(_ _ _)

21. (M0220) Conditions prior to medical or treatment regimen change or inpatient stay within past 14 days: If this patient experienced an inpatient facility discharge or change in medical or treatment regimen within the past 14 days, indicate any conditions that existed <u>prior to</u> the inpatient stay or change in medical or treatment regimen. (Mark all that apply.)
    - ☒ 1 - Urinary incontinence
    - ☐ 2 - Indwelling/suprapubic catheter
    - ☐ 3 - Intractable pain
    - ☒ 4 - Impaired decision-making
    - ☐ 5 - Disruptive or socially inappropriate behavior
    - ☒ 6 - Memory loss to the extent that supervision required
    - ☐ 7 - None of the above
    - ☐ NA - No inpatient facility discharge <u>and</u> no change in medical or treatment regimen in past 14 days
    - ☐ UK - Unknown

(continued)

BETTER CHARTING

Using the OASIS-B form *(continued)*

22. (M0230/M0240) Diagnoses and severity index: List each medical diagnosis or problem for which the patient is receiving home care and ICD code category (no surgical or V-codes), and rate them using the following severity index. (Choose one value that represents the most severe rating appropriate for each diagnosis.)

0 - Asymptomatic, no treatment needed at this time
1 - Symptoms well controlled with current therapy
2 - Symptoms controlled with difficulty, affecting daily functioning; patient needs ongoing monitoring
3 - Symptoms poorly controlled; patient needs frequent adjustment in treatment and dose monitoring
4 - Symptoms poorly controlled, history of rehospitalizations

	Primary diagnosis (M0230)	ICD	Severity rating				
a.	*Heart failure*	(*4 2 8*)	☐ 0	☐ 1	☐ 2	☒ 3	☐ 4
	Other diagnosis (M0240)	**ICD**	**Severity rating**				
b.	*Sacral decubitus*	(*7 0 7*)	☐ 0	☐ 1	☒ 2	☐ 3	☐ 4
c.	*Urinary retention*	(*7 8 8*)	☐ 0	☒ 1	☐ 2	☐ 3	☐ 4
d.		(_ _ _)	☐ 0	☐ 1	☐ 2	☐ 3	☐ 4
e.		(_ _ _)	☐ 0	☐ 1	☐ 2	☐ 3	☐ 4
f.		(_ _ _)	☐ 0	☐ 1	☐ 2	☐ 3	☐ 4

23. (M0250) Therapies the patient receives at home: (Mark all that apply.)
    - ☐ 1 - Intravenous or infusion therapy (excludes TPN)
    - ☐ 2 - Parenteral nutrition (TPN or lipids)
    - ☒ 3 - Enteral nutrition (nasogastric, gastrostomy, jejunostomy, or any other artificial entry into the alimentary canal)
    - ☐ 4 - None of the above

24. (M0260) Overall prognosis: BEST description of patient's overall prognosis for recovery from this episode of illness:
    - ☐ 0 - Poor: little or no recovery is expected and/or further decline is imminent
    - ☒ 1 - Good/Fair: partial to full recovery is expected
    - ☐ UK - Unknown

25. (M0270) Rehabilitative prognosis: BEST description of patient's prognosis for functional status:
    - ☒ 0 - Guarded: minimal improvement in functional status is expected; decline is possible
    - ☐ 1 - Good: marked improvement in functional status is expected
    - ☐ UK - Unknown

26. (M0280) Life expectancy: (Physician documentation is not required.)
    - ☒ 0 - Life expectancy is greater than 6 months
    - ☐ 1 - Life expectancy is 6 months or fewer

27. (M0290) High risk factors characterizing this patient: (Mark all that apply.)
    - ☐ 1 - Heavy smoking
    - ☒ 2 - Obesity
    - ☐ 3 - Alcohol dependency
    - ☐ 4 - Drug dependency
    - ☐ 5 - None of the above
    - ☐ UK - Unknown

LIVING ARRANGEMENTS

28. (M0300) Current residence:
    - ☒ 1 - Patient's owned or rented residence (house, apartment, or mobile home owned or rented by patient/couple/significant other)
    - ☐ 2 - Family member's residence
    - ☐ 3 - Boarding home or rented room
    - ☐ 4 - Board and care or assisted living facility
    - ☐ 5 - Other (specify) ____________

29. (M0310) Structural barriers in the patient's environment limiting independent mobility: (Mark all that apply.)
    - ☐ 0 - None
    - ☐ 1 - Stairs inside home that must be used by the patient (e.g., to get to toileting, sleeping, eating areas)
    - ☐ 2 - Stairs inside the home that are used optionally (e.g., to get to laundry facilities)
    - ☒ 3 - Stairs leading from inside house to outside
    - ☐ 4 - Narrow or obstructed doorways

DOCUMENTATION IN HOME CARE

Using the OASIS-B form *(continued)*

30. (M0320) Safety hazards found in the patient's current place of residence: (Mark all that apply.)
    - ☐ 0 - None
    - ☐ 1 - Inadequate floor, roof, or windows
    - ☒ 2 - Inadequate lighting
    - ☐ 3 - Unsafe gas/electric appliance
    - ☒ 4 - Inadequate heating
    - ☐ 5 - Inadequate cooling
    - ☒ 6 - Lack of fire safety devices
    - ☐ 7 - Unsafe floor coverings
    - ☐ 8 - Inadequate stair railings
    - ☐ 9 - Improperly stored hazardous materials
    - ☒ 10 - Lead-based paint
    - ☐ 11 - Other (specify) ____________________

31. (M0330) Sanitation hazards found in the patient's current place of residence: (Mark all that apply.)
    - ☐ 0 - None
    - ☐ 1 - No running water
    - ☐ 2 - Contaminated water
    - ☐ 3 - No toileting facilities
    - ☐ 4 - Outdoor toileting facilities only
    - ☐ 5 - Inadequate sewage disposal
    - ☐ 6 - Inadequate/improper food storage
    - ☐ 7 - No food refrigeration
    - ☐ 8 - No cooking facilities
    - ☒ 9 - Insects/rodents present
    - ☐ 10 - No scheduled trash pickup
    - ☒ 11 - Cluttered/soiled living area
    - ☐ 12 - Other (specify) ____________________

32. (M0340) Patient lives with: (Mark all that apply.)
    - ☐ 1 - Lives alone
    - ☒ 2 - With spouse or significant other
    - ☐ 3 - With other family member
    - ☐ 4 - With friend
    - ☐ 5 - With paid help (other than home care agency staff)
    - ☐ 6 - With other than above

SUPPORTIVE ASSISTANCE

33. (M0350) Assisting person(s) other than home care agency staff: (Mark all that apply.)
    - ☐ 1 - Relatives, friends, or neighbors living outside the home
    - ☒ 2 - Person residing in the home (excluding paid help)
    - ☐ 3 - Paid help
    - ☐ 4 - None of the above (If none of the above, go to M0390)
    - ☐ UK - Unknown (If unknown, go to M0390)

34. (M0360) Primary caregiver taking <u>lead</u> responsibility for providing or managing the patient's care, providing the most frequent assistance, etc. (other than home care agency staff):
    - ☐ 0 - No one person (If no one person, go to M0390)
    - ☒ 1 - Spouse or significant other
    - ☐ 2 - Daughter or son
    - ☐ 3 - Other family member
    - ☐ 4 - Friend or neighbor or community or church member
    - ☐ 5 - Paid help
    - ☐ UK - Unknown (If unknown, go to M0390)

35. (M0370) How often does the patient receive assistance from the primary caregiver?
    - ☐ 1 - Several times during day and night
    - ☒ 2 - Several times during day
    - ☐ 3 - Once daily
    - ☐ 4 - Three or more times per week
    - ☐ 5 - One to two times per week
    - ☐ 6 - Less often than weekly
    - ☐ UK - Unknown

36. (M0380) Type of primary caregiver assistance: (Mark all that apply.)
    - ☐ 1 - ADL assistance (bathing, dressing, toileting, bowel/bladder, eating/feeding)
    - ☒ 2 - IADL assistance (meds, meals, housekeeping, laundry, telephone, shopping, finances)
    - ☐ 3 - Environmental support (housing, home maintenance)
    - ☒ 4 - Psychosocial support (socialization, companionship, recreation)
    - ☐ 5 - Advocates or facilitates patient's participation in appropriate medical care
    - ☐ 6 - Financial agent, power of attorney, or conservator of finance
    - ☐ 7 - Health care agent, conservator of person, or medical power of attorney
    - ☐ UK - Unknown

(continued)

BETTER CHARTING

Using the OASIS-B form *(continued)*

SENSORY STATUS

37. (M0390) Vision with corrective lenses if the patient usually wears them:
    - ☐ 0 - Normal vision: sees adequately in most situations; can see medication labels, newsprint
    - ☐ 1 - Partially impaired: cannot see medication labels or newsprint, but can see obstacles in path and the surrounding layout; can count fingers at arm's length
    - ☒ 2 - Severely impaired: cannot locate objects without hearing or touching them or patient nonresponsive

38. (M0400) Hearing and ability to understand spoken language in patient's own language (with hearing aids if the patient usually uses them):
    - ☐ 0 - No observable impairment; able to hear and understand complex or detailed instructions and extended or abstract conversation
    - ☐ 1 - With minimal difficulty, able to hear and understand most multi-step instructions and ordinary conversation; may need occasional repetition, extra time, or louder voice
    - ☐ 2 - Has moderate difficulty hearing and understanding simple, one-step instructions and brief conversation; needs frequent prompting or assistance
    - ☒ 3 - Has severe difficulty hearing and understanding simple greetings and short comments; requires multiple repetitions, restatements, demonstrations, additional time
    - ☐ 4 - Unable to hear and understand familiar words or common expressions consistently, or patient nonresponsive

39. (M0410) Speech and oral (verbal) expression of language (in patient's own language):
    - ☐ 0 - Expresses complex ideas, feelings, and needs clearly, completely, and easily in all situations with no observable impairment
    - ☐ 1 - Minimal difficulty in expressing ideas and needs (may take extra time, makes occasional errors in word choice, grammar or speech intelligibility; needs minimal prompting or assistance)
    - ☐ 2 - Expresses simple ideas or needs with moderate difficulty (needs prompting or assistance, errors in word choice, organization or speech intelligibility); speaks in phrases or short sentences
    - ☒ 3 - Has severe difficulty expressing basic ideas or needs and requires maximal assistance or guessing by listener; speech limited to single words or short phrases
    - ☐ 4 - Unable to express basic needs even with maximal prompting or assistance but is not comatose or unresponsive (e.g., speech is nonsensical or unintelligible)
    - ☐ 5 - Patient nonresponsive or unable to speak

40. (M0420) Frequency of pain interfering with patient's activity or movement:
    - ☐ 0 - Has no pain or pain does not interfere with activity or movement
    - ☐ 1 - Less often than daily
    - ☒ 2 - Daily, but not constantly
    - ☐ 3 - All of the time

41. (M0430) Intractable pain: Is the patient experiencing pain that is not easily relieved, occurs at least daily, and affects the patient's sleep, appetite, physical or emotional energy, concentration, personal relationships, emotions, or ability or desire to perform physical activity?
    - ☒ 0 - No
    - ☐ 1 - Yes

DOCUMENTATION IN HOME CARE

Using the OASIS-B form *(continued)*

INTEGUMENTARY STATUS

42. (M0440) Does this patient have a skin lesion or an open wound? This excludes "ostomies."
    - ☐ 0 - No (If No, go to M0490)
    - ☒ 1 - Yes

43. (M0445) Does this patient have a pressure ulcer?
    - ☐ 0 - No (If No, got to M0468)
    - ☒ 1 - Yes

    43a. (M0450) Current number of pressure ulcers at each stage: (Circle one response for each stage.)

Pressure ulcer stages

a) Stage 1: Nonblanchable erythema of intact skin; the heralding of skin ulceration. In darker pigmented skin, warmth, edema, hardness, or discolored skin may be indicators.

Number of pressure ulcers

(0) 1 2 3 4 or more

b) Stage 2: Partial-thickness skin loss involving epidermis and/or dermis. The ulcer is superficial and presents clinically as an abrasion, blister, or shallow crater.

Number of pressure ulcers

0 1 (2) 3 4 or more

c) Stage 3: Full-thickness skin loss involving damage or necrosis of subcutaneous tissue that may extend down to, but not through, underlying fascia. The ulcer presents clinically as a deep crater with or without undermining of adjacent tissue.

Number of pressure ulcers

0 (1) 2 3 4 or more

d) Stage 4: Full-thickness skin loss with extensive destruction, tissue necrosis, or damage to muscle, bone, or supporting structures (e.g., tendon, joint capsule, etc.)

Number of pressure ulcers

(0) 1 2 3 4 or more

e) In addition to the above, is there at least one pressure ulcer that cannot be observed due to the presence of eschar or a nonremovable dressing, including casts?

☒ 0 - No ☐ 1 - Yes

43b. (M0460) Stage of most problematic (observable) pressure ulcer:
- ☐ 1 - Stage 1
- ☐ 2 - Stage 2
- ☒ 3 - Stage 3
- ☐ 4 - Stage 4
- ☐ NA - No observable pressure ulcer

43c. (M0464) Status of most problematic (observable) pressure ulcer:
- ☐ 1 - Fully granulating
- ☐ 2 - Early/partial granulation
- ☒ 3 - Not healing
- ☐ NA - No observable pressure ulcer

44. (M0468) Does this patient have a stasis ulcer?
    - ☒ 0 - No (If no, go to M0482)
    - ☐ 1 - Yes

    44a. (M0470) Current number of observable stasis ulcer(s):
    - ☐ 0 - Zero
    - ☐ 1 - One
    - ☐ 2 - Two
    - ☐ 3 - Three
    - ☐ 4 - Four or more

    44b. (M0474) Does this patient have at least one stasis ulcer that cannot be observed due to the presence of a nonremovable dressing?
    - ☐ 0 - No
    - ☐ 1 - Yes

    44c. (M0476) Status of most problematic (observable) stasis ulcer:
    - ☐ 1 - Fully granulating
    - ☐ 2 - Early/partial granulation
    - ☐ 3 - Not healing
    - ☐ NA - No observable stasis ulcer

45. (M0482) Does this patient have a surgical wound?
    - ☒ 0 - No (If no, go to M0490)
    - ☐ 1 - Yes

(continued)

BETTER CHARTING

Using the OASIS-B form *(continued)*

45a. (M0484) Current number of (observable) surgical wounds: (If a wound is partially closed but has more than one opening, consider each opening as a separate wound.)
- ☐ 0 - Zero
- ☐ 1 - One
- ☐ 2 - Two
- ☐ 3 - Three
- ☐ 4 - Four or more

45b. (M0486) Does this patient have at least one surgical wound that cannot be observed due to the presence of a nonremovable dressing?
- ☐ 0 - No
- ☐ 1 - Yes

45c. (M0488) Status of most problematic (observable) surgical wound:
- ☐ 1 - Fully granulating
- ☐ 2 - Early/partial granulation
- ☐ 3 - Not healing
- ☐ NA - No observable surgical wound

RESPIRATORY STATUS

46. (M0490) When is the patient dyspneic or noticeably short of breath?
- ☐ 0 - Never; patient is not short of breath
- ☐ 1 - When walking more than 20 feet, climbing stairs
- ☐ 2 - With moderate exertion (e.g., while dressing, using commode or bedpan, walking distances less than 20 feet)
- ☐ 3 - With minimal exertion (e.g., while eating, talking, or performing other ADLs) or with agitation
- ☒ 4 - At rest (during day or night)

47. (M0500) Respiratory treatments utilized at home: (Mark all that apply.)
- ☒ 1 - Oxygen (intermittent or continuous)
- ☐ 2 - Ventilator (continually or at night)
- ☐ 3 - Continuous positive airway pressure
- ☐ 4 - None of the above

ELIMINATION STATUS

48. (M0510) Has this patient been treated for a urinary tract infection in the past 14 days?
- ☐ 0 - No
- ☒ 1 - Yes
- ☐ NA - Patient on prophylactic treatment
- ☐ UK - Unknown

49. (M0520) Urinary incontinence or urinary catheter presence:
- ☐ 0 - No incontinence or catheter (includes anuria or ostomy for urinary drainage) (If no, go to M0540)
- ☒ 1 - Patient is incontinent
- ☐ 2 - Patient requires a urinary catheter (i.e., external, indwelling, intermittent, suprapubic) (Go to M0540)

50. (M0530) When does urinary incontinence occur?
- ☐ 0 - Timed voiding defers incontinence
- ☐ 1 - During the night only
- ☒ 2 - During the day and night

51. (M0540) Bowel incontinence frequency:
- ☐ 0 - Very rarely or never has bowel incontinence
- ☐ 1 - Less than once weekly
- ☐ 2 - One to three times weekly
- ☐ 3 - Four to six times weekly
- ☐ 4 - On a daily basis
- ☒ 5 - More often than once daily
- ☐ NA - Patient has ostomy for bowel elimination
- ☐ UK - Unknown

52. (M0550) Ostomy for bowel elimination: Does this patient have an ostomy for bowel elimination that (within the last 14 days): a) was related to an inpatient facility stay, or b) necessitated a change in medical or treatment regimen?
- ☒ 0 - Patient does <u>not</u> have an ostomy for bowel elimination
- ☐ 1 - Patient's ostomy was <u>not</u> related to an inpatient stay and did not necessitate change in medical or treatment regimen
- ☐ 2 - Ostomy <u>was</u> related to an inpatient stay or <u>did</u> necessitate change in medical or treatment regimen

Using the OASIS-B form *(continued)*

NEURO/EMOTIONAL/BEHAVIORAL STATUS

53. (M0560) Cognitive functioning: (patient's current level of alertness, orientation, comprehension, concentration, and immediate memory for simple commands)
    - ☐ 0 - Alert/oriented, able to focus and shift attention, comprehends and recalls task directions independently
    - ☐ 1 - Requires prompting (cuing, repetition, reminders) only under stressful or unfamiliar conditions
    - ☐ 2 - Requires assistance and some direction in specific situations (e.g., on all tasks involving shifting of attention), or consistently requires low-stimulus environment due to distractibility
    - ☒ 3 - Requires considerable assistance in routine situations; is not alert and oriented or is unable to shift attention and recall directions more than half the time
    - ☐ 4 - Totally dependent due to disturbances such as constant disorientation, coma, persistent vegetative state, or delirium

54. (M0570) When confused (reported or observed):
    - ☐ 0 - Never
    - ☐ 1 - In new or complex situations only
    - ☐ 2 - On awakening or at night only
    - ☐ 3 - During the day and evening, but not constantly
    - ☒ 4 - Constantly
    - ☐ NA - Patient nonresponsive

55. (M0580) When anxious (reported or observed):
    - ☐ 0 - None of the time
    - ☒ 1 - Less often than daily
    - ☐ 2 - Daily, but not constantly
    - ☐ 3 - All of the time
    - ☐ NA - Patient nonresponsive

56. (M0590) Depressive feelings reported or observed in patient: (Mark all that apply.)
    - ☒ 1 - Depressed mood (e.g., feeling sad, tearful)
    - ☐ 2 - Sense of failure or self-reproach
    - ☒ 3 - Hopelessness
    - ☐ 4 - Recurrent thoughts of death
    - ☐ 5 - Thoughts of suicide
    - ☐ 6 - None of the above feelings observed or reported

57. (M0600) Patient behaviors (reported or observed): (Mark all that apply.)
    - ☐ 1 - Indecisiveness, lack of concentration
    - ☐ 2 - Diminished interest in most activities
    - ☐ 3 - Sleep disturbances
    - ☐ 4 - Recent change in appetite or weight
    - ☒ 5 - Agitation
    - ☐ 6 - A suicide attempt
    - ☐ 7 - None of the above behaviors observed or reported

58. (M0610) Behaviors demonstrated <u>at least once a week</u> (reported or observed): (Mark all that apply.)
    - ☒ 1 - Memory deficit: failure to recognize familiar persons/places, inability to recall events of past 24 hours, significant memory loss so that supervision is required
    - ☒ 2 - Impaired decision-making: failure to perform usual ADLs or IADLs, inability to appropriately stop activities, jeopardizes safety through actions
    - ☐ 3 - Verbal disruption: yelling, threatening, excessive profanity, sexual references, etc.
    - ☐ 4 - Physical aggression: aggressive or combative to self and others (e.g., hits self, throws objects, punches, performs dangerous maneuvers with wheelchair or other objects)
    - ☐ 5 - Disruptive, infantile, or socially inappropriate behavior (excludes verbal actions)
    - ☒ 6 - Delusional, hallucinatory, or paranoid behavior
    - ☐ 7 - None of the above behaviors demonstrated

59. (M0620) Frequency of behavior problems (reported or observed) (e.g., wandering episodes, self-abuse, verbal disruption, physical aggression, etc.):
    - ☐ 0 - Never
    - ☐ 1 - Less than once a month
    - ☐ 2 - Once a month
    - ☐ 3 - Several times each month
    - ☐ 4 - Several times a week
    - ☒ 5 - At least daily

(continued)

BETTER CHARTING

Using the OASIS-B form *(continued)*

60. (M0630) Is this patient receiving psychiatric nursing services at home provided by a qualified psychiatric nurse?
    - ☒ 0 - No
    - ☐ 1 - Yes

ADLs/IADLs

> For Questions 61 to 77, complete the "current" column for all patients. For these same items, complete the "prior" column at the start of care or resumption of care; mark the level that corresponds to the patient's condition 14 days prior to the start of (or resumption of) care. In all cases, record what the patient is able to do.

61. (M0640) Grooming: Ability to tend to personal hygiene needs (i.e., washing face and hands, hair care, shaving or makeup, teeth or denture care, fingernail care):

Prior	Current	
☐	☐	0 - Able to groom self unaided, with or without the use of assistive devices or adapted methods
☐	☐	1 - Grooming utensils must be placed within reach before able to complete grooming activities
☒	☐	2 - Someone must assist the patient to groom self
☐	☒	3 - Depends entirely upon someone else for grooming needs
☐		UK - Unknown

62. (M0650) Ability to dress upper body (with or without dressing aids), including pullovers, undergarments, front-opening shirts and blouses, managing zippers, buttons, and snaps:

Prior	Current	
☐	☐	0 - Able to get clothes out of closets and drawers, put them on, and remove them from the upper body without assistance
☐	☐	1 - Able to dress upper body without assistance if clothing is laid out or handed to the patient
☒	☐	2 - Someone must help the patient put on upper body clothing
☐	☒	3 - Depends entirely upon another person to dress the upper body
☐		UK - Unknown

63. (M0660) Ability to dress lower body (with or without dressing aids), including slacks, undergarments, socks or nylons, shoes:

Prior	Current	
☐	☐	0 - Able to obtain, put on, and remove clothing and shoes without assistance
☐	☐	1 - Able to dress lower body without assistance if clothing and shoes are laid out or handed to patient
☒	☐	2 - Someone must help the patient put on undergarments, slacks, socks or nylons, and shoes
☐	☒	3 - Depends entirely upon another person to dress lower body
☐		UK - Unknown

Using the OASIS-B form *(continued)*

64. (M0670) Bathing: Ability to wash entire body; excludes grooming (washing face and hands only):

Prior	Current	
☐	☐	0 - Able to bathe self in shower or tub independently
☐	☐	1 - With the use of devices, able to bathe self in shower or tub independently
☐	☐	2 - Able to bathe in shower or tub with the assistance of another person: (a) for intermittent supervision or encouragement or reminders or (b) to get in and out of the shower or tub or (c) for washing difficult-to-reach areas
☒	☐	3 - Participates in bathing self in shower or tub, but requires presence of another person throughout the bath for assistance or supervision
☐	☐	4 - Unable to use the shower or tub and is bathed in bed or bedside chair
☐	☒	5 - Unable to effectively participate in bathing and is totally bathed by another person
☐		UK - Unknown

65. (M0680) Toileting: Ability to get to and from the toilet or bedside commode:

Prior	Current	
☐	☐	0 - Able to get to and from the toilet independently with or without a device
☐	☐	1 - When reminded, assisted, or supervised by another person, able to get to and from the toilet
☐	☐	2 - Unable to get to and from the toilet but is able to use a bedside commode (with or without assistance)
☒	☐	3 - Unable to get to and from the toilet or bedside commode but is able to use a bedpan/urinal independently
☐	☒	4 - Totally dependent in toileting
☐		UK - Unknown

66. (M0690) Transferring: Ability to move from bed to chair, on and off toilet or commode, into and out of tub or shower, and ability to turn and position self in bed if patient is bedfast:

Prior	Current	
☐	☐	0 - Able to transfer independently
☐	☐	1 - Transfers with minimal human assistance or with use of an assistive device
☐	☐	2 - Unable to transfer self but able to bear weight and pivot during the transfer process
☒	☐	3 - Unable to transfer self and unable to bear weight or pivot when transferred by another person
☐	☒	4 - Bedfast, unable to transfer but able to turn and position self in bed
☐	☐	5 - Bedfast, unable to transfer and unable to turn and position self
☐		UK - Unknown

67. (M0700) Ambulation/Locomotion: Ability to walk SAFELY, once in a standing position, or use a wheelchair, once in a seated position, on a variety of surfaces:

Prior	Current	
☐	☐	0 - Able to walk independently on even and uneven surfaces and climb stairs with or without railings (i.e., needs no human assistance or assistive device)
☐	☐	1 - Requires use of a device (e.g., cane, walker) to walk alone or requires human supervision or assistance to negotiate stairs or steps or uneven surfaces
☐	☐	2 - Able to walk only with the supervision or assistance of another person at all times
☐	☐	3 - Chairfast, unable to ambulate but able to wheel self independently
☒	☐	4 - Chairfast, unable to ambulate and unable to wheel self
☐	☒	5 - Bedfast, unable to ambulate or be up in a chair
☐		UK - Unknown

(continued)

BETTER CHARTING

Using the OASIS-B form *(continued)*

68. (M0710) Feeding or eating: Ability to feed self meals and snacks: (Note: This refers only to the process of eating, chewing, and swallowing, not preparing the food to be eaten.)

Prior	Current	
☐	☐	0 - Able to feed self independently
☒	☐	1 - Able to feed self independently but requires: (a) meal set-up or (b) intermittent assistance or supervision from another person; or (c) a liquid, pureed, or ground meat diet
☐	☒	2 - Unable to feed self and must be assisted or supervised throughout the meal/snack
☐	☒	3 - Able to take in nutrients orally and receives supplemental nutrients through a nasogastric tube or gastrostomy
☐	☐	4 - Unable to take in nutrients orally and is fed nutrients through a nasogastric tube or gastrostomy
☐	☐	5 - Unable to take in nutrients orally or by tube feeding
☐		UK - Unknown

69. (M0720) Planning and preparing light meals (e.g., cereal, sandwich) or reheat delivered meals:

Prior	Current	
☐	☐	0 - (a) Able to independently plan and prepare all light meals for self or reheat delivered meals; or (b) Is physically, cognitively, and mentally able to prepare light meals on a regular basis but has not routinely performed light meal preparation in the past (i.e., prior to this home care admission)
☒	☐	1 - Unable to prepare light meals on a regular basis due to physical, cognitive, or mental limitations
☐	☒	2 - Unable to prepare any light meals or reheat any delivered meals
☐		UK - Unknown

70. (M0730) Transportation: Physical and mental ability to safely use a car, taxi, or public transportation (bus, train, subway):

Prior	Current	
☐	☐	0 - Able to independently drive a regular or adapted car, or uses a regular or handicap-accessible public bus
☒	☐	1 - Able to ride in a car only when driven by another person; or able to use a bus or handicap van only when assisted or accompanied by another person
☐	☒	2 - Unable to ride in a car, taxi, bus, or van, and requires transportation by ambulance
☐		UK - Unknown

71. (M0740) Laundry: Ability to do own laundry — to carry laundry to and from washing machine, to use washer and dryer, to wash small items by hand:

Prior	Current	
☐	☐	0 - (a) Able to take care of all laundry tasks independently; or (b) Physically, cognitively, and mentally able to do laundry and access facilities, but has not routinely performed laundry tasks in the past (i.e., prior to this home care admission)
☒	☐	1 - Able to do only light laundry, such as minor hand wash or light washer loads; due to physical, cognitive, or mental limitations, needs assistance with heavy laundry such as carrying large loads of laundry
☐	☒	2 - Unable to do any laundry due to physical limitation or needs continual supervision and assistance due to cognitive or mental limitation
☐		UK - Unknown

Using the OASIS-B form *(continued)*

72. (M0750) Housekeeping: Ability to safely and effectively perform light housekeeping and heavier cleaning tasks:

Prior	Current	
☐	☐	0 - (a) Able to independently perform all housekeeping tasks; <u>or</u> (b) Physically, cognitively, and mentally able to perform all housekeeping tasks but has not routinely participated in housekeeping tasks in the past (i.e., prior to this home care admission)
☐	☐	1 - Able to perform only <u>light</u> housekeeping (e.g., dusting, wiping kitchen counters) tasks independently
☐	☐	2 - Able to perform housekeeping tasks with intermittent assistance or supervision from another person
☒	☐	3 - <u>Unable</u> to consistently perform any housekeeping tasks unless assisted by another person throughout the process
☐	☒	4 - <u>Unable</u> to effectively participate in any housekeeping tasks
☐		UK - Unknown

73. (M0760) Shopping: Ability to plan for, select, and purchase items in a store and to carry them home or arrange delivery:

Prior	Current	
☐	☐	0 - (a) Able to plan for shopping needs and independently perform shopping tasks, including carrying packages; <u>or</u> (b) Physically, cognitively, and mentally able to take care of shopping, but has not done shopping in the past (i.e., prior to this home care admission)
☐	☐	1 - Able to go shopping, but needs some assistance: (a) By self is able to do only light shopping and carry small packages, but needs someone to do occasional major shopping; <u>or</u> (b) <u>Unable</u> to go shopping alone, but can go with someone to assist
☒	☐	2 - <u>Unable</u> to go shopping, but is able to identify items needed, place orders, and arrange home delivery
☐	☒	3 - Needs someone to do all shopping and errands
☐		UK - Unknown

(continued)

BETTER CHARTING

Using the OASIS-B form *(continued)*

74. (M0770) Ability to use telephone: Ability to answer the phone, dial numbers, and effectively use the telephone to communicate:

Prior	Current	
☐	☐	0 - Able to dial numbers and answer calls appropriately and as desired
☐	☐	1 - Able to use a specially adapted telephone (i.e., large numbers on the dial, teletype phone for the deaf) and call essential numbers
☐	☐	2 - Able to answer the telephone and carry on a normal conversation but has difficulty placing calls
☐	☐	3 - Able to answer the telephone only some of the time or is able to carry on only a limited conversation
☒	☐	4 - Unable to answer the telephone at all but can listen if assisted with equipment
☐	☐	5 - Totally unable to use the telephone
☐	☒	NA - Patient does not have a telephone
☐		UK - Unknown

MEDICATIONS

75. (M0780) Management of oral medications: Patient's ability to prepare and take all prescribed oral medications reliably and safely, including administration of the correct dosage at the appropriate times/intervals; excludes injectable and I.V. medications: (Note: This refers to ability, not compliance or willingness.)

Prior	Current	
☐	☐	0 - Able to independently take the correct oral medication(s) and proper dosage(s) at the correct times
☒	☐	1 - Able to take medication(s) at the correct times if: (a) individual dosages are prepared in advance by another person; or (b) given daily reminders; or (c) someone develops a drug diary or chart
☐	☒	2 - Unable to take medication unless administered by someone else
☐	☐	NA - No oral medications prescribed
☐		UK - Unknown

76. (M0790) Management of inhalant/mist medications: Patient's ability to prepare and take all prescribed inhalants/mist medications (nebulizers, metered dose devices) reliably and safely, including administration of the correct dosage at the appropriate times/intervals; excludes all other forms of medication (oral tablets, injectable and I.V. medications):

Prior	Current	
☐	☐	0 - Able to independently take the correct medication and proper dosage at the correct times
☒	☐	1 - Able to take medication at the correct times if: (a) individual dosages are prepared in advance by another person; or (b) given daily reminders.
☐	☒	2 - Unable to take medication unless administered by someone else
☐	☐	NA - No inhalants/mist medications prescribed
☐		UK - Unknown

Using the OASIS-B form *(continued)*

77. (M0800) Management of injectable medications: Patient's ability to prepare and take all prescribed injectable medications reliably and safely, including administration of correct dosages at appropriate times/intervals; excludes I.V. medications:

Prior	Current	
☐	☐	0 - Able to independently take the correct medication and proper dosage at the correct times
☐	☐	1 - Able to take injectable medication at the correct times if: (a) individual syringes are prepared in advance by another person, or (b) given daily reminders
☐	☐	2 - Unable to take injectable medications unless administered by someone else
☐	☒	NA - No injectable medications prescribed
☒		UK - Unknown

EQUIPMENT MANAGEMENT

78. (M0810) Patient management of equipment (includes only oxygen, I.V./infusion therapy, enteral/parenteral nutrition equipment or supplies): Patient's ability to set up, monitor, and change equipment reliably and safely; to add appropriate fluids or medication; and to clean/store/dispose of equipment or supplies using proper technique: (Note: This refers to ability, not compliance or willingness.)
    - ☐ 0 - Manages all tasks related to equipment completely independently
    - ☐ 1 - If someone else sets up equipment (i.e., fills portable oxygen tank, provides patient with prepared solutions), is able to manage all other aspects of equipment
    - ☐ 2 - Requires considerable assistance from another person to manage equipment, but completes portions of the task independently
    - ☐ 3 - Only able to monitor equipment (e.g., liter flow, fluid in bag) and must call someone else to manage the equipment
    - ☒ 4 - Is completely dependent on someone else to manage all equipment
    - ☐ NA - No equipment of this type used in care (If NA, go to M0830)

79. (M0820) Caregiver management of equipment (includes only oxygen, I.V./infusion equipment, enteral/parenteral nutrition, ventilator therapy equipment or supplies): Caregiver's ability to set up, monitor, and change equipment reliably and safely, to add appropriate fluids or medication, and to clean/store/dispose of equipment or supplies using proper technique. (Note: This refers to ability, not compliance or willingness.)
    - ☐ 0 - Caregiver manages all tasks related to equipment independently
    - ☐ 1 - If someone else sets up equipment, caregiver is able to manage all other aspects
    - ☐ 2 - Caregiver requires considerable assistance from another person to manage equipment, but completes signifigant portions of the task independently
    - ☐ 3 - Caregiver is only able to complete small portions of task (e.g., administer nebulizer treatment, clean/store/dispose of equipment and supplies)
    - ☒ 4 - Caregiver is completely dependent on someone else to manage all equipment
    - ☐ NA - No caregiver
    - ☐ UK - Unknown

EMERGENT CARE

80. (M0830) Emergent care: Since the last time OASIS data were collected, has the patient utilized any of the following services for emergent care (other than home care agency services)? (Mark all that apply.)
    - ☐ 0 - No emergent care services (If no emergent care and patient discharged, go to M0855)
    - ☒ 1 - Hospital emergency room (includes 23-hour holding)
    - ☒ 2 - Doctor's office emergency visit/house call
    - ☐ 3 - Outpatient department/clinic emergency (includes urgicenter sites)
    - ☐ UK - Unknown

(continued)

BETTER CHARTING

Using the OASIS-B form *(continued)*

81. (M0840) Emergent care reason: For what reason(s) did the patient/family seek emergent care? (Mark all that apply.)
    - ☐ 1 - Improper medication administration, medication adverse effects, toxicity, anaphylaxis
    - ☐ 2 - Nausea, dehydration, malnutrition, constipation, impaction
    - ☐ 3 - Injury caused by fall or accident at home
    - ☒ 4 - Respiratory problems (e.g., shortness of breath, tracheobronchial obstruction, respiratory infection)
    - ☒ 5 - Wound infection, deteriorating wound status, new lesion/ulcer
    - ☒ 6 - Cardiac problems (e.g., fluid overload, exacerbation of heart failure, chest pain)
    - ☐ 7 - Hypoglycemia/hyperglycemia, diabetes out of control
    - ☐ 8 - GI bleeding, obstruction
    - ☐ 9 - Other than above reasons
    - ☐ UK - Reason unknown

DATA ITEMS COLLECTED AT INPATIENT FACILITY ADMISSION OR DISCHARGE ONLY

82. (M0855) To which inpatient facility has the patient been admitted?
    - ☐ 1 - Hospital (Go to M0890)
    - ☐ 2 - Rehabilitation facility (Go to M0903)
    - ☐ 3 - Nursing home (Go to M0900)
    - ☐ 4 - Hospice (Go to M0903)
    - ☒ NA - No inpatient facility admission

83. (M0870) Discharge disposition: Where is the patient after discharge from your agency? (Choose only one answer.)
    - ☒ 1 - Patient remained in the community (not in hospital, nursing home, or rehab facility)
    - ☐ 2 - Patient transferred to a noninstitutional hospice (Go to M0903)
    - ☐ 3 - Unknown because patient moved to a geographic location not served by this agency (Go to M0903)
    - ☐ UK - Other unknown (Go to M0903)

84. (M0880) After discharge, does the patient receive health, personal, or support services or assistance? (Mark all that apply.)
    - ☐ 1 - No assistance or services received
    - ☒ 2 - Yes, assistance or services provided by family or friends
    - ☐ 3 - Yes, assistance or services provided by other community resources (e.g., Meals-on-Wheels, home health services, homemaker assistance, transportation assistance, assisted living, board and care)

    (Go to M0903)

85. (M0890) If the patient was admitted to an acute care hospital, for what reason was he/she admitted?
    - ☐ 1 - Hospitalization for emergent (unscheduled) care
    - ☒ 2 - Hospitalization for urgent (scheduled within 24 hours of admission) care
    - ☐ 3 - Hospitalization for elective (scheduled more than 24 hours before admission) care
    - ☐ UK - Unknown

86. (M0895) Reason for hospitalization: (Mark all that apply.)
    - ☐ 1 - Improper medication administration, medication adverse effects, toxicity, anaphylaxis
    - ☐ 2 - Injury caused by fall or accident at home
    - ☒ 3 - Respiratory problems (shortness of breath, infection, obstruction)
    - ☒ 4 - Wound or tube site infection, deteriorating wound status, new lesion/ulcer
    - ☐ 5 - Hypoglycemia/hyperglycemia, diabetes out of control
    - ☐ 6 - GI bleeding, obstruction
    - ☒ 7 - Exacerbation of heart failure, fluid overload, heart failure
    - ☐ 8 - Myocardial infarction, stroke
    - ☐ 9 - Chemotherapy
    - ☐ 10 - Scheduled surgical procedure
    - ☒ 11 - Urinary tract infection
    - ☐ 12 - I.V. catheter–related infection
    - ☐ 13 - Deep vein thrombosis, pulmonary embolus
    - ☐ 14 - Uncontrolled pain
    - ☐ 15 - Psychotic episode
    - ☐ 16 - Other than above reasons

    (Go to M0903)

Using the OASIS-B form *(continued)*

87. (M0900) For what reason(s) was the patient admitted to a nursing home? (Mark all that apply.)
   - ☐ 1 - Therapy services
   - ☐ 2 - Respite care
   - ☐ 3 - Hospice care
   - ☐ 4 - Permanent placement
   - ☐ 5 - Unsafe for care at home
   - ☐ 6 - Other
   - ☐ UK - Unknown

88. (M0903) Date of last (most recent) home visit:
   0 2 / 0 1 / 1 9 9 9
   month day year

89. (M0906) Discharge/transfer/death date: Enter the date of the discharge, transfer, or death (at home) of the patient.
   __ __ / __ __ / __ __ __ __
   month day year
   - ☐ UK - Unknown

A20: Teaching tracheostomy care
A21: Administration of tracheostomy care
A22: Teaching inhalation treatment
A23: Administration of inhalation treatment
A24: Teaching administration of injection
A25: Teaching diabetic care
A26: Disimpaction and follow-up enema
A27: Other treatments not listed above but ordered by a doctor
A28: Wound care dressing (closed incision or suture line)
A29: Decubitus care other than A5
A30: Teaching indwelling catheter care
A31: Management and evaluation of patient's plan of care
A32: Teaching and training of other skilled nursing services ordered by a doctor.

Progress notes

Each time you visit a patient, you must write a progress note, which documents:

- any changes in the patient's condition
- skilled nursing interventions performed related to the plan of care
- the patient's responses to services provided
- any event or incident in the home that would affect the treatment plan
- vital signs
- education of the patient and home caregiver (includes written instructional materials and brochures as well as the patient's response to the instruction and any return demonstrations).

Nursing summaries

As a home health care nurse, you must compile a summary of the patient's progress (and discharge from home health care, when appropriate). You must also submit a patient progress report to the attending doctor every 62 days and to the reimburser to confirm the need for continuing services.

When writing these summaries, include the following information:

- current problems, treatments, interventions, and instructions
- care provided by other home caregivers, such as physical therapists, speech pathologists, occupational therapists, social workers, and home health aides

BETTER CHARTING

Providing updated medical and patient information

To continue providing reimbursable skilled nursing care to a patient at home, Medicare requires that the home health care agency submit a Medical Update and Patient Information form (also known as Form 486) after the first 62 days of home care. A sample of this form appears below.

Department of Health and Human Services
Health Care Financing Administration

Form Approved
OMB No. 0938-0357

MEDICAL UPDATE AND PATIENT INFORMATION

1. Patient's HI Claim No. 48-7850
2. SOC Date 06/08/98
3. Certification Period From: 11/08/98 To: 01/07/99
4. Medical Record No. 75-4099
5. Provider No. 98-7654
6. Patient's Name and Address James Dole, 412 Main Street, Newark, NJ
7. Provider's Name Home Health Agency
8. Medicare Covered: ☑ Y ☐ N
9. Date Physician Last Saw Patient: 10/24/99
10. Date Last Contacted Physician: 10/25/98
11. Is the Patient Receiving Care in an 1861 (J)(1) Skilled Nursing Facility or Equivalent? ☐ Y ☑ N ☐ Do Not Know
12. ☐ Certification ☑ Recertification ☐ Modified
13. Dates of Last Inpatient Stay: Admission 05/31/98 Discharge 06/05/98
14. Type of Facility: A
15. Updated information: New Orders/Treatments/Clinical Facts/Summary from Each Discipline

Discipline	Visits (this bill)	Frequency and duration	Treatment codes	Total visits projected this cert.
SN	00	2 times a week X 3 weeks	A1	06
Aide	00	3 times a week X 4 weeks	A6	12

SN: A&O x 3. Skin warm, dry, pale, slight dyspnea noted with activity. Trace bilat. pedal edema, lungs clear. No complaints. Improved & increased feeling of well-being demonstrated. Peg tube patent and functioning well. Correctly demonstrates checking for residual, peg tube site care.
Aide: pt seen 3x/wk. Increased difficulty ambulating. Expressed feelings of despair and hopelessness associated with physical condition.

16. Functional Limitations (Expand From 485 and Level of ADL) Reason Homebound/Prior Functional Status Interaction between pt and daughter who wants pt to strive to live. Pt increasingly fearful of institutional care. Pt agrees to join gastrostomy support group. CCSW to facilitate. Needs more encouragement to perform ADLs. Daughter more involved with care.

17. Supplementary Plan of Care on File from Physician Other than Referring Physician: ☐ Y ☐ N
(If Yes, Please Specify Giving Goals/Rehab. Potential/Discharge Plan)

18. Unusual Home/Social Environment N/A

19. Indicate Any Time When the Home Health Agency Made a Visit and Patient was Not Home and Reason Why if Ascertainable

20. Specify Any Known Medical and/or Non-Medical Reasons the Patient Regularly Leaves Home and Frequency of Occurrence

21. Nurse or Therapist Completing or Reviewing Form M. Hoffner, RN
Date (Mo., Day, Yr.) 10/26/98

Form HCFA-486 (C3) (02-94) (Print Aligned)

PROVIDER

- reason for any change in services
- patient outcomes and responses—both physical and emotional—to services provided.

Patient or caregiver teaching

Correct documentation will help justify to your agency and to third-party payers your visits to teach the patient or caregiver. Find out about the patient's and family's needs, resources, and support systems. This will help you outline the basic plan for teaching.

Remember that teaching is usually an ongoing process requiring more than one visit. Until the patient becomes independent, your documentation will help other nurses continue the teaching and identify additional areas of teaching.

Keep a list of teaching and reference materials you have supplied to the patient or caregiver. Also document modifications made to accommodate the patient's or caregiver's literacy skills and native language.

If the patient isn't physically or mentally able to perform the skills himself and no caregiver is available, report this in your documentation. Never leave a patient alone to perform a procedure until he can express understanding of it and perform it competently.

Be careful to call equipment by the same names used on the packages and in teaching literature. Consider providing a glossary of terms. Make sure that the patient can identify devices when speaking on the telephone. Document all teaching materials given to the patient, and keep copies in your records.

Most agencies require patients to sign a teaching documentation record indicating that they accept responsibility for learning self-care activities. This is a critical piece of documentation for the home care chart.

Recertification

To ensure continued home health services for patients who need them, you'll have to prove that the patient still requires home care. Medicare and many managed care plans certify an initial 62-day period during which your agency can receive reimbursement for the patient's home care. When that period is over, the insurer may certify an additional 62 days. This period is called the recertification period.

Naturally, your documentation requesting recertification must clearly support the patient's need for continued care within the insurer's guidelines. A clinical summary of care must be compiled and sent to the patient's doctor and then to the insurer. For Medicare, you'll need to submit a new plan of care on Form 485 as well as a medical update on Form 486. Make sure this form includes data as amended by verbal order since the start of care.

Finally, when you record the primary diagnosis, make sure that it reflects the patient's current needs, not the original reason for the home care.

Discharge summary

You'll prepare a discharge summary for the doctor's approval to discharge, for notifying reimbursers that services have been terminated, and for officially closing the case. When preparing this document, summarize:

- the services provided
- the clinical and psychosocial conditions of the patient at discharge
- recommendations for further care
- the patient's response to and comprehension of patient-teaching efforts
- outcomes attained.

Community referrals

If you work in the home health setting, you'll want to think about local community resources that can help maintain and promote your patients' health and well-being. Such resources may consist of a free mobile health unit or services to provide emotional support. Whenever you make a referral for community services, be sure to document your actions and the reasons for the referral.

Documentation guidelines

Update the record with any changes in the patient's condition or plan of care and document that you reported these changes to the doctor. Keep in mind that Medicare and Medicaid will not reimburse for skilled services implemented but not reported to the doctor.

Be certain to state in your documentation that the patient is housebound and provide the reason for this. A example of a valid reason for being housebound is dyspnea on minimal activity; an invalid reason would be not having a car. Again, keep in mind that Medicare requires that a patient receiving skilled care in the home must be housebound (although some commercial insurers do not).

If an emergency arises in the home during your presence, accompany the patient to the hospital or emergency unit and stay with him until another professional caregiver takes over. Document all assessments and interventions performed for the patient until you're relieved. Note the date and time of transfer and the name of the caregiver who assumes responsibility for the patient.

To prevent your patient from feeling neglected, don't spend a lot of time charting in his home. Instead, complete your records while he sleeps or is otherwise occupied.

Be sure that documentation reflects consistent adherence to the plan of care by all caregivers involved.

Whenever possible, use flow sheets and checklists to record vital signs, intake and output measurements, and nutritional data. Encourage the patient or home caregiver to fill out these forms when appropriate. Doing so involves the patient and family in the patient's progress and increases their feeling of control.

At least once a week, remove documentation materials completed and left in the patient's home. This keeps volumes of paper from piling up or becoming misplaced. It also makes the records available for review by the agency supervisor.

Selected references

Galloway, P.L. "Designing a Discharge Planning Program that Fits," *Caring* 16(10):42-44, 46, October 1997.

Kluka, M. "Home Care Today: Fifteen Common Errors to Avoid When Completing a Skilled Home Care Referral," *Home Healthcare Nurse* 15(11):793-95, November 1997.

"Make Transition to New Documentation System," *Home Care Case Management* 3(8):106-107, August 1996.

"This OASIS Is No Mirage, and It's Heading Your Way," *Home Care Case Management* 4(10):131-34, October 1997.

Using Performance Improvement Tools in Home Care. Oakbrook Terrace, Ill.: Joint Commission on Accreditation of Healthcare Organizations, 1996.

8

Documentation of the Nursing Process

Five-step nursing process

This flowchart shows the five steps of the nursing process and lists the forms you should use to document them.

Step 1
ASSESSMENT
Gather data from the patient's health history, physical examination, medical record, and diagnostic test results.

Documentation tools
Initial assessment form, flow sheets

Step 2
NURSING DIAGNOSIS
Make judgments based on assessment data.

Documentation tools
Nursing plan of care, patient care guidelines, clinical pathway, progress notes, problem list

Regardless of which documentation system you use, your documentation must reflect the nursing process. In the current accreditation manual of the Joint Commission on Accreditation of Healthcare Organizations (JCAHO), the updated charting guidelines reaffirm this emphasis.

Based on theories of nursing and other disciplines, the nursing process follows the scientific method. This problem-solving process systematically organizes nursing activities to ensure the highest quality of care. It allows you to determine which problems you can help alleviate and which potential problems you can help prevent. The nursing process also helps you identify what kind of and how much assistance a patient requires, who can best provide that assistance, which desired outcomes the patient can achieve, and whether he achieves them.

To get such a complete picture of the patient's situation, you'll need to systematically follow the five steps of the nursing process—assessment, nursing diagnosis, planning, intervention, and evaluation—and document them effectively. (See *Five-step nursing process.*)

Fundamentals of nursing documentation

To ensure clear communication and complete, accurate documentation of your nursing care, you must keep in mind the fundamentals of documentation. Follow these guidelines.

Write neatly and legibly

One important reason to document your nursing care is to communicate with other members of the health care team. Sloppy or illegible handwriting confuses people and wastes their time as they try to decipher it. More seriously, the patient might be injured if other caregivers can't understand crucial information.

If you don't have room to chart something legibly, leave that section blank, put a bracket

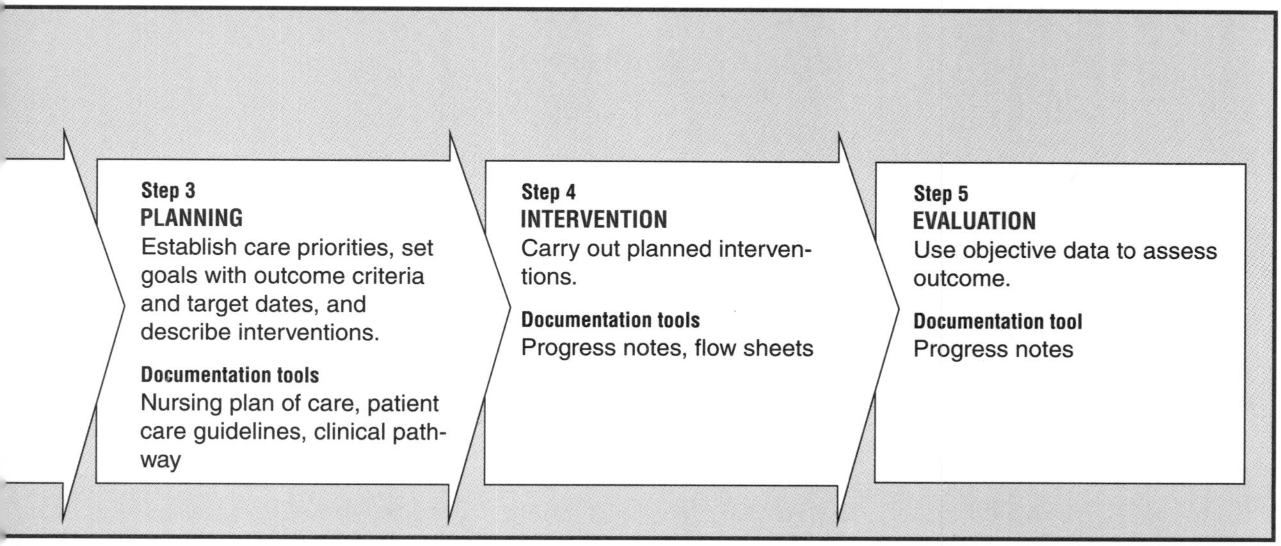

Step 3
PLANNING
Establish care priorities, set goals with outcome criteria and target dates, and describe interventions.

Documentation tools
Nursing plan of care, patient care guidelines, clinical pathway

Step 4
INTERVENTION
Carry out planned interventions.

Documentation tools
Progress notes, flow sheets

Step 5
EVALUATION
Use objective data to assess outcome.

Documentation tool
Progress notes

around it, and write, "See progress notes." Then record the information fully and legibly in the notes.

Write in ink

Because it's a permanent document, the clinical record should be completed in ink or printed out from a computer. Use black or blue ink because other colors may not photocopy well. Also, don't use felt-tipped pens on forms containing carbon paper; the pens may not produce sufficient pressure for copies.

Use correct spelling and grammar

Notes filled with misspelled words and incorrect grammar create the same negative impression as illegible handwriting. To avoid spelling and grammatical errors:

- keep a dictionary in charting areas
- post a list of commonly misspelled words, especially terms and medications regularly used on the unit.

Use standard abbreviations

JCAHO standards and many state regulations require health care facilities to use an approved abbreviation list to prevent confusion. Make sure that you know and use your facility's approved abbreviations. (See the appendix Commonly Accepted Abbreviations.)

Using unapproved abbreviations can result in ambiguity, which may endanger a patient's health. For example, if you use "o.d." for "once a day," another nurse may misinterpret it as "oculus dexter" (right eye) and mistakenly instill medication into the patient's eye instead of giving it once a day. (See *Abbreviations to avoid,* pages 210 and 211.)

Write clear, concise sentences

Avoid using a long word when a short word will do. Clearly identify the subject of the sentence. Don't be afraid to use "I," as in "I contacted the patient's family at 1300 hours, and I explained the change in his condition." Doing so differentiates your actions from those of the patient, doctor, or another staff member.

(Text continues on page 212.)

Abbreviations to avoid

The Joint Commission on Accreditation of Healthcare Organizations requires every health care facility to develop a list of approved abbreviations for staff use. Certain abbreviations should be avoided because they're easily misunderstood, especially when handwritten. Here's a list of abbreviations to avoid.

ABBREVIATION	INTENDED MEANING	MISINTERPRETATION	CORRECTION
Apothecaries' symbols			
f℥	fluidounce	Frequently misinterpreted	Use the metric equivalents.
ʒ	fluidram	Frequently misinterpreted	Use the metric equivalents.
♏	minim	Frequently misinterpreted	Use the metric equivalents.
℈	scruple	Frequently misinterpreted	Use the metric equivalents.
Drug names			
MTX	methotrexate	mustargen (mechlorethamine hydrochloride)	Use the complete spelling for drug names.
CPZ	Compazine (prochlorperazine)	chlorpromazine	Use the complete spelling for drug names.
HCl	hydrochloric acid	potassium chloride ("H" is misinterpreted as "K")	Use the complete spelling for drug names.
DIG	digoxin	digitoxin	Use the complete spelling for drug names.
MVI	multivitamins *without* fat-soluble vitamins	multivitamins *with* fat-soluble vitamins	Use the complete spelling for drug names.
HCTZ	hydrochlorothiazide	hydrocortisone (HCT)	Use the complete spelling for drug names.
ara-a	vidarabine	cytarabine (ara-C)	Use the complete spelling for drug names.
Dosage directions			
au	*auris uterque* (each ear)	Frequently misinterpreted as "OU" (*oculus uterque*—each eye)	Write it out.
μg	microgram	Frequently misinterpreted as "mg"	Use "mcg."

Abbreviations to avoid *(continued)*

ABBREVIATION	INTENDED MEANING	MISINTERPRETATION	CORRECTION
Dosage directions *(continued)*			
OD	once daily	Frequently misinterpreted as "OD" (*oculus dexter*— right eye)	Don't abbreviate "daily." Write it out.
OJ	orange juice	Frequently misinterpreted as "OD" (*oculus dexter*— right eye) or "OS" (*oculus sinister*— left eye). Medications that were meant to be diluted in orange juice and given orally have been given in a patient's right or left eye.	Write it out.
ṫID	once daily	Misinterpreted as "t.i.d." (three times daily)	Write it out.
Per os	orally	The "os" is frequently misinterpreted as "OS" (*oculus sinister*— left eye).	Use "P.O.," "by mouth," or "orally."
q.d.	every day	The period after the "q" has sometimes been misinterpreted as "i," and the drug has been given q.i.d. rather than daily.	Write it out.
qn	nightly or at bedtime	Misinterpreted as "qh" (every hour)	Use "h.s." or "nightly."
qod	every other day	Misinterpreted as "q.d." (daily) or "q.i.d."	Use "q other day" or "every other day."
subq	subcutaneous	The "q" has been misinterpreted as "every." For example, a prophylactic heparin dose meant to be given 2 hours before surgery may be given every 2 hours before surgery.	Use "S.C.," "S.Q.," or write out "subcutaneous."
U or u	unit	Misinterpreted as a "0" or a "4," causing a tenfold or greater overdose.	Write it out.

Say what you mean

Many nurses were taught that nurses don't make diagnoses, so you may sometimes qualify your observations with such words as "appears" or "apparently" when describing symptoms. However, if you use these inexact qualifiers, anyone reading the patient's chart may conclude that you weren't sure what you were describing or doing. The best approach is to state clearly and succinctly what you see, hear, and do. Don't sound tentative.

Chart promptly

Do your charting as soon as possible after you make an observation or provide care because that's when you'll recollect the circumstances most clearly. If you leave your charting until the end of the shift, you may forget important details.

Bedside flow sheets facilitate charting throughout the shift. Some facilities also place progress notes at the bedside. Of course, bedside computers also allow you to document promptly.

However, some nurses are uncomfortable about leaving written flow sheets or notes at the bedside — and understandably so. Although flow sheets don't usually contain confidential information, progress notes do. Unless the records can be kept in a secure place, confidentiality could be breached. Fold-down desks outside the patient's room are one solution: In addition to giving you a handy writing surface, they provide a secure place for keeping the chart.

If bedside flow sheets or computers aren't available, consider making notes on worksheets or pads that you keep in your pocket. Jot down key phrases and times; then transcribe the information into the chart later. Use these notes as a reminder, not as part of the medical record.

Note the time

Be specific about times in the chart. In particular, note the exact time of all sudden changes in the patient's condition, significant events, and nursing actions. Avoid block charting such as "0700 to 1500." This sounds vague and implies inattention to the patient.

Chart in chronological order

Most assessments and observations are useful only as part of a *pattern* of assessments and observations. When isolated, most assessments tell us very little; in chronological order, they reveal a pattern of improvement or deterioration.

If you take the time to note your observations and assessments when you make them, they'll be recorded in chronological order. Too often, nurses wait until the end of the shift, then record groups of assessments that omit important variations.

Document accurately and completely

Record the facts, not opinions or assumptions. Although you don't need to chart routine tasks, such as changing bed linens, you do need to chart all relevant information relating to patient care and reflecting the nursing process.

Document objectively

Record exactly what you see, hear, and do. When you record a patient's statement, use his exact words. Avoid making subjective statements such as "Patient's level of cooperation has deteriorated since yesterday." Instead, include the facts that led you to this

CHARTING GUIDELINES

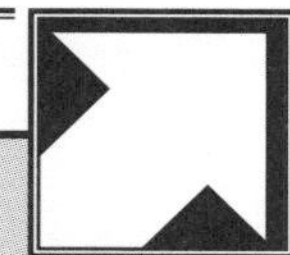

Watch your charting language

At times, some of us may speak and write in a vague or judgmental manner without being aware of it. However, when you're charting, you should conscientiously avoid including ambiguous statements or subjective judgments.

Ambiguous time periods
"Mrs. Brown asks for pain medication *every so often.*" How would you interpret "every so often" — once an hour, once a shift, or once a day? Although you can't time each and every interaction or occurrence precisely, you should document time relationships when appropriate. In this case, for example, you might chart, "Mrs. Brown asked for pain medication at 0800 and again at 1300."

Of course, such precision isn't always necessary. For example, you can write, "The patient was quiet for most of the shift"; you don't have to note the exact number of minutes she was quiet.

Ambiguous quantities
"A *large amount* of bloody drainage drained from the nasogastric tube" could mean 75 ml of fluid to you, 150 ml to the next nurse. Chart a specific measurement.

Subjective judgments
"Mr. Russo has a *good attitude.*" How do you know? Support your judgment with an objective rationale — for example, "Mr. Russo states that he intends to learn insulin injection techniques before discharge."

Don't be afraid to give your impressions of the patient; just make sure that you support your observations — for example, "Leslie was frustrated, voicing dismay at being unable to walk around the room without help." Avoid using words such as "seems" or "appears" — they make you sound unsure of your observations.

conclusion. For example, write "The patient stated, 'I don't want to learn how to inject insulin. I tried yesterday, but I'm not going to do it today.'" In some cases, you may include your conclusion, as long as you record the objective assessment data that supports it.

Remember to document only data you witness yourself or data from a reliable source — such as the patient or another nurse. When you include information reported by someone else, cite your source. (See *Watch your charting language.*)

Sign each entry

Sign each entry you make in your progress notes with your first name or initial, full last name, and professional licensure (such as RN or LPN). If you find the last entry unsigned, immediately contact the nurse who made the entry and have her sign her name. If you can't locate her, simply write and sign your progress notes. The different times and handwriting on the chart should dispel confusion as to the author. (See *Signing nurses' notes,* page 214.)

Assessment

Your assessment of a patient begins when you first encounter him and continues throughout his hospitalization as you obtain more information about his changing condition. The

BETTER CHARTING

Signing nurses' notes

To discourage others from adding information to the nurses' notes, draw a line through any blank spaces and sign your name at the far right of the column.

1/5/99	1200	Will continue plan and request enterostomal
		therapist to assess patient's knowledge and
		acceptance of colostomy on the 2nd postop
		day. ——————— Nora Martin, RN

If you don't have enough room to sign your name after the last word of your entry, draw a line from the last word to the end of the line. Then go to the next line and draw a line from the left margin toward the right margin, leaving room to sign your name on the far right side.

1/5/99	0900	Pt.'s respiratory status markedly improved after
		diuretic and O_2 therapy. Continue to monitor
		ABGs, urine output, weight, and breath sounds.
		Continue diuretic therapy as prescribed. ———
		——————— Nora Martin, RN

If you want to record a lot of information but think you'll run out of room on the page, leave space at the bottom of the page to write "Continued on next page," and add your signature. Start the next page with "Continued from previous page." Then finish your notes and sign the second page as usual.

		Medication effective. Patient drowsy and
		(continued on next page) ——— Nora Martin, RN

1/5/99	1500	(continued from previous page)
		relaxed. States that pain is now 2 on a scale of
		1 to 10. ——————— Nora Martin, RN

initial step of the nursing process, assessment includes collecting relevant information from various sources and analyzing it to form a complete picture of your patient.

As you obtain assessment information, you need to document it accurately for several reasons. First of all, accurately recorded assessment information helps guide you through the rest of the nursing process. Using reliable assessment documentation, you can formulate nursing diagnoses, create patient problem lists, and write nursing plans of care. Properly documented assessment information also serves as a vital communication tool for other health care team members, forming a baseline from which to evaluate a patient's progress.

You also need to document your assessments accurately to meet the requirements of JCAHO and other regulatory agencies. Good documentation provides a means of indicating that quality care has been given. Peer review organizations and other quality assurance reviewers often look to the nursing assessment data as proof of quality care. Finally, in case of litigation, your record of your assessments can be used as evidence in court.

Initial assessment

You'll perform your initial assessment when you first meet a patient. Before getting started, consider two questions:

- Which information will be most relevant for this patient?
- How much time do I have to gather the information?

Your answers will help you collect meaningful information during your assessment. This in turn makes comprehensive, goal-directed nursing interventions possible.

Collecting relevant information

Your initial assessment of a patient may begin with his signs and symptoms, chief complaint, or medical diagnosis. It also may focus on the type of care he received in another unit, such as the critical care unit (CCU) or the emergency department (ED).

Start by finding out some basic information: Why has the patient sought health care? What are his immediate problems? Are these problems life-threatening? Does a potential for injury exist? What other influences — such as advanced age, fear, cultural differences, or lack of understanding — might affect treatment outcomes? Does he have a latex allergy? (See *Handling latex allergy*, page 216.)

Complying with the time frame

Your time limit for completing the initial assessment depends on the policy of your health care facility. JCAHO requires facilities to establish an assessment time frame for each type of patient they serve. Thus, depending on the unit where you work, the time frame for initiating the first assessment may range from 15 minutes to 8 hours. On medical-surgical units, for example, the initial assessment should usually be completed within 1 hour of the patient's arrival on the unit.

Because many facilities offer a wide variety of care, they must establish individual assessment time frames for units or groups of units that share similar patient populations. Thus, a nurse on a CCU or a trauma emergency unit would have a much shorter time frame for completing an initial assessment than a nurse on an elective surgical unit would have.

Handling latex allergy

Allergy to latex, a material derived from natural rubber, is a large and growing problem in the United States. Reactions range from mild dermatitis to anaphylactic shock. As part of the initial patient evaluation, you should ask each patient if he has an allergy to latex or natural rubber.

When caring for a patient with a known or suspected latex allergy, clearly document the allergy in the computer and Kardex, and document latex precautions in the body of the chart, including precautions you've taken to create a latex-safe environment for the patient. Also, place a "Latex precautions" label across the front of the patient's chart, place latex signs over the patient's bed and at the door to the room, and apply a latex identification bracelet to the patient's wrist.

Latex allergy policies may vary from one institution to another, so follow your facility's protocol. If your facility has a latex-free supply cart, be sure to document that it was placed in or outside the patient's room, according to your facility's protocol.

Categorizing assessment data

When you collect and analyze assessment information, you need to distinguish between two types—subjective and objective. Subjective information represents the patient's perception of his problem. A patient's complaint of chest pain, for example, is subjective information. Objective information, on the other hand, is something you can observe and verify—such as a patient's blood pressure reading. During your assessment, you'll gather both types of information from primary and secondary sources.

Subjective data

Subjective data collected during the patient history generally include the patient's chief complaint or concern, current health status, health history, family history, psychosocial history, activities of daily living (ADLs), and a review of body systems.

The patient's history, embodying his perception of his problems, is your most important source of assessment information. However, it's also subjective, so you must interpret it carefully.

Suppose, for instance, that a patient complains of frequent stomach pain. To find out what he considers "frequent," ask if the pain occurs once a week, once a day, twice a day, or all day. To find out what he means by "stomach," have him point to the specific area affected. This also tells you if the pain is localized or generalized. To find out how he defines "pain," have him describe the sensation. Is it stabbing or dull, twisting or nagging? How does he rate its severity on a scale of 1 to 10?

When documenting subjective data, be sure to record it as such. Whenever possible, write the patient's own words in quotation marks. Introduce patient statements with a phrase such as "Patient states." For instance, you'd document the previous example like this: "Patient states that he has frequent stomach pain. He describes pain as dull and nagging. Patient rates pain as 4 on a scale of 1 to 10. The pain occurs after eating, is relieved by antacids, and is located in the left lower quadrant."

If the patient uses unfamiliar words or phrases, such as slang words, ask him to define them. For clarity, record both the phrase and the patient's definition of it.

Objective data

Unlike subjective data, objective data involve no interpretation. If another practitioner were to make the same observations under the same circumstances, she'd obtain the same information. That's why it's important to be specific and avoid using subjective descriptions, such as "large," "small," or "moderate," when documenting your findings.

Whenever possible, use measurements to record data clearly. Specify color, size, and location when appropriate. For instance, "small amount of abdominal wound drainage" could be more specifically described as "serosanguineous nonodorous abdominal wound drainage that completely saturated three 4″ × 4″ pads."

Also, avoid interpreting the data and reflecting your opinion. For example, don't write, "patient is in shock." Instead, document the findings: "pale skin, pulse rate of 140, blood pressure of 90/60 mm Hg."

Sources of data

Usually, information gathered directly from the patient (primary source data) is the most valuable because it reflects his situation most accurately. Additional data about a patient can be obtained from secondary sources, including family members, friends, and other members of the health care team. Written records — past clinical records, transfer summaries, and personal documents such as a living will — also provide important information about the patient.

Information from secondary sources often gives you alternative viewpoints to the patient's. In addition, because of a patient's condition or age, secondary sources may be essential to establish a complete profile. For example, a child or a patient who's profoundly confused may be able to answer only the simplest questions.

Besides providing essential data, family members and friends give important indications of family dynamics, educational needs, and available support systems. Also, including persons close to the patient helps alleviate their feelings of helplessness during the hospitalization.

Performing the initial assessment

An initial assessment consists of your general observations, the health history, and the physical examination.

General observations

You can obtain a wealth of information simply by observing the patient. These observations can begin as soon as you meet him. You may, for instance, observe him while taking him to his room or helping him change into a hospital gown.

Continue to make general observations during the interview and physical examination as well as throughout the patient's hospitalization. By looking critically at the patient, you can collect valuable information about his emotional state, immediate comfort level, and general physical condition. (See *Making general observations*, pages 218 and 219.)

Keep your observations objective and don't draw conclusions. Just document the facts. Remember, initial conclusions are frequently wrong because they're based on too little evidence.

Suppose, for example, that your patient is a middle-aged man who's brought to the ED by ambulance after being found lying in a deserted alley. His clothes are soiled and torn and he smells of urine and feces. He babbles

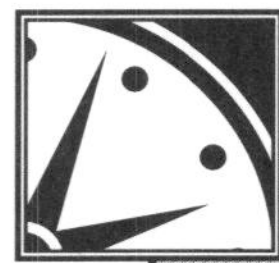

CHARTING TIMESAVER

Making general observations

Your general observations of the patient's appearance, mobility, communication ability, and cognitive function form an important part of your initial assessment. To save you time, here are some specific characteristics to look for and to document.

Appearance

Age

- Appears to be stated age
- Appears older or younger than stated age

Physical condition

- Physically fit, strong, and appropriate weight for height
- Deconditioned, weak, and either underweight or overweight
- Apparent limitations, such as an amputation or paralysis
- Obvious scars or rash

Dress

- Dressed appropriately or inappropriately for season
- Clean and well-kept clothes
- Soiled or torn clothes; smell of alcohol, urine, or feces

Personal hygiene

- Clean and well-groomed
- Unkempt; unshaved; dirty skin, hair, and nails
- Body odor or unusual breath odor

Skin color

- Appropriate for race
- Pale, ruddy, cyanotic, jaundiced, or tanned

Mobility

Ambulation

- Walks independently; steady gait
- Uses a cane, crutches, or walker
- Unsteady, slow, hesitant, or shuffling gait; leans toward one side; can't support own weight
- Transfers from chair to bed independently
- Needs assistance (from one, two, or three people) to transfer from chair to bed

Movement

- Moves all extremities
- Has right- or left-sided weakness; paralysis
- Can't turn in bed independently
- Has jerky or spastic movements of body parts (specify)

Communication

Speech

- Speaks clearly in English or other language
- Speaks only with one-word responses; doesn't respond to verbal stimuli
- Speech is slurred, hoarse, loud, soft, incoherent, hesitant, slow, fast, or nonsensical
- Has difficulty completing sentences because of shortness of breath or pain

Hearing

- Hears well enough to respond to questions
- Hard of hearing; wears hearing aid; must speak loudly into left or right ear
- Deaf; reads lips or uses sign language

incoherently, although obscenities are clearly discernible.

To document properly, you should record these facts, but you shouldn't conclude that the patient is drunk. He may have diabetes mellitus and be suffering from acute hypoglycemia.

Vision
- Sees well enough to read instructions in English or other language
- Wears glasses to see or to read
- Can't read
- Blind

Cognitive functions
Awareness
- Oriented; aware of surroundings
- Disoriented; unaware of person, place, time

Mood
- Responds appropriately; talkative
- Answers in one-word responses; offers information only in response to direct questions
- Hesitates in answering questions; looks to family member before answering
- Angry; states "Leave me alone" (or similar response); speaks loudly and abruptly to family members
- Maintains or avoids eye contact

Thought processes
- Maintains a conversation; makes relevant statements; follows commands appropriately
- Mind wanders; makes irrelevant statements; follows commands inappropriately

Health history

A guide to subsequent physical assessment, the health history organizes pertinent physiologic, psychological, cultural, and psychosocial information. It consists of subjective data about the patient's current health status and provides clues that point to actual or potential health problems. It also reveals the patient's ability to comply with health care interventions and his expectations for treatment outcomes. Finally, the health history yields details about the patient's lifestyle, family relationships, and cultural influences — all of which may affect his health care needs.

Use the health history to identify patient problems that your nursing interventions can help resolve. Then formulate your nursing diagnoses and subsequent plan of care based on these problems.

Preparing to take the health history

Obtain the patient's health history by interviewing him in a comfortable environment and recording his answers to your questions. If appropriate, also interview the patient's family members and close friends.

Before the interview, consider the patient's ability and readiness to participate. For example, if he's sedated or confused, hostile or angry, or experiencing pain or dyspnea, ask only the most essential questions. You can perform a more in-depth interview later, when his condition improves. In the meantime, secondary sources can often provide much of the needed information.

Try to alleviate as much of the patient's discomfort and anxiety as possible. Also attempt to create a quiet, private environment for your talk. Avoid interruptions by arranging for another nurse to cover your other patients during the interview. Your efforts let your patient know that you're interested in what he tells you and that you respect the confidentiality of the information he shares.

Tell the patient how long the interview will last — usually from 15 to 30 minutes for a medical-surgical patient. Explain the purpose of the history so he understands why you'll be asking him personal questions. Finally, be calm, relaxed, and unhurried. Your actions will convey to the patient the importance of the health history interview.

Conducting the interview

You'll need to show empathy, compassion, self-awareness, and objectivity to promote a trusting relationship with your patient — the first step toward a successful interview. To obtain a comprehensive health history, you'll also need to use a variety of interviewing techniques. Here are some examples.

USING GENERAL LEADS. Broad opening questions allow the patient to relate information that he deems essential. Asking such questions as "What brought you to the hospital?" or "What concerns do you have?" encourages the patient to discuss what's most important to him.

RESTATING (SUMMARIZING) INFORMATION. To help clarify the patient's meaning, restate the essence of his comments. For instance, suppose a patient says, "I have pain after I eat" and you respond, "So, you have pain about three times a day." This might prompt the patient to reply, "Oh no, I only eat breakfast and then the pain is so severe that I don't eat for the rest of the day."

USING REFLECTION. Asking a question in a different way offers the patient an opportunity to reconsider his response. A patient might say, "I've told you everything about my home life." Using reflection, you might respond, "Do you have any other concerns about your situation after you leave the hospital?"

STATING THE IMPLIED MEANING. A patient may hint at difficulties or problems. By stating what he has left unspoken, you give him an opportunity to clarify his thoughts and accurately interpret the meaning of his statements. For example, a patient who remarks, "I'm sure my wife is glad that I'm in the hospital" may be implying several things. To clarify this statement, you might respond, "By saying your wife is glad, do you mean she has been concerned about your condition, or do you feel you've been a burden to her at home?"

FOCUSING THE DISCUSSION. Patients often stray from the topic at hand to relate other information they feel you should know. You need to get the conversation back on track without insulting the patient or making him feel that the information isn't important. To help him refocus the conversation, you might say, "That's very interesting, but first I'd like to get back to our discussion about your last hospitalization."

ASKING OPEN-ENDED QUESTIONS. Questions that encourage the patient to express himself elicit more information than questions that call for a one-word response. If you ask, "Do you take your medications?" the patient may respond with a simple "Yes." But if you ask, "How do you take your medications?" you might discover that the patient takes his antihypertensive pills sporadically because they make him feel dizzy.

Techniques to avoid

To avoid alienating the patient during the interview and thus hindering communication, don't use the following techniques.

JUDGMENTAL OR THREATENING QUESTIONS. A patient shouldn't have to justify his feelings or actions. Questions such as "Why did you do that?" or demanding statements such as "Explain your behavior" may be perceived as a threat or challenge. They force the patient to defend himself. What's more, when a patient doesn't have a specific answer to this type of question, he may invent an appropriate response merely to satisfy you.

PROBING AND PERSISTENT QUESTIONS. This style of questioning can make the patient feel manipulated and defensive. Make only one or two attempts to obtain information about a particular subject. If the patient seems to be avoiding the topic or is reluctant to answer, reevaluate the relevance of the information. Respect his right to privacy.

INAPPROPRIATE LANGUAGE. Don't use technical terms or jargon when interviewing the patient. Questions such as "Do you take that med q.i.d. or p.r.n.?" can intimidate or alienate the patient and his family. Using unfamiliar language can make the patient feel you're unwilling to share information about his condition or to converse on his level.

ADVICE. Giving advice implies that you know what's best for the patient. Instead, you should encourage the patient and family members to participate in health care decisions. If the patient asks for advice, inform him about available options and then help him explore his own opinions about them.

FALSE REASSURANCES. Statements such as "You'll be all right" or "Everything will work out fine" tend to devalue a person's feelings. By recognizing those feelings, you can open communication channels. Saying something such as "You seem worried or frightened" encourages the patient to speak candidly. Always try to be honest and sensitive. Even when a patient asks, "Am I going to die?" you can honestly state, "I don't know. Tell me what makes you ask that."

Timesaving measures

Although increased patient acuity and staff shortages sometimes make conducting a thorough patient interview difficult, certain strategies can help you make the most of the time you have without compromising quality. For example, in some cases, you can ask the patient to complete a questionnaire about his past and present health status instead of conducting a patient interview. Then you can quickly and easily document his health history by reviewing the information on the questionnaire. This method tends to be most successful in short procedure units and before admission for elective procedures. Unfortunately, although it saves time, this method doesn't give you an opportunity to develop a positive relationship with your patient. (See *When interview time is limited,* page 222.)

Physical examination

Perform the physical examination by using the assessment techniques of inspection, palpation, percussion, and auscultation. During this phase of the assessment, you'll obtain objective data that may confirm or rule out suspicions raised during the health history interview. Your findings will enable you to plan care and start teaching your patient about his

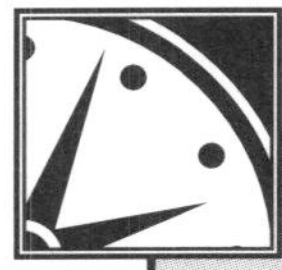

CHARTING TIMESAVER

When interview time is limited

When you're pressed for time, the following tips will help you obtain a health history more quickly.

- Before the interview, fill in as much of the health history information as you can from secondary sources, such as admission forms, transfer summaries, and the medical history. This avoids duplication of effort and reduces interview time. If some of this information needs clarification, you can ask the patient to give you a fuller explanation. For instance, you might say something such as "You told Dr. Smith that you have periodic dizzy spells. Could you tell me more about those spells?"
- Check your facility's policy regarding who can gather assessment data. You may be able to have a nursing assistant collect routine information, such as allergies and past hospitalizations. Remember, however, that you must review the information and verify it, as necessary.
- Begin by asking about the patient's chief complaint and the reason for his hospitalization. Then, if the interview is interrupted, you'll have some initial information on which to base a plan of care.
- Use your facility's nursing assessment documentation form only as a guide to organize information. Ask your patient only pertinent questions from the form.
- Take only brief notes during the interview to avoid interrupting the flow of conversation. Write a longer summation or expand on information as soon as possible after the interview. You can always go back to the patient if you need to clarify or verify information.
- Record your findings using concise, specific phrases and approved abbreviations.

condition. For example, an elevated blood pressure reading tells you that a patient may need a sodium-restricted diet and, possibly, patient teaching on how to control hypertension.

The scope of the physical examination depends on the patient's condition, the clinical setting, and the policies and procedures established by your health care facility. A routine neurologic examination on a medical- surgical unit, for example, may include assessments of level of consciousness, orientation, muscle strength, and pupillary response. Abnormal findings would then call for you to perform a more in-depth assessment — an assessment that would be routine on a neurologic unit or CCU.

The major components of the physical examination include height, weight, vital signs, and a review of the major body systems. A routine review for an adult patient on a medical-surgical unit includes the following body systems.

Respiratory system

Note the rate and rhythm of respirations, and auscultate the lung fields. Inspect the lips, mucous membranes, and nail beds. Also inspect any sputum, noting color, consistency, and other characteristics.

Cardiovascular system

Auscultate for heart sounds. Note heart rate and rhythm. Document the color and temperature of the extremities, and assess the peripheral pulses. Also check for edema. Inspect the neck veins, noting their appearance — for example, flat or distended.

Neurologic system

Inspect the patient's head for evidence of trauma. Then assess his level of consciousness, noting his orientation to time, place, and person and his ability to follow commands. Also assess his pupillary reactions and cranial nerve function. Check his extremities for movement and sensation.

Eyes, ears, nose, and throat

Assess the patient's ability to see objects with or without corrective lenses as appropriate. Also assess his ability to hear spoken words clearly. Inspect the eyes and ears for discharge; the nasal mucous membranes for dryness, irritation, and the presence of blood; and the teeth for cleanliness.

If appropriate, note how well the patient's dentures fit. Observe the condition of the oral mucous membranes, and palpate the lymph nodes in the neck.

GI system

Auscultate for bowel sounds in all quadrants. Note any abdominal distention or ascites. Palpate the abdomen to assess for tenderness.

Musculoskeletal system

Assess the range of motion of major joints. Look for any swelling at the joints as well as for any contractures, muscular atrophy, or obvious deformity.

Genitourinary system

Check for any bladder distention or incontinence. If indicated, inspect the genitalia for rashes, edema, or deformity. (Inspection of the genitalia may be waived at the patient's request or if no dysfunction was reported during the interview.)

Reproductive system

If indicated, inspect the genitalia for sexual maturity. Also, perform a breast examination if permitted, noting any abnormalities.

Integumentary system

Note any sores, lesions, scars, pressure ulcers, rashes, bruises, or petechiae. Also note the patient's skin turgor.

Meeting JCAHO requirements

JCAHO requires that health care professionals in accredited facilities meet certain standards for performing patient assessments. By reviewing the documentation of patient assessments, JCAHO determines whether these standards have been met. (See chapter 3, Quality Management and Reimbursement, for more information on JCAHO requirements.)

One key JCAHO requirement is that you obtain assessment information from the patient's family or friends when appropriate. When you interview someone close to the patient who isn't part of his family, make sure that you note the nature of the relationship and the length of time the person has known the patient. For instance, in your documentation, you might write something such as "Information supplied by Daniel Rosenberger, a friend who has lived with the patient for 3 years."

Assessment requirements

Current JCAHO standards mandate that each patient's initial assessment include three key categories: physical, psychological, and social status. The standards go on to state that the scope and intensity of any further assessments are based on the patient's diagnosis, the care setting, the patient's desire for care, and his response to previous care. If appropriate, the patient's nutritional status and functional status are also assessed. The patient's learning needs and discharge planning needs should be assessed early in the admission process.

Physical factors
These include physical examination findings from your review of the major body systems.

Psychological factors
These include the patient's fears, anxieties, and other concerns related to his hospitalization. To find out what support systems the patient has, you might ask something such as "How does being in the hospital affect your home situation?" or "How is your family coping while you're hospitalized?" A patient's concerns about these matters may impair his willingness or ability to comply with health care interventions.

Social status factors
These include family structure and the patient's role or roles within that structure. Questions regarding work status, income level, and socioeconomic concerns may also be included as indicated.

Nutritional status
Questions regarding food and fluid intake, use of nutritional supplements or vitamins (or both), elimination patterns, and any recent weight gain or loss are included. A registered dietitian should be consulted as warranted by the patient's needs or condition.

Functional status
Because a patient's ability to perform ADLs affects how well he complies with his treatment regimen both before and after discharge, you must assess his ability to eat, wash, dress, use the bathroom, turn in bed, get out of bed, and get around. At some health care facilities, you'll use a checklist to indicate if a patient can perform these tasks independently or if he needs partial or total assistance. The use of any assistive devices should be noted.

Learning needs
An early assessment of what the patient needs to know about his condition leads to effective patient teaching. During the initial assessment, evaluate your patient's knowledge of the disease process, self-care, diet, medications, lifestyle changes, treatment measures, and any limitations resulting from the disease or its treatment.

One way to evaluate your patient's educational needs is to ask open-ended questions such as "What do you know about the medicine you take?" His response will tell you if he understands and complies with his medication regimen or if he needs more teaching.

You should also assess factors that may hinder learning. These include the nature of the patient's illness or injury as well as his health beliefs, religious beliefs, educational level, sensory deficits (such as hearing difficulties), language barriers, stress level, age, and any pain or discomfort he may be experiencing.

Discharge planning needs
As with patient teaching, discharge planning should begin as soon as possible. You must identify the discharge planning needs of every patient — especially those who are most likely to require help after discharge.

Find out where the patient will go after discharge. Will follow-up care be accessible? Are community resources, such as visiting nurse services and Meals on Wheels, available where the patient lives? Answers to such questions will help you plan effectively for your patient's discharge.

Documenting the initial assessment

Depending on where you work, you may hear the initial assessment information referred to by any of several names, including the "nursing admission assessment" and the "nursing database." Some institutions have adopted initial assessment forms that include information gathered from different members of the health care team, such as doctors, nurses, social workers, physical or occupational therapists, nutritionists, and pastoral care workers. These forms may be called "integrated," "interdisciplinary," or "multidisciplinary" care team assessment forms. (See *Integrated admission database form,* pages 226 to 229.)

Documentation styles and formats vary, depending on the facility's policy and the patient population. What's more, health care facilities have different policies for documenting learning needs, discharge planning, and incomplete initial assessment data. So you must be familiar with your facility's standards to document your initial assessment findings appropriately.

Documentation styles

Initial assessment findings are documented in one of three basic styles: narrative notes, standardized open-ended style, and standardized closed-ended style. Many assessment forms use a combination of all three styles.

Narrative notes

Narrative notes consist of handwritten accounts in paragraph form, summarizing information obtained by general observation, interview, and physical examination.

Although narrative notes allow you to list your findings in order of importance, they also pose problems. In many cases, the notes mimic the medical model by focusing on a review of body systems. They're also time-consuming — both to write and to read. Plus, narrative notes require you to remember and record all significant information in a detailed, logical sequence — often an unrealistic goal in today's hectic world of health care. Finally, difficulty in interpreting handwriting can easily lead to misinterpretation of findings.

Narrative notes are most practical for independent practitioners. Within health care institutions, however, exclusive use of narrative notes wastes time and may jeopardize quality monitoring.

Standardized open-ended style

The typical "fill-in-the blanks" assessment form comes with preprinted headings and questions. This form saves you time in a couple of ways. Information is categorized under specific headings, so you can easily record and retrieve it. And the form can be completed using partial phrases and approved abbreviations. (See *Documenting assessment on an open-ended form,* page 230.)

Unfortunately, however, open-ended forms don't always provide enough space or instructions to encourage thorough descriptions. Thus, under the heading *type of dwelling,* one nurse may write "apartment" whereas another may write "apartment in four-flight walk-up, without heat or hot water."

Nonspecific responses can lead to misinterpretation. For instance, a nurse may write

(Text continues on page 230.)

BETTER CHARTING

Integrated admission database form

Most health care facilities use a multidisciplinary admission form. The sample form below has spaces that can be filled in by the nurse, doctor, and other health care providers.

Name *Beatrice Perry*
Address *2 Clayton Street*
Dallas, Texas
Admission Date *2/26/99* Time *1345*
Admitted per: ____ Ambulatory ✔ Stretcher ____ Wheelchair
T *97* P *92* R *24* BP *98/52*
Ht. *5'2"* Wt. *225 lb*
(estimated/actual) — actual circled

ORIENTATION TO ROOM/UNIT POLICIES EXPLAINED

- ✔ Call light
- ✔ Bed oper.
- ✔ Phone
- ✔ Television
- ✔ Meals
- ___ Advance directive explained
- ___ Valuables form completed
- ✔ Elec.
- ✔ Smoking
- ___ Side rails
- ✔ ID bracelet on
- ___ Visiting hours

SECTION COMPLETED BY: *P. Lippman, CST* **TIME:** *1350*

Name and phone numbers of two people to call if necessary:

Name	Relationship	Phone#
Mary Ryan	*daughter*	*665-2190*
Thomas Perry	*son*	*630-4785*

REASON FOR HOSPITALIZATION (patient quote:) *I go numb in my rt. arm and leg*
ANTICIPATED DATE OF DISCHARGE: *2/28/99*
PREVIOUS HOSPITALIZATIONS: SURGERY/ILLNESS — DATE
TIA — *1/15/99*

HEALTH PROBLEM	Yes	No	?
Arthritis		✔	
Blood problem (anemia, sickle cell, clotting, bleeding)		✔	
Cancer		✔	
Diabetes	✔		
Eye problems (cataracts, glaucoma)		✔	
Heart problem		✔	
Liver problem		✔	
Hiatal hernia		✔	
High blood pressure	✔		
HIV/AIDS		✔	
Kidney problem		✔	

Comments: ____

HEALTH PROBLEM	Yes	No	?
Lung problem (Emphysema, Asthma, Bronchitis, TB, Pneumonia, Shortness of breath) — Emphysema circled, Pneumonia struck through	✔		
Stroke		✔	
Ulcers		✔	
Thyroid problem		✔	
Psychological disorder		✔	
Alcohol abuse		✔	
Drug abuse / Drug(s) ____		✔	
Smoking	✔		
Other			

ALLERGIES: ☐ TAPE ☐ IODINE ☐ LATEX ☐ no known allergies
☐ FOOD ____ ☑ DRUG: *Penicillin*
☐ BLOOD REACTION: ____ ☐ OTHER: ____

MEDICATIONS: ____

Information received from:
☑ Patient ☐ Relative ____ ☐ Friend ____ ☐ Other ____

Section completed by: *Jill O'Brien, RN* Date *2/26/99* Time *1405*

DOCUMENTATION OF THE NURSING PROCESS

Integrated admission database form *(continued)*

All assessment sections are to be completed by a professional nurse. Date 2/26/99

Addressograph

GENERAL PHYSICAL APPEARANCE

✔ Clean ___ Disheveled

SKIN INTEGRITY: Indicate the location of any of the following on the chart to the right using the designated letter: a = rashes, b = lesions, c = significant bruises/ abrasions, d = burns, e = pressure sores, f = recent scars, g = presence of tubes/ appliances, h = other

Comments: b: ischemic leg ulcer (2cm – healing)

PRESSURE SORE POTENTIAL ASSESSMENT

PARAMETERS	0	1	2	3	Score
Mental status	(Alert)	Lethargic	Semi-Comatose	Comatose	0
			Count These Conditions As Double		
Activity	Ambulatory	(Needs help)	Chairfast	Bedfast	1
Mobility	~~Full~~	(Limited)	Very limited	Immobile	1
Incontinence	(None)	Occasional	Usually of urine	Total of urine and feces	0
Oral nutrition intake	~~Good~~	(Fair)	Poor	None	1
Oral fluid intake	(Good)	Fair	Poor	~~None~~	0
Predisposing diseases (diabetes, neuropathies, vascular disease, anemias)	Absent	Slight	Moderate	(Severe)	6
	Patients with scores of 10 or above should be considered at risk.			Total	9

FALL-RISK ASSESSMENT

Impaired:
___ Sensory function
___ Urinary/GI function
___ Mobility function
___ Mental status

✔ General debility/weakness
✔ History of recent falls/dizziness/blackouts (automatically designates patient as prone-to-fall)
✔ Prone-to-fall risk (indicated on nursing Kardex ✔)

NEUROLOGICAL

___ Dizziness ___ Syncope ___ Headache ___ Blurred vision
___ Recent seizure ✔ Numbness/tingling location: Rt. arm and leg

LOC: ✔ Alert ___ Lethargic ___ Semi-comatose ___ Comatose
Mental Status: ✔ Oriented ___ Confused ___ Disoriented
Speech: ✔ Clear ___ Slurred ___ Garbled ___ Aphasic

Neurological Checklist

Right Arm / Left Arm	Right Leg / Left Leg	R.Pupil / L. Pupil	Pupil Reaction	Coma Scale: Eyes Open	Best Verbal Response	Best Motor Response	Total
+2/+4	+2/+4	5/6	+	4	5	6	15

COMA SCALE CODE	1	2	3	4	5	6
Response	1	2	3	4	5	6
EYES OPEN	Never	To Pain	To Sound	Sponta-neously		
VERBAL	None	Incompre-hensible Sounds	Inappro-priate words	Confused Conversa-tion	Oriented	
MOTOR	None	Extension	Flexion Abnormal	Flexion Withdrawal	Localizes Pain	

+1: cannot move
+2: cannot move against gravity
+3: move against gravity
+4: move strongly against gravity

CODE

Pupil Reaction
R Reactive
N Nonreactive
D Dilated
C Constricted
> Greater than
< Less than
= Equal
S Sluggish

Pupils (mm): 1 2 3 4 5 6 7 8

Comments: numbness transient Signature: B. Mayer, MD

BEHAVIORAL

Behavior: ✔ Cooperative ___ Uncooperative ___ Depressed ___ Restless
___ Combative ✔ Anxious ___ Unresponsive ___ Other

Comments:

Religious/Spiritual beliefs: Lutheran

P. request to contact minister/priest/rabbi? ___ Y ✔ N

Name Rev. William Lacy Phone # 726-8039

(continued)

DOCUMENTATION OF THE NURSING PROCESS

Integrated admission database form *(continued)*

Addressograph | Date 2/26/99

CARDIOVASCULAR

Skin Color: ___Normal ___Flushed ___Pale ✔ Cyanotic
Apical Pulse: ___Regular ✔ Irregular ___Pacemaker: Type ___ Rate ___
Peripheral Pulses: ✔ Present ___ Equal ✔ Weak ___Absent
Comments: bilat. weak lower extremities
Specify: R ___radial ___ pedal L ___radial ___pedal
Comments:
Edema: ___No ✔ Yes +1 bilat. pretibial Numbness: ___No ✔ Yes Site: Rt. arm and leg
Chest Pain: ✔ No ___Yes ___ P ___ Q ___ R ___ S ___ T ___
Family Cardiac History: ___No ✔ Yes Telemetry Monitor: ___No ✔ Yes rhythm normal sinus
Comments:

PULMONARY

Respirations: ✔ Regular ___Irregular ___Shortness of breath ___Dyspnea on exertion
O_2 use at home? ___Yes ✔ No
Chest expansion: ✔ Symmetrical ___Asymmetrical (explain:
Breath sounds: ___Clear ___Crackles ___Rhonchi ✔ Wheezing ___ Location bilat upper lobe, inspiratory
Cough: None ✔ Nonproductive ___ Productive ___ Describe
Comments: pulse oximetry 98% on 2 L; sleeps with 2 pillows

GASTROINTESTINAL

Stool: ✔ Formed, ___ Loose, ___ Liquid, ___ Mucus, ___ Ostomy, ___ Incontinent
Color: ✔ Brown, ___ Black, ___ Red tinged, ___ Bloody

Diarrhea ___
Constipation ___
Abdomen: ✔ Soft, ___ Rigid, ✔ Nontender, ___ Tender (Location)
Bowel Sounds: ✔ Present, ___ Absent, ___ Hypoactive, ___ Hyperactive

Obese ✔
Thin ___
Emaciated ___
Nourished ___

*NUTRITION:
✔ Special Diet 1800 ADA
___ Tube feeding
___ Chewing problem
___ Swallowing problems
___ Nausea/vomiting
___ Poor appetite
___ Wt. loss/gain ___ lb
*Refer to dietitian if any ✔

GENITOURINARY/ REPRODUCTIVE

Color of Urine: ✔ Yellow ___Amber ___Pink/Red tinged ___Brown ___Orange ___Clear ___Cloudy
___Ileo-Conduit ___Incontinent ___Catheter in place ___Frequency ___Urgency
___Difficulty in initiating stream ___Pain ___Burning ___Oliguria ___Anuria
___Dialysis Access site: ___ Date of last Dialysis:
Comments:
Date of LMP 1977 Date of last PAP 5/98 Breast self-exam ___Yes ✔ No
Use of contraceptives: ___Yes (type ___) ___No ✔ N/A
Vaginal Discharge: ___Yes (describe ___) ✔ No
Bleeding: ___Yes (amount ___) ✔ No
Pregnancies: Pregnant ___Yes ___Weeks gravida ___ Para ✔ No
Date of last Prostate Exam ___ Testicular self-exam ___Yes ___No
Comments:

ACTIVITY/ MOBILITY PATTERNS

___Ambulates independently ___Full ROM ___Limited ROM (explain:)
✔ Ambulates with assistance (explain: ___) ✔ cane ___walker ___crutches
___Gait steady/unsteady ___Mobility in bed (ability to turn self) ___
Musculoskeletal ___Pain ___Weakness ___Contractures ___Joint swelling
___Paralysis ___Deformity ___Joint stiffness ___Cast ___Amputation
Describe:
Comments:

REST/ SLEEP PATTERNS

___Use of sleeping aids ___ Sleeps 6 hr/day
Comments:

Additional assessment comment: On arrival, diaphoretic and Ⓛ hand tremors. Vital signs stable. glucose 56 mg/dl. Orange juice and lunch given to patient. 2 hr postprandial glucose 204. Symptoms subsided with juice. Nutrition and diabetes educator consulted. — Jill O'Brien, RN
MRI shows no cerebral lesions. Carotid doppler ultrasound pending. — B. Mayer MD

Integrated admission database form *(continued)*

EDUCATION/DISCHARGE SECTION
Instructions: Assessment sections must be completed within 8 hours of admission. Discharge planning and summary must be completed by day of discharge.

Addressograph

EDUCATIONAL ASSESSMENT

Yes	No	
✔		Patient understands current diagnosis
✔		Family/significant other understands diagnosis
✔		Patient able to read English
✔		Patient able to write English
✔		Patient able to communicate
	✔	Patient/family understands pre-hospital medication/treatment regimen

Yes	No	**Emotional factors:**
✔		Patient appears to be coping*
✔		Family appears to be coping*
	✔	Any suspicion of family violence
	✔	Any suspicion of family abuse
	✔	Any suspicion of family neglect

Comment: *diabetic teaching*

Language spoken, written, and read (other than English): ____
Interpreter services needed: ✔ No ___ Yes
Are there any barriers to learning (e.g., emotional, physical, cognitive)? *No*
Religious or cultural practices that may alter care or teaching needs? ___ Yes ✔ No Describe: ____
Is pt/family motivated to learn? ✔ Yes ___ No describe: ____

DISCHARGE ASSESSMENT

Living arrangements/caregiver (relationship): *lives alone*
Type of dwelling: ___ Apartment ✔ House ___ Nursing home ___ More than 1 floor? ✔ Yes ___ No Describe: ____
___ Boarding home ___ Other ____
Physical barriers in home: ✔ No ___ Yes (explain: ____)
Access to follow-up medical care: ✔ Yes ___ No (explain: ____)
Ability to carry out ADL: ___ Self-care ✔ Partial assistance ___ Total assistance
Needs help with: ✔ Bathing ___ Feeding ___ Ambulation ___ Other ____
Anticipated discharge destination: ___ Home ___ Rehab. ✔ Nursing home ___ SNF ___ Boarding home
___ Other ____
Currently receiving services from a community agency? ___ Yes ✔ No
If yes, check which one ___ visiting nurses ___ Meals on Wheels
Concerned about returning home? ___ Being alone ___ Financial problems ___ Homemaking ___ Meal prep.
___ Managing ADLs ___ Other ____
Assessment completed by: *J. O'Brien, RN* Date *2/26/99* Time *1430*
Assessment completed by: *B. Mayer, MD* Date *2/26/99* Time *1445*

DISCHARGE PLANNING

Resources notified	Name	Date	Time	Signature
Social worker				
Home care coordinator	*M. Murphy, RN*	*2/28/99*	*0900*	
Other____				

Equipment/Supplies needed: *stair chair*
Arranged for by: *M. Murphy, RN* Date *2/28/99* Time *0930*
Comment: *Daughter to stay with pt at home*

DISCHARGE SUMMARY

Alterations in patterns (If yes, explain.)	Yes	No	**Explanation**
Nutrition	✔		*adherence to ADA diet regimen*
Elimination		✔	
Self-care		✔	
Skin integrity		✔	
Mobility	✔		*needs help with stairs*
Comfort pain		✔	
Mental status/behavior		✔	
Vision/Hearing/Speech		✔	

Discharge instructions given (specify): *standard hosp. discharge instruction sheet*
Effects of illness on employment/lifestyle: ____
Central venous line removed: *N/A* By whom: ____
Belongings sent with patient: ✔ clothes ✔ dentures ✔ eyeglasses ___ hearing aid ___ prosthesis ___ valuables
✔ prescriptions ✔ other *cane*
Follow-up medical supervision to be provided by: *Dr. Schneider*
✔ Patient/family instructed to call for follow-up appointment Discharge destination: *pt's home with daughter*
Section completed by: *C. Rafferty, RN* Date *2/28/99* Time *1130*

BETTER CHARTING

Documenting assessment on an open-ended form

At some health care facilities, you may use a standardized open-ended form to document initial assessment information. Below you'll find a portion of such a form.

Reason for hospitalization "My blood sugar is high"

Expected outcomes By discharge, the patient and his family will understand the disease process of diabetes mellitus, demonstrate correct insulin administration techniques, and identify signs and symptoms of hyperglycemia and hypoglycemia.

Last hospitalization

Date 3/95 Reason high blood pressure

Medical history hypertension, diabetes mellitus

Medications and allergies

Drug	Dose	Time of last dose	Patient's statement of drug's purpose
Humulin N	30 units	0730	for sugar
Humulin R	5 units	0730	for sugar
furosemide	20 mg	1000	water pill
atenolol	50 mg	0800	for BP

Allergy	Reaction
shellfish	hives

that a patient performs a task "within normal limits." But unless normal limits have been defined, this notation is neither clear nor legally sound.

Standardized closed-ended style

This type of assessment form provides preprinted headings, checklists, and questions with specific responses. You simply check off the appropriate response. (See *Documenting assessment on a closed-ended form.*)

In addition to saving time, the closed-ended form eliminates the problem of illegible handwriting and makes checking documented information easy. In addition, the form can be easily incorporated into most computerized systems.

This kind of form also clearly establishes the type and amount of information required by the health care facility. And even though the closed-ended forms usually use nonspecific terminology, such as "within normal limits"

BETTER CHARTING

Documenting assessment on a closed-ended form

At some health care facilities, you may use a standardized closed-ended form to document initial assessment information. Below you'll find a portion of such a form.

SELF-CARE ABILITY

Activity	1	2	3	4	5	6
Bathing		✔				
Cleaning		✔				
Climbing stairs			✔			
Cooking	✔					
Dressing and grooming		✔				
Eating and drinking	✔					
Moving in bed	✔					
Shopping					✔	
Toileting			✔			
Transferring			✔			
Walking		✔				
Other home functions			✔			

Key
1 = Independent
2 = Requires assistive device
3 = Requires personal assistance
4 = Requires personal assistance and assistive device
5 = Dependent
6 = Experienced change in last week

Assistive devices
- ☑ Bedside commode
- ☐ Brace or splint
- ☐ Cane
- ☐ Crutches
- ☐ Feeding device
- ☐ Trapeze
- ☑ Walker
- ☐ Wheelchair
- ☐ Other
- ☐ None

Activity tolerance
- ☐ Normal
- ☑ Weakness
- ☐ Dizziness
- ☑ Exertional dyspnea
- ☐ Dyspnea at rest
- ☐ Angina
- ☐ Pain at rest
- ☐ Oxygen needed
- ☐ Intermittent claudication
- ☐ Unsteady gait
- ☐ Other

Rest pattern

Sleep habits
- ☑ Less than 8 hours
- ☐ 8 hours
- ☐ More than 8 hours
- ☐ Morning nap
- ☑ Afternoon nap

Sleep difficulties
- ☐ Insomnia
- ☑ Early awakening
- ☐ Unrefreshing sleep
- ☐ Nightmares
- ☐ None

or "no alteration," guidelines clearly define these responses.

Closed-ended forms also have some disadvantages. For instance, many of them provide no place to record relevant information that doesn't fit the preprinted choices. In addition, the forms tend to be lengthy, especially when a facility's policy calls for recording in-depth physical assessment data.

Documentation formats

Historically, nursing assessment has followed a medical format, emphasizing the patient's initial symptoms and a comprehensive review of body systems. Although many health care facilities still use a medical format to organize their nursing assessment forms, some facilities have adopted formats that more readily reflect the nursing process.

Most facilities that use a nursing format for assessment base it on either human response patterns or functional health care patterns. Other documentation formats are modeled on specific conceptual frameworks based on published nursing theories.

Human response patterns

As you know, the North American Nursing Diagnosis Association (NANDA) has developed a classification system for nursing diagnoses based on human response patterns. These patterns relate directly to actual or potential health problems, as indicated by assessment data.

Thus, when you use an assessment form organized by these patterns, you can easily establish appropriate diagnoses while you record assessment data — especially if a listing of diagnoses is included with the form. The main drawback is that these forms tend to be lengthy.

Functional health care patterns

Some health care facilities organize their assessment data according to functional health care patterns. Developed by Marjory Gordon, this system classifies nursing data according to the patient's ability to function independently. Many nurses consider functional health care patterns easier to understand and remember than human response patterns.

Conceptual frameworks

At some health care facilities, assessment forms have been modeled on the nursing philosophies that the nursing departments follow. Some examples include Dorothea Orem's self-care model, Imogene King's theory of goal attainment, and Sister Callista Roy's adaptation model. Assessment forms based on these nursing philosophies reflect the individual theory's approach to nursing care.

Documenting learning needs

Most initial assessment forms have a separate section for documenting a patient's learning needs. When you reassess your patient's learning needs, you can document your findings in the progress notes, on an open-ended patient education flow sheet, or on a structured patient education flow sheet designed for a specific problem such as diabetes mellitus.

Documenting discharge planning needs

Effective discharge planning begins when you identify and document the patient's needs during the initial assessment. Depending on the policy at your health care facility, you'll record the patient's discharge needs on the initial assessment form (in a designated section), on a specially designed discharge planning form, in a separate section on the patient care card file, in the progress notes, or on a discharge planning flow sheet. (See *Documenting discharge planning needs.*)

Documenting incomplete initial data

No matter which assessment tool you use, you may not always be able to obtain a complete health history during the initial assessment. For instance, the patient may be too ill to participate, and secondary sources may be unavailable.

BETTER CHARTING

Documenting discharge planning needs

How and where you document your discharge planning will depend on the policy at the health care facility where you work. Here's one of the more common ways of documenting this information.

DISCHARGE PLANNING NEEDS

Occupation *Retired college professor* **Language spoken** *English*
Patient lives with *Wife*
Self-care capabilities *Needs extensive assistance*
Assistance available

- [ ] Cooking
- [ ] Cleaning
- [x] Shopping
- [x] Dressing changes/treatments *Irrigate Ⓛ lower leg wound b.i.d. with 1/2 strength H_2O_2, followed by rinse with normal saline solution. Pack with 1/2" iodoform gauze. Apply dry sterile dressing.*

Medication administration routes

- [x] P.O.
- [ ] I.V.
- [ ] I.M.
- [ ] S.C.
- [ ] Other: ______

Dwelling

- [ ] Apartment
- [x] Private home
- [ ] Single room
- [ ] Institution
- [ ] Elevator
- [x] Outside steps (number) *6*
- [x] Inside steps (number) *12*
- [x] Kitchen
  - (gas stove) — circled
  - electric stove
  - wood stove
- [ ] other ______
- [x] Bathrooms (number) *2* (location) *one upstairs, one downstairs*
- [x] Telephones (number) *1* (location) *kitchen*

Transportation

- [ ] Drives own car
- [ ] Takes public transportation
- [x] Relies on family member or friend

After discharge, patient will be:

- [ ] Home alone
- [x] Home with family
- [ ] Other: ______

Patient has had help from:

- [x] Visiting nurse
- [x] Housekeeper
- [x] Other: *social worker*

Anticipated needs *Nurse for dressing changes, transportation for groceries, etc.*
Social service requests *VNA*
Date contacted *1/10/99* **Reason** *Contacted VNA for dressing changes and transportation needs.*

DOCUMENTATION OF THE NURSING PROCESS

JCAHO reassessment guidelines

- Reassessment occurs at regular intervals in the course of care.
- Reassessment determines a patient's response to care.
- Significant change in a patient's condition results in reassessment.
- Significant change in a patient's diagnosis results in reassessment.

When this occurs, base your initial assessment on your observations and physical examination of the patient. When documenting your findings, be sure to write something such as "Unable to obtain complete data at this time." Otherwise, it might appear that you failed to perform a complete assessment.

Try to obtain missing information as soon as possible, either when the patient's condition improves or when family members or other secondary sources are available. Be sure to record how and when you obtained the missing data. Depending on your facility's policy, you may record the information on the progress notes, or you may return to the initial assessment form and add the new information along with the date and your signature. Both methods have advantages and disadvantages.

Adding to the initial assessment form makes it easy to retrieve the data when it's needed — either during the patient's hospitalization or after discharge for quality assurance. Putting the information into the nursing progress notes aids in the day-to-day communication with others who read the notes but makes it difficult to retrieve the data later.

Remember, when you add information to complete an initial assessment, be sure to revise your nursing plan of care accordingly.

Ongoing assessment

Your assessment of a patient, of course, is a continuous process. Reassessment lets you evaluate the effectiveness of your nursing interventions and determine your patient's progress toward the desired outcomes. Effective documentation of your assessment findings facilitates communication with other health care practitioners, allowing you to plan the most appropriate patient care.

How often should you reassess a patient? That depends primarily on his condition. However, JCAHO requires that each patient be reassessed at appropriate intervals, as designated by the institution's policy. You need to be aware of your facility's policy on reassessing patients and plan your care accordingly. (See *JCAHO reassessment guidelines.*)

Planned reassessment

A planned reassessment provides the routine data you need to evaluate a patient on a daily basis. On a medical-surgical unit, this may include reviewing the patient's mental status, respiratory status, vital signs, skin integrity, self-care capabilities, appetite, and fluid balance as well as psychosocial factors. You'll also need to regularly reassess environmental factors and his learning and discharge needs. Based on the patient's condition, your nursing plan of care may specify other reassessments as well.

At some facilities, health care team members must meet every 2 or 3 days during a patient's hospital stay to discuss and update discharge plans. At these meetings, staff representatives from various departments —

including nursing, medicine, social services, physical therapy, and dietary — evaluate the patient's progress toward established goals and revise the plan of care as needed. Records of these meetings are maintained in the medical record to ensure communication with other team members.

Unplanned reassessment

An unplanned reassessment occurs whenever the patient's condition or circumstances change unexpectedly. For example, suppose a patient with no previous cardiac dysfunction suddenly develops severe chest pain and shortness of breath. You'd perform a complete assessment and schedule future cardiac reassessments according to the revised plan of care.

Or suppose you're caring for an elderly patient whose wife is his primary home caregiver. If his wife suddenly becomes incapacitated, you'd need to perform an unplanned reassessment of the patient's discharge needs to accommodate this change.

Documenting ongoing assessment

You'll usually document ongoing assessment data on flow sheets or in narrative notes on the patient's progress report. Ideally, you should use flow sheets to document all routine assessment data and nursing interventions. That way, you can shorten the narrative notes to include only information regarding the patient's progress toward achieving desired outcomes as well as any unplanned assessments.

Flow sheets come in many varieties, including temperature graphs and intake and output forms. When used to record routine assessment data, flow sheets are a quick and consistent way to highlight trends in the patient's condition. A flow sheet for documenting information about a patient's skin integrity, for instance, will clearly show the progression of any pressure ulcers or reddened areas.

Because flow sheets are legally accepted components of the patient's medical record, they must be documented correctly. Give yourself enough time to evaluate each piece of information on the flow sheet. And keep in mind that it must accurately reflect the patient's current clinical status.

In some cases, you'll find that recording only the information requested on a flow sheet is not be sufficient to give a complete picture of the patient's status. When this occurs, record additional information in the space provided on the flow sheet. If additional information isn't necessary, draw a line through the space. Doing so indicates that, in your judgment, further information isn't required. If your flow sheet doesn't have additional space and you need to record more information, use the progress notes.

Nursing diagnosis and plan of care

When you formulate nursing diagnoses and write a plan of care for a patient, you're playing a key role in his recovery. To build a solid foundation for your plan of care, you need to identify nursing diagnoses carefully. Then you must write a plan that not only fits your nursing diagnoses, but also fits your patient—taking into account his needs, age, developmental level, culture, strengths and weaknesses, and willingness and ability to take part in his care.

Your plan should help the patient reach his highest functional level with minimal risk and without new problems. If a complete recovery is unlikely or impossible, your plan of care should help him cope physically and emotionally with his impaired or declining health. And, of course, you need to document all of this — carefully and completely.

That's a tall order. But this section will help you fill it by explaining the nursing diagnosis and planning processes and showing you how to document them most effectively. The first section discusses how to formulate nursing diagnoses. Next comes a section on how to rank these diagnoses so you treat your patient's most urgent problems first.

The third section reviews how to develop realistic expected outcomes — goals your patient should reach by or before discharge so he can function as effectively as possible. In the fourth section, you'll learn how to choose the nursing interventions that will help your patient reach those expected outcomes.

The next section explains how to write plans of care, including how to use practice guidelines to make planning and documentation more efficient and how to document your patient teaching and discharge planning. The final section looks at case management, a comprehensive way of caring for a patient that attempts to meet both clinical and financial goals.

Formulating nursing diagnoses

Unlike a medical diagnosis, which focuses on the patient's pathophysiology or illness, a nursing diagnosis focuses on the patient's responses to illness. (See *Nursing diagnoses: Avoiding the pitfalls.*)

Types of nursing diagnoses

Depending on the policy of your health care facility, you'll either use standardized diagnoses or formulate your own diagnoses.

Using standardized diagnoses

To make nursing diagnoses consistent, several organizations have developed standardized lists, which are used by a growing number of health care facilities. NANDA has developed the most widely accepted taxonomy of nursing diagnoses. (See the appendix NANDA Taxonomy I, Revised, for a complete list.) NANDA categorizes nursing diagnoses according to these human response patterns: exchanging, communicating, relating, valuing, choosing, moving, perceiving, knowing, and feeling. The association meets every 2 years to consider new diagnoses.

Diagnoses can also be categorized according to nursing models, such as the one developed by Marjory Gordon, in which nursing diagnoses correspond to functional health patterns. Other ways of categorizing diagnoses — for instance, according to Orem's self-care model — may also be used. Or your health care facility or unit can establish its own list of nursing diagnoses, categorizing them according to medical diagnoses and surgical procedures, for example.

No accrediting organization requires the use of standardized diagnoses. By using nationally accepted nursing diagnoses such as the NANDA taxonomy, however, health care facilities help establish a common language for nursing diagnoses — making communication easier and diagnoses more precise.

Formulating your own nursing diagnoses

Developing your own diagnoses takes more effort than using standardized ones. Even so, some nurses prefer this approach because they find the standardized diagnoses incomplete or their language overly formal or abstract. Such an approach can also help you characterize a problem that standardized diagnoses don't readily address.

Deciding on a diagnosis

Before developing or using nursing diagnoses, you must evaluate relevant assessment data. You'll usually find this data on a standardized assessment form that groups related information into categories. Looking at the data in these groupings lets you determine which patient needs require nursing intervention. (See *Evaluating assessment data,* page 238.) Some assessment forms list relevant nursing diagnoses next to specific assessment findings. (See *Relating assessment data to nursing diagnoses,* page 239.)

Components of the diagnosis

Once you've examined the assessment data, you're ready to formulate your nursing diagnoses. A diagnosis usually has three components: the human response or problem, related factors, and signs and symptoms.

HUMAN RESPONSE OR PROBLEM. The first part of the diagnosis, the human response, identifies an actual or a potential problem that can be affected by nursing care. For instance, if assessment information on a patient with osteoarthritis shows that he has trouble moving, you might turn to the NANDA taxonomy, look under the human response pattern of moving, and identify the problem as impaired physical mobility. If the NANDA taxonomy doesn't provide a label that fits a patient's problem or if your facility doesn't use standardized diagnoses, create your own label for the patient's condition.

Nursing diagnoses: Avoiding the pitfalls

To avoid making common mistakes when formulating your nursing diagnoses, follow these guidelines.

Use nursing diagnoses
Don't use medical diagnoses or interventions. Terms such as *angioplasty* and *coronary artery disease* belong in a medical diagnosis—not in a nursing diagnosis.

Use all relevant assessment data
If you focus on only the physical assessment, for instance, you might miss psychosocial or cultural information relevant to your diagnoses.

Take your time
Take enough time to analyze the assessment data. If you rush, you might easily miss something important.

Interpret the assessment data accurately
Make sure that you follow established norms, professional standards, and interdisciplinary expectations in interpreting the assessment data. In addition, don't permit your biases to interfere with your interpretation of information.

For instance, don't assume your patient is exaggerating if he states that he feels pain during what you would consider a painless procedure. If possible, have the patient verify your interpretation.

Keep data up-to-date
Don't stop assessing and updating your diagnoses after the initial examination. As the patient's condition changes, so should your evaluation.

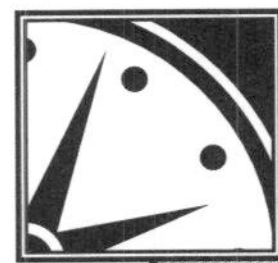

CHARTING TIMESAVER

Evaluating assessment data

To formulate your nursing diagnoses, you must evaluate the essential assessment information. These questions will help you quickly zero in on the appropriate data.

- Which signs and symptoms does the patient have?
- Which assessment findings are abnormal for this patient?
- How do particular behaviors affect the patient's well-being?
- What strengths or weaknesses does the patient have that affect his health status?
- Does he understand his illness and treatment?
- How does the patient's environment affect his health?
- Does he want to change his state of health?
- Do I need to gather any further information for my diagnoses?

RELATED FACTORS. The second part of the nursing diagnosis identifies related factors. Such factors may precede, contribute to, or simply be associated with the human response. But no matter how they relate, these factors make your diagnosis more closely fit the particular patient and help you choose the most effective interventions.

For example, for your patient with osteoarthritis you could write "Impaired physical mobility related to pain" or "Impaired physical mobility related to depression." Depending on these related factors, your interventions would probably differ.

When you can't determine the related factors, write "related to unknown etiology" and modify your diagnosis as you obtain more information. To save charting time, use the standard abbreviation "R/T" for "related to" when writing your nursing diagnoses.

SIGNS AND SYMPTOMS. Finally, a complete nursing diagnosis includes the signs and symptoms that led you to the diagnosis—what NANDA calls the "defining characteristics." You'll draw these from the assessment data. Not all nurses include signs and symptoms in their diagnoses but, like related factors, they help tailor the nursing diagnosis to the particular patient.

To help keep the nursing diagnosis brief, choose only the key characteristics. You can list them after the human response and related factors. For instance, you might write "Impaired thought processes R/T uncompensated perceptual or cognitive impairment. Defining characteristics: short attention span during conversation; minimal speech; confused, oriented to person."

Alternatively, you can join the signs and symptoms to the first part of the nursing diagnosis with the words "as evidenced by," abbreviated "AEB." For example, you'd write "Fluid volume excess R/T increased sodium intake AEB edema, weight gain, shortness of breath, and S_3 heart sounds."

Setting priorities

Once you've determined your nursing diagnoses, you'll need to rank them based on which problems require immediate attention. Whenever possible, you should include the patient in this process. Maslow's hierarchy of needs is generally accepted as the basis for setting priorities. (See *Maslow's hierarchy of needs,* page 240.)

BETTER CHARTING

Relating assessment data to nursing diagnoses

Some assessment forms group assessment information and relevant nursing diagnoses together so that you can immediately relate one to the other. This saves you from looking back through the form for assessment data when determining the nursing diagnosis. Here's a section of this type of form.

Patient *Michael Ramsey* **Age** *72*
Medical diagnosis: *Heart failure*

ASSESSMENT FINDINGS			NURSING DIAGNOSES
Cardiopulmonary			
Breath sounds *crackles, bilateral bases*			☑ Impaired gas exchange
Breathing pattern	☐ cough *dry*	☐ smoker	☐ Ineffective airway clearance
Dyspnea	☐ on exertion	☐ nocturnal	☐ Inability to sustain spontaneous ventilation
Sputum	color		☑ Ineffective breathing pattern
	consistency		☑ Decreased cardiac output
Heart sounds *S_3 and S_4 present*			☐ Altered peripheral tissue perfusion
Peripheral pulses *all peripheral pulses +1*			☐ Altered cardiopulmonary tissue perfusion
Edema	☑ Extremities *ankles*		
	☐ Other		
Cyanosis	☑ Extremities *nail beds*		
	☑ Other *lips*		
Nutrition			
Diet *2G Na, low cholesterol*			
Appetite			
☐ normal	☐ increased	☑ decreased	☑ Altered nutrition: less than body requirements
☐ vomiting	☐ nausea		☐ Altered nutrition: more than body requirements
			☐ Altered nutrition: risk for more than body requirements

Typically, the first nursing diagnosis will stem from the primary medical diagnosis or from the patient's chief complaint. This nursing diagnosis points out a threat to the patient's physical well-being — sometimes to his life. For a patient who has a primary medical diagnosis of heart failure, for instance, you'd give first priority to the nursing diagnosis of "Decreased cardiac output R/T decreased contractility and altered heart rhythm."

Related nursing diagnoses come next. These define problems that pose less immediate threats to the patient's well-being. For instance, you may have also selected for the heart failure patient the nursing diagnosis of

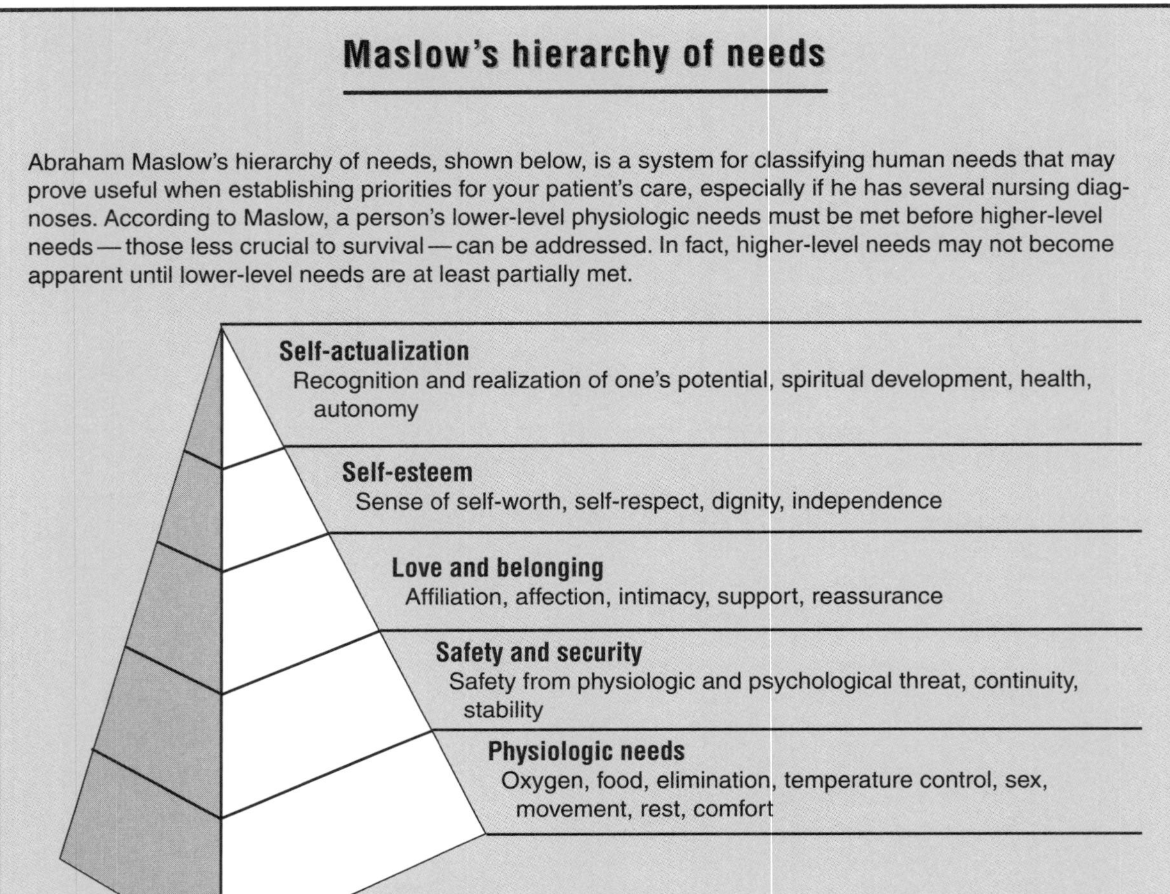

"Fluid volume excess R/T compromised regulatory mechanism."

Then you'll usually list nursing diagnoses that pertain to the patient's psychosocial, emotional, or spiritual needs. For the heart failure patient, a nursing diagnosis of "Anxiety R/T possible loss of employment" doesn't carry the same urgency as the previous two nursing diagnoses.

However, although a nursing diagnosis may have a lower priority, you shouldn't wait to intervene until you've resolved all the higher-priority problems. Helping the heart failure patient cope with anxiety about losing his job, for example, may speed his recovery because psychological problems can have an impact on physical well-being.

Developing expected outcomes

After you've established and ranked nursing diagnoses, you're ready to develop relevant expected outcomes, an increasingly important planning step. Based on the nursing diagnoses, expected outcomes are goals that the patient should reach as a result of planned nursing interventions. (Once achieved, an expected outcome is called a patient outcome.) You may find that one nursing diagnosis requires more than one expected outcome.

An outcome can specify an improvement in the patient's ability to function, such as an increase in the distance he can walk, or an amelioration of a problem, such as a reduction of pain. Each outcome should call for the maximum realistic improvement for a particular patient.

Writing outcome statements

Ideally, an outcome statement should include four components: the specific behavior that will demonstrate the patient has reached his goal, criteria for measuring the behavior, the conditions under which the behavior should occur, and the time by which the behavior should occur. (See *Writing an outcome statement,* page 242.)

When you're writing outcome statements, follow the guidelines listed below.

Make your statements specific

Use action verbs, such as *walks, demonstrates, consumes,* and *expresses.* A vague statement, such as "Patient improves nutritional intake," gives you and your colleagues little to go on. Instead, clearly state which behaviors you expect the patient to exhibit and when — for example, "Patient will consume 1,200 calories daily by 3/10/99."

Focus on the patient

Make sure that the outcome statement reflects the patient's behavior — not your intervention. The statement "Medication brings chest pain relief" doesn't say anything about the patient's behavior. A proper statement would be "Patient will express relief of chest pain within 1 hour of receiving medication."

Let the patient help you

A patient who takes part in developing outcome statements is more motivated to achieve his goals. And his input — and the input of family members — can help you set realistic goals.

Take medical orders into account

Make sure that you don't write outcome statements that ignore or contradict medical orders. For example, before writing the outcome statement "Patient will ambulate 10 feet unassisted twice a day by 1/10/99," make sure that the medical orders don't call for more restricted activity.

Adapt the outcome to the circumstances

Take into account the patient's coping ability, age, educational level, cultural influences, support systems, living conditions, and socioeconomic status. Also consider his anticipated length of stay when you're deciding on time limits for achieving goals. In some cases, you'll need to consider the health care setting itself. For instance, an outcome statement such as "Patient will ambulate outdoors with assistance for 20 minutes t.i.d. by 2/15/99" may be unrealistic in a large city hospital.

Change your statements as necessary

Sometimes, you may need to revise even the most carefully written outcome statements. For example, if the patient has trouble reaching his goal, you may have to choose a later target date or change the goal to one the patient can reach more easily.

Writing an outcome statement

An outcome statement should consist of four components:

B	M	C	T
Behavior A desired behavior for the patient. This behavior must be observable.	**Measure** Criteria for measuring the behavior. The criteria should specify how much, how long, how far, and so on.	**Condition** The conditions under which the behavior should occur.	**Time** The time by which the behavior should occur.

As indicated, the two outcome statements below have these four components.

Limit sodium intake	2 g/day	using hospital menu	by 1/10/99
Eat	50% of all meals	unassisted	by 1/10/99

Use shortcuts

You can save charting time by including only the essentials in your outcome statements. For example, in many cases, you can omit the words "Patient will" from your outcomes because "patient" is understood. Thus, rather than writing "Patient will demonstrate insulin self-administration by 1/18/99," you can simply write "Demonstrate insulin self-administration by 1/18/99."

Many facilities also use abbreviations for target dates, such as "HD2" for "hospital day 2" and "POD3" for postoperative day 3."

Selecting interventions

Now you're ready to select interventions—nursing actions that you and your patient agree will help him reach the expected outcomes. Base these interventions on the second part of your nursing diagnosis, the related factors. With a nursing diagnosis of "Impaired physical mobility R/T arthritic morning stiffness," for example, you'd select interventions that reduce or eliminate the patient's stiffness, such as mild stretching exercises. You'll need to write at least one intervention for each outcome statement.

You can determine interventions in several ways. Start by considering ones that your patient or you have successfully tried before. Say your patient is having trouble sleeping. He knows he sleeps better at home if he has a glass of warm milk at bedtime. That could work as an intervention for the expected outcome "Patient will sleep through the night without medication by 1/16/99."

You can also select interventions from standardized plans of care, talk with your colleagues about interventions they've used successfully, or check nursing journals that discuss interventions for standardized nursing diagnoses. If these methods don't yield anything useful, try brainstorming.

Writing intervention statements

Your intervention statements must communicate your ideas clearly to other staff members. When writing your interventions, follow the guidelines listed below.

Clearly state the necessary action

To ensure continuity of care, include as much specific detail as possible in your interventions. Note how and when to perform the intervention as well as any special instructions. An intervention such as "Promote comfort" doesn't tell another nurse what specific actions she should take. But "Administer ordered analgesic ½ hr before dressing change" lets her know exactly what to do and when to do it.

Tailor the intervention to the patient

Keep in mind the patient's age, condition, developmental level, environment, and value system when writing your interventions. For instance, if your patient is a vegetarian, you shouldn't write an intervention that requires him to eat lean meat to gain extra protein for healing. Instead, your intervention could call for him to eat legumes and dairy products.

Keep the patient's safety in mind

Take into account the patient's physical and mental limitations so that your interventions don't worsen existing problems or create new ones. For example, if the patient needs the support of two nurses during ambulation, include that information in your intervention. If you're teaching a patient how to perform a new exercise, make sure that he's physically capable of doing it without hurting or straining himself.

Follow the rules of your health care facility

If your facility has a rule that only nurses may administer medications, you obviously would not write an intervention calling for the patient to "administer hemorrhoidal suppositories as needed."

Take other health care activities into account

Sometimes, other necessary activities may interfere with interventions you want to use. For example, you may want your patient to get plenty of rest on a day he has several diagnostic tests scheduled. In this case, you'd need to adjust your interventions.

Include available resources

To help carry out interventions effectively, make full use of your facility's resources and outside sources. For example, if your patient needs to learn about his cardiac problem, provide him with literature from your facility's education department, brochures and videotapes from the American Heart Association, and referrals to local support groups. Then write the intervention to reflect the use of these resources.

Writing your plan of care

A good plan of care is the blueprint for concise, meaningful charting. If you write a good plan of care, your nurses' notes will practically write themselves. A good plan consists of the following:

- patient problems identified during the admission interview and hospitalization
- realistic, measurable expected outcomes and target dates
- nursing interventions that will help the patient or his family achieve these outcomes.

To document your nursing diagnoses, expected outcomes, and interventions, you can use either a traditional or a standardized plan of care. You also may decide to use protocols along with one of these plans. In some cases, you can use protocols alone to demonstrate planned care. The plan of care will also include your patient-teaching and discharge plans.

Types of nursing plans of care

Two basic types of plans of care exist: traditional and standardized. No matter which you use, your plan should cover all nursing care from admission to discharge and should be a permanent part of the patient's medical record. Be sure to write the plan of care and put it into action as soon as possible after the initial assessment. Then you can revise and update it throughout the patient's hospitalization.

Traditional plan of care

Also called the *individually developed plan of care,* the traditional plan of care is written from scratch for each patient. After analyzing the assessment data, you'll either write the plan or enter it into a computer. Although the traditional plan of care is now rarely used because of the time required to write one for each patient, it is worthwhile to understand how it's developed.

The basic form can vary, depending on the needs of the health care facility or department. Most forms have three main columns: one for nursing diagnoses, another for expected outcomes, and a third for interventions. Other columns allow you to enter the date you initiated the plan of care, the target dates for expected outcomes, and the dates for review, revisions, and resolution. Most forms also have a place for you to sign or initial when you make an entry or a revision.

What you must include on these forms also varies. With shorter stays brought on by the advent of diagnosis-related groups (DRGs), most facilities require you to write only short-term outcomes that the patient should reach by or before discharge. However, some facilities — particularly long-term care facilities —also want you to include long-term outcomes that reflect the maximum functional level the patient can reach. Such facilities frequently use forms that provide separate places for the two types of outcomes. (See *Using a traditional plan of care.*)

Standardized plan of care

Developed to save documentation time and improve the quality of care, standardized plans of care provide a series of standard interventions for patients with similar diagnoses. These standardized plans of care can be computer generated or preprinted, and become a part of the permanent patient record. Most standardized plans also supply root outcome statements. Some of these plans are classified by medical diagnoses or DRGs; others, by nursing diagnoses.

The early versions of standardized plans of care made no allowances for differences in

BETTER CHARTING

Using a traditional plan of care

Here's an example of a traditional plan of care. It shows how these forms are typically organized. Remember that a traditional plan is written from scratch for each patient.

DATE	NURSING DIAGNOSIS	EXPECTED OUTCOMES	INTERVENTIONS	REVISION (INITIALS AND DATE)	RESOLUTION (INITIALS AND DATE)
1/8/99	Decreased cardiac output R/T reduced stroke volume secondary to fluid volume overload	Lungs clear on auscultation by 1/10/99. BP will return to baseline by 1/10/99	Monitor for signs and symptoms of hypoxemia, such as dyspnea, confusion, arrhythmias, restlessness, and cyanosis. Ensure adequate oxygenation by placing patient in semi-Fowler's position and administering supplemental O_2 as ordered. Monitor breath sounds q 4 hr. Administer cardiac medications as ordered and document pt's response, drugs' effectiveness, and any adverse reactions. Monitor and document heart rate and rhythm, heart sounds, and BP. Note the presence or absence of peripheral pulses. ———— KK		

REVIEW DATES		
Date	Signature	Initials
1/8/99	Karen Kramer, RN	KK

BETTER CHARTING

Using a standardized plan of care

The standardized plan of care below is for a patient with a nursing diagnosis of decreased cardiac output. To customize it to your patient, you'd complete the diagnosis—including related factors and signs and symptoms—and fill in the expected outcomes. You'd also modify, add, or delete interventions as necessary.

Date *1/8/99*

Nursing diagnosis

Decreased cardiac output *R/T reduced stroke volume secondary to fluid volume overload*

Target date *1/9/99*

Expected outcomes

Adequate cardiac output (AEB): *>4.0 L/min*
Heart rate: *Apical rate <90*
BP: *140/80 mm Hg*
Pedal pulse: *palpable and regular*
Radial pulse: *palpable and regular*
Cardiac rhythm: *normal sinus rhythm*
Cardiac index: *2.2 to 4.0 L/min/m²*
Pulmonary artery wedge pressure (PAWP): *10 mm Hg*
Pulmonary artery pressure (PAP): *20/12 mm Hg*
$S\bar{v}O_2$: *Between 60% and 80%*
Urine output in ml/hr: *>30 ml/hr*

Date *1/8/99*

Interventions

- Monitor ECG for rate and rhythm; note ectopic beats. If arrhythmias occur, note patient's response. Document and report findings and follow appropriate arrhythmia protocol.
- Monitor $S\bar{v}O_2$, T, R, and central pressures continuously.
- Monitor other hemodynamic pressures q *1* hr and p.r.n.
- Auscultate for heart sounds and palpate peripheral pulses q *2* hr and p.r.n.
- Monitor I & O q *1* hr. Notify doctor if output < 30 ml/hr x 2 hr.
- Administer medications and fluids as ordered, noting effectiveness and adverse reactions. Titrate vasoactive drugs p.r.n. Follow appropriate vasoactive drug protocol to wean pt. as tolerated.
- Monitor O_2 therapy or other ventilatory assistance.
- Decrease patient's activity to reduce O_2 demands. Increase as tolerated.
- Assess and document LOC. Assess for changes q *1* hr and p.r.n.
- Additional interventions:
  Inspect for pedal and sacral edema q 2 hr

patient needs. But current versions allow you to customize the plan to fit your patient's specific needs. In fact, they require you to explain how you've individualized the plan of care. To use such a plan, you'll usually fill in the following information:

- related factors and signs and symptoms for a nursing diagnosis. For instance, the form will provide a root diagnosis such as "Pain R/T. . . ." You might fill in "inflammation as exhibited by grimacing, expressions of pain."
- time limits for the outcomes. To a root outcome statement of "Patient will perform postural drainage without assistance," you might add "for 15 minutes immediately upon awakening in the morning by 2/8/99."
- frequency of interventions. You can complete an intervention such as "Perform passive range-of-motion exercises" with "twice a day: 1 × each in the morning and evening."
- specific instructions for interventions. For a standard intervention of "Elevate patient's head," you might specify "Before sleep, elevate the patient's head on three pillows."

When a patient has more than one diagnosis, the resulting combination of standardized plans of care can be long and cumbersome; computerized documentation can help. With computerized plans, you can pull only what you need from each one and combine them to make one manageable plan. Some computer programs simply provide a checklist of interventions you can use to build your own plan.

Keep in mind that standardized plans usually include only essential information. However, most provide space for you to add further nursing diagnoses, expected outcomes,and interventions. (See *Using a standardized plan of care.*)

Practice guidelines

A newer documentation tool, practice guidelines give specific sequential instructions for treating patients with particular problems. Developed to help nurses manage equipment and provide specific treatments, practice guidelines now are also used to manage patients with specific nursing diagnoses. (See *Practice guidelines for acute pulmonary edema,* pages 248 and 249, and *Managing ineffective breathing pattern,* page 250.)

Practice guidelines offer several advantages. Because they spell out the steps to follow for a patient with a particular nursing diagnosis, they can help you provide thorough care and ensure that the patient receives consistent care from all caregivers. Many detailed practice guidelines even specify what to teach the patient and what to document, and they include a reference section that lets you quickly determine how up-to-date they are.

Some practice guidelines also spell out the role of other health care professionals, helping all team members coordinate their efforts. By supplying such comprehensive instruction, practice guidelines also help teach inexperienced staff members. Used in conjunction with other plans of care or alone, practice guidelines can also save documentation time.

Using practice guidelines

Use the practice guidelines that best fit your patient. You'll probably use some practice guidelines, such as the generic one for pain, for many patients and others rarely. For example, the practice guideline *Potential for violence: self-directed* applies mainly to patients in psychiatric settings. If you find that a practice guideline doesn't exist for a patient problem, you can help develop a new one.

(Text continues on page 251.)

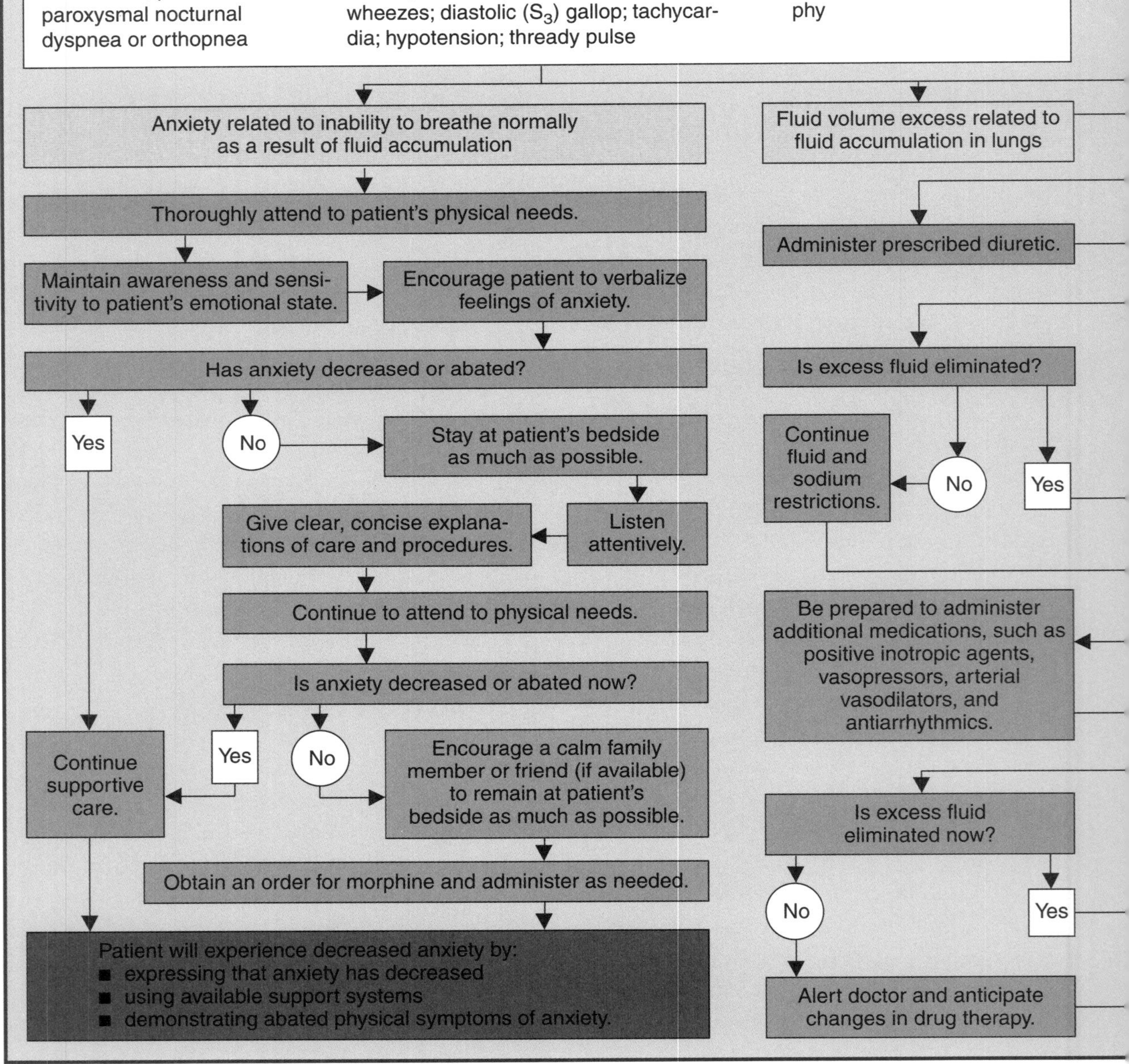

Practice guidelines for acute pulmonary edema
Presence of predisposing factors, such as cardiovascular diseases, persistent cough, dyspnea on exertion, possible paroxysmal nocturnal dyspnea or orthopnea
Physical findings, including restlessness; anxiety; labored, rapid respirations; frothy, bloody sputum; decreased level of consciousness; neck vein distention; cold, clammy skin; crepitant crackles and wheezes; diastolic (S_3) gallop; tachycardia; hypotension; thready pulse
Results of chest X-ray, arterial blood gas (ABG) analysis, pulse oximetry, pulmonary artery catheterization, electrocardiography
Anxiety related to inability to breathe normally as a result of fluid accumulation
Thoroughly attend to patient's physical needs.
Maintain awareness and sensitivity to patient's emotional state.
Encourage patient to verbalize feelings of anxiety.
Has anxiety decreased or abated?
Yes
No
Stay at patient's bedside as much as possible.
Listen attentively.
Give clear, concise explanations of care and procedures.
Continue to attend to physical needs.
Is anxiety decreased or abated now?
Yes
No
Continue supportive care.
Encourage a calm family member or friend (if available) to remain at patient's bedside as much as possible.
Obtain an order for morphine and administer as needed.
Patient will experience decreased anxiety by:
■ expressing that anxiety has decreased
■ using available support systems
■ demonstrating abated physical symptoms of anxiety.
Fluid volume excess related to fluid accumulation in lungs
Administer prescribed diuretic.
Is excess fluid eliminated?
Continue fluid and sodium restrictions.
No
Yes
Be prepared to administer additional medications, such as positive inotropic agents, vasopressors, arterial vasodilators, and antiarrhythmics.
Is excess fluid eliminated now?
No
Yes
Alert doctor and anticipate changes in drug therapy.

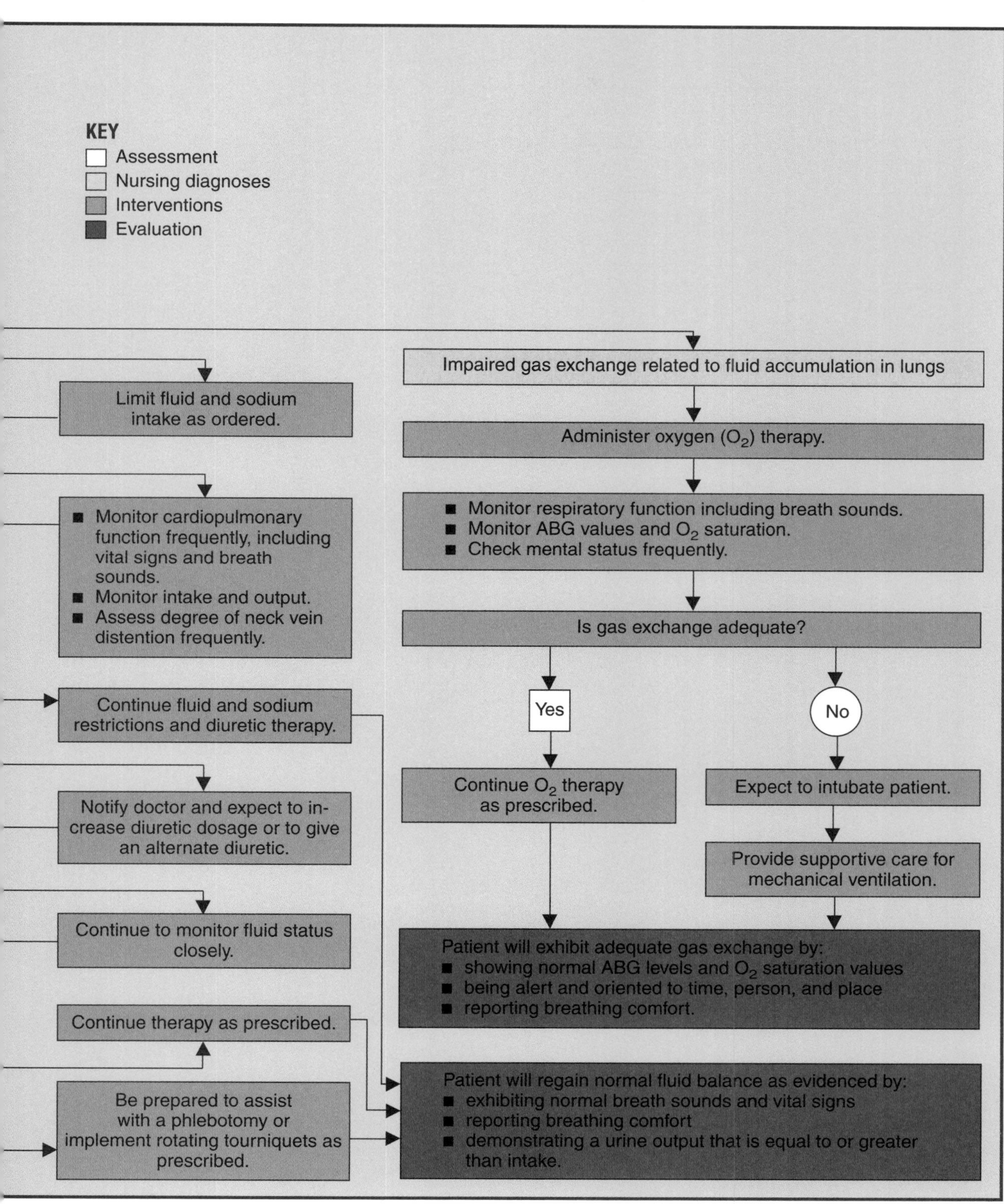
KEY
Assessment
Nursing diagnoses
Interventions
Evaluation
Limit fluid and sodium intake as ordered.
Monitor cardiopulmonary function frequently, including vital signs and breath sounds.
Monitor intake and output.
Assess degree of neck vein distention frequently.
Continue fluid and sodium restrictions and diuretic therapy.
Notify doctor and expect to increase diuretic dosage or to give an alternate diuretic.
Continue to monitor fluid status closely.
Continue therapy as prescribed.
Be prepared to assist with a phlebotomy or implement rotating tourniquets as prescribed.
Impaired gas exchange related to fluid accumulation in lungs
Administer oxygen (O_2) therapy.
Monitor respiratory function including breath sounds.
Monitor ABG values and O_2 saturation.
Check mental status frequently.
Is gas exchange adequate?
Yes
No
Continue O_2 therapy as prescribed.
Expect to intubate patient.
Provide supportive care for mechanical ventilation.
Patient will exhibit adequate gas exchange by:
showing normal ABG levels and O_2 saturation values
being alert and oriented to time, person, and place
reporting breathing comfort.
Patient will regain normal fluid balance as evidenced by:
exhibiting normal breath sounds and vital signs
reporting breathing comfort
demonstrating a urine output that is equal to or greater than intake.

Managing ineffective breathing pattern

Below you'll find a portion of a practice guideline for a patient who has chronic obstructive pulmonary disease (COPD) and a nursing diagnosis of ineffective breathing pattern.

NURSING DIAGNOSIS AND PATIENT OUTCOMES	IMPLEMENTATION	EVALUATION
Ineffective breathing pattern related to decreased lung compliance and air trapping By 3/10/99 the patient will: ■ demonstrate a respiratory rate within ± 5 of baseline ■ maintain arterial blood gas (ABG) levels within acceptable ranges ■ verbalize his understanding of the disease process, including its causes and risk factors ■ demonstrate diaphragmatic pursed-lip breathing ■ take all medication as prescribed ■ use oxygen as prescribed.	■ Monitor respiratory function. Auscultate for breath sounds, noting improvement or deterioration. Obtain ABG levels and pulmonary function tests as ordered. ■ Explain lung anatomy and physiology, using illustrated teaching materials, if possible. ■ Explain COPD, its physiologic effects, and its complications. ■ Review the most common signs and symptoms associated with the disease: dyspnea, especially with exertion; fatigue; cough; occasional mucus production; weight loss; rapid heart rate; irregular pulse; and use of accessory muscles to help with breathing because of limited diaphragm function. ■ Explain the purpose of diaphragmatic pursed-lip breathing for patients with COPD; demonstrate the correct technique and have the patient perform a return demonstration. ■ If the patient smokes, provide information about smoking cessation groups in the community. ■ Explain the importance of avoiding fumes, respiratory irritants, temperature extremes, and exposure to upper respiratory tract infections. ■ Review the patient's medications and explain the rationale for their use, their dosages, and possible adverse effects. Advise him to report any adverse reactions to the doctor immediately. ■ For the patient receiving oxygen, explain the rationale for therapy and the safe use of equipment. Explain that the oxygen flow rate should never be increased above the prescribed target.	■ Patient's respiratory rate remains within ± 5 of baseline. ■ ABG levels return to and remain within established limits. ■ Patient verbalizes an understanding of his disease. ■ Patient properly demonstrates diaphragmatic pursed-lip breathing. ■ Patient takes all medication as prescribed. ■ Patient demonstrates the appropriate use of oxygen as prescribed.

When you've selected a practice guideline, make sure that you tailor it to fit your patient's needs. Record any modifications you made on the patient's plan of care.

Documenting practice guidelines

To document a practice guideline on a plan of care, note in the interventions section that you'll follow the guideline—for instance, "Follow impaired gas exchange guideline." Or list the practice guidelines you plan to use on a flow sheet. Be sure to document any modifications you'll need to make.

After you intervene, simply write in your progress notes that you followed the practice guidelines, or check off the practice guidelines box on your flow sheet and initial it. The guidelines themselves usually remain at the nurses' station.

Clinical pathways

One of the newest documentation tools is the clinical pathway, also known as a critical pathway or care map. This tool uses input from all disciplines involved in caring for a group of similar patients (usually those with the same diagnosis) and defines the care to be provided on each anticipated day of stay. For a more detailed explanation of clinical pathways, with examples, see the "Case Management" section later in this chapter.

Patient-teaching plan

You'll also need to include a patient-teaching plan as part of your plan of care. You may include this on your main plan or write a separate plan. Today, many health care facilities require a separate plan because of the emphasis placed on patient teaching by accrediting and regulatory organizations. The need to control costs and the current practice of discharging patients earlier also calls for more extensive teaching plans.

Besides identifying what the patient needs to learn and how he'll be taught, a teaching plan sets criteria for evaluating how well he learns. The plan also helps all the patient's educators coordinate their teaching. Plus, it serves as legal proof that the patient received appropriate instruction and satisfies the requirements of regulatory agencies such as JCAHO.

To make sure that your teaching plan does all that it should, carefully organize what the patient needs to learn and how you'll provide the instruction and measure the results. Work closely with other health care team members as well as with the patient and his family to make the plan's content realistic and attainable during his stay. Include provisions for follow-up teaching at home.

Also, keep your patient-teaching plan flexible. Take into account such variables as the patient being unreceptive because of a poor night's sleep as well as your own daily time limits.

Components of the plan

Although the scope of each teaching plan differs, all should contain the same elements:

- patient-learning needs
- expected learning outcomes
- teaching content, organized from the simplest concepts to the most complex
- teaching methods and tools
- barriers to learning and readiness to learn.

PATIENT-LEARNING NEEDS. Identifying learning needs helps you decide which outcomes you should establish for your patient. Be sure to take into account not only what you, the doctor, and other health care team members want the patient to learn, but also what he wants to learn.

EXPECTED LEARNING OUTCOMES. As with your other expected outcomes, expected learning outcomes should focus on the patient and be readily measurable.

Your patient's learning behaviors and the outcomes you develop fall into three categories:

- cognitive, relating to understanding
- psychomotor, covering manual skills
- affective, dealing with attitudes.

For a patient learning to give himself subcutaneous injections, identifying an injection site would be the cognitive outcome; giving the injection, the psychomotor outcome; and coping with the need for injections, the affective outcome. (See *Writing clear learning outcomes.*)

To help formulate precise, measurable outcomes, decide which evaluation techniques will best reveal the patient's progress. For cognitive learning, you might use questions and answers; for psychomotor learning, you might use return demonstration. To measure affective learning, which can be difficult because changes in attitudes develop slowly, you can use several evaluation techniques. For example, to determine whether a patient has overcome his anxiety about giving himself an injection, you can ask him if he still feels anxious, you can assess his willingness to perform the procedure, and you can observe whether he hesitates or shows other signs of stress while doing it.

TEACHING CONTENT. Next, you'll need to select what to teach the patient to help him achieve the expected outcomes. As you make these decisions, be sure to include family members and other caregivers in your plan. Even if a patient will learn to care for himself, you can teach a family member how to provide physical and emotional support or how to serve as a source of information in case the patient forgets some aspect of his care.

Once you've decided what to teach, carefully organize it. Start with the simplest concepts and work toward the more complex ones. You'll find this especially helpful for teaching a patient with little education or one who doesn't learn well by listening.

TEACHING METHODS. You'll also need to select the appropriate teaching method for your patient. You can probably plan to do most of your teaching on a one-on-one basis. This method gives you a chance to learn about your patient, build a relationship with him, and tailor your teaching to his learning needs.

But you can use other methods too — either in place of or in conjunction with one-on-one teaching. For instance, you may want to incorporate demonstration, practice, and return demonstration in your teaching plan. Role playing can help involve your patient in learning, as can case studies, which call for him to evaluate how someone else with his disorder responds to different situations. Self-monitoring also involves the patient because he must assess his situation and determine which aspects of his environment or behavior need correction. If you have several patients who need similar instruction, you can also try group teaching or lecturing.

TEACHING TOOLS. Teaching tools — ranging from printed pamphlets to closed-circuit television programs — can help familiarize the patient with a specific topic.

Writing clear learning outcomes

The patient's learning behaviors fall into three categories: cognitive, psychomotor, and affective. With these categories in mind, you can write clear, concise, expected learning outcomes. Remember, your outcomes should clarify what you're going to teach, indicate the behavior you expect to see, and set criteria for evaluating what the patient has learned.

Review the two sets of sample learning outcomes for a patient with chronic renal failure. Notice that the outcomes in the well-phrased set start with a precise action verb, confine themselves to one task, and describe measurable and observable learning. In contrast, the poorly phrased outcomes may encompass many tasks and describe learning that's difficult or even impossible to measure.

WELL-PHRASED LEARNING OUTCOMES	POORLY PHRASED LEARNING OUTCOMES
Cognitive domain The patient with chronic renal failure will be able to:	
■ state when to take each prescribed drug	■ know his medication schedule
■ describe symptoms of elevated blood pressure	■ know when his blood pressure is elevated
■ list permitted and prohibited foods on his diet.	■ know his dietary restrictions.
Psychomotor domain The patient with chronic renal failure will be able to:	
■ take his blood pressure accurately, using a stethoscope and a sphygmomanometer	■ take his blood pressure
■ read a thermometer correctly	■ use a thermometer
■ collect a urine specimen, using sterile technique.	■ bring in a urine specimen for laboratory studies.
Affective domain The patient with chronic renal failure will be able to:	
■ comply with dietary restrictions to maintain normal electrolyte values	■ appreciate the relationship of diet to renal failure
■ verbally express his feelings about adjustments to be made in the home environment	■ adjust successfully to limitations imposed by chronic renal failure
■ keep scheduled doctors' appointments.	■ understand the importance of seeing his doctor.

When choosing your tools, focus on what will work best for the particular patient. For instance, if your patient likes to watch how something is done, he may respond best to a videotape of a procedure, a closed-circuit television demonstration, or a slide show. For a patient who prefers a hands-on approach, you might use a working model or let him handle the equipment he'll use. A computerized patient-teaching program may be best for a patient who likes to work interactively at his own pace. And some patients may simply want to read about a treatment or procedure.

Keep your patient's abilities and limitations in mind as you choose teaching tools. For instance, if you plan to provide written materials to reinforce your instructions, make sure that he can understand them. (The average adult has only a seventh-grade reading level.)

To get the tools you need, consult the staff-development instructors on your unit, the health care facility's librarian, or staff specialists. If your facility doesn't have what you need, you might try pharmaceutical and medical supply companies in your community. Don't overlook national associations and foundations such as the American Cancer Society. These organizations usually have large supplies of patient-education materials written specifically for laymen.

BARRIERS TO LEARNING AND READINESS TO LEARN. Another important aspect of the teaching plan is assessing any barriers to learning and the patient's readiness to learn. The patient's physical condition may impede the learning process — he may be experiencing fatigue, pain, physical disability, communication problems, cognitive or sensory impairment, or lack of motivation. Initially, the patient may be unwilling or unable to learn because he's overwhelmed by his illness, frightened, in denial, or all three. That's why it's important to assess your patient's response to teaching. If the patient is not receptive to the information you're giving him, wait, if possible, until he's ready. In any event, always document the presence of any learning barriers as well as the patient's willingness to learn.

Documenting the patient-teaching plan

Several forms are available for documenting your patient-teaching plan. Many of them include the phases of the nursing process as they relate to patient education. (See *Documenting patient teaching.*) Health care facilities are also being encouraged to create systematic interdisciplinary approaches to patient teaching.

Patient-teaching plans come in two basic types. Like the traditional plan of care, one type provides only the format and calls for you to come up with the plan. When a patient requires extensive teaching, you may be able to use a standardized plan instead, checking off or dating steps as you complete them and adding or deleting information.

Depending on the plan's format, it may include space for problems that may hinder learning, comments and evaluations, and dates and signatures. You may also be instructed to include this information in the progress notes. Whichever plan you use becomes a permanent part of the medical record.

Discharge planning

The final part of the planning process, the discharge plan has gained importance recently because of the trend toward shorter hospital stays. To help avert problems, start your discharge planning the day your patient is admitted — or sooner for a planned admission.

Responsibility for discharge planning

In some health care facilities, the social services department carries the major responsibility for discharge planning. Larger organizations may hire a nurse discharge planner to facilitate home care planning. But staff nurses still play a major role in preparing patients and caregivers to assume responsibility for ongoing care.

Even if you don't have the primary responsibility for discharge planning, you still play an important part. You and other health care team members need to coordinate your efforts with the discharge planners or social ser-

BETTER CHARTING

Documenting patient teaching

Below you'll find the first page of a patient-teaching flow sheet. Such flow sheets let you quickly and easily tailor your teaching plan to fit your patient's needs.

PATIENT-TEACHING FLOW SHEET

DIABETES MELLITUS

Problems affecting learning

- ☐ None
- ☑ Fatigue or pain
- ☐ Communication problem
- ☐ Cognitive or sensory impairment
- ☐ Physical disability
- ☐ Lack of motivation
- ☐ Other ______

LEARNING OUTCOMES	INITIAL TEACHING						REINFORCEMENT					
	Date	Time	Learner	Techniques and tools	Evaluation	Initials	Date	Time	Learner	Techniques and tools	Evaluation	Initials
Basic knowledge ■ Define diabetes mellitus (DM).	3/10/99	1000	P	E,W	S	JM	3/11/99	1000	P	E,W	S	JM
■ List four symptoms of DM.	3/10/99	1000	P	E,W	S	JM	3/11/99	1000	P	E,W	S	JM
Medication ■ State the action of insulin and its effects on the body.	3/10/99	1000	P	E,W	S	JM						
■ List the three major classifications of insulin. Give their onsets, peaks, and durations.	3/10/99	1000	P	E,W,V	Dv	JM						
■ Demonstrate the ability to draw up insulin in a syringe and mix the correct amount.	3/10/99	1000	P	E,W	S	JM						

KEY

Learner
- P = patient
- S = spouse
- M = mother
- F = father
- D1 = daughter 1
- D2 = daughter 2
- S1 = son 1
- S2 = son 2
- O = other

Teaching techniques
- D = demonstration
- E = explanation
- R = role-playing

Teaching tools
- F = filmstrip
- P = physical model
- S = slide
- V = videotape
- W = written material

Evaluation
- S = states understanding
- D = demonstrates understanding
- Dp = demonstrates understanding with physical coaching
- Dv = demonstrates understanding with verbal coaching
- T = passes written test
- N = no indication of learning
- NE = not evaluated

vices department. Typically, you'll do this at a multidisciplinary discharge conference, in which team members evaluate the patient's discharge needs, discuss appropriate plans, and evaluate his progress.

Components of the plan

A discharge plan should note the anticipated length of stay and specify what the patient needs to learn, including:

- diet
- medications
- treatments
- physical activity limitations
- signs and symptoms to report to the doctor
- follow-up medical care
- equipment
- appropriate community resources.

As part of your plan, make sure that the patient receives an instruction sheet to reinforce what he learns and what he needs to remember about follow-up care. The discharge plan should also spell out future care, including the setting for it, the patient's intended caregiver and support systems, actual or potential barriers to care, and any referrals.

Documenting the discharge plan

How you document the discharge plan will depend on the policy at your health care facility. Some policies require you to include your assessment of discharge needs on the initial assessment form, then document the discharge plan itself on a separate form. At many facilities you must include the discharge plan as a component of the discharge summary. Some forms used for discharge planning allow several members of the health care team to include information.

Case management

A method of delivering health care that controls costs while still ensuring quality care, case management goes a step beyond planned care to managed care. It came into being after the federal government introduced the prospective payment system in 1983. Under this system, Medicare pays the facility based on the patient's diagnosis — not on his length of stay or the number or types of services he receives. Thus, the facility loses money if the patient has a lengthy stay or develops complications.

Such a system forces health care facilities to deliver cost-effective care — without compromising the quality of care. And the case management system proposes to help them do that by managing each patient's care to meet both clinical and financial goals.

Your role in case management

If you become a case manager, your role will expand beyond giving nursing care. You'll learn to manage a closely controlled system of multidisciplinary care. You'll also take on responsibility for outcomes, length of stay, and use of resources throughout the patient's illness — not just during your shift.

How the system works

When a patient is assigned a particular DRG, he's also assigned a case manager. (In some facilities, a patient isn't assigned a DRG until after discharge — in which case, you'll need to make an educated guess about which DRG he'll be assigned to.) Each DRG case management plan has standard outcome criteria and includes medical and nursing interventions as well as interventions from other disciplines.

As the case manager for a patient, you'll discuss the outcomes with the patient and his family, using the established time line for the patient's DRG. This time line should cover all the processes that must occur for the patient to reach the expected outcome, including tests, procedures, and patient teaching, and the resources the patient will need, such as social services. If it doesn't, you'll adapt it as necessary to fit the patient's needs. If possible, you should do all this before the patient is even admitted, but you must complete these steps within the time limit set by your facility—usually 24 hours.

Once the patient is admitted, the multidisciplinary team evaluates his progress and suggests any necessary revisions, keeping in mind the need for continuity of care and the best use of resources. You'll document any variations in the time line, processes, or outcomes, along with the reasons for the changes. Plus, you'll keep a lookout for duplication of services and medical orders.

You must also start discharge planning, beginning an assessment of the patient's discharge needs at or before admission. You're also responsible for activating home health care services—including obtaining personnel and equipment—well before discharge.

Types of case management systems

Several case management systems and various adaptations exist, and health care facilities continue to create new systems. But most facilities pattern their systems after the one developed at the New England Medical Center (NEMC), one of the first centers to use case management in an acute care setting. Facilities typically adapt this system to meet their own needs and philosophy of care.

Tools for case management

Most facilities also pattern their case management tools after those of the NEMC system. Called the *case management plan* and the *clinical pathway,* they allow you to direct, evaluate, and revise patient progress and outcomes.

Case management plan

The basic tool of case management systems, the case management plan spells out the standardized care that a patient with a specific DRG should receive. The plan covers:

- nursing-related problems
- patient outcomes
- intermediate patient outcomes
- nursing interventions
- medical interventions
- target times.

Each subsection of the plan covers a care unit to which the patient may be admitted during his illness. For instance, a patient with a myocardial infarction may go to both the critical care and medical-surgical units.

Clinical pathway

Because of the length of case management plans, you probably won't use them on a daily basis. Instead, you'll turn to an abbreviated form of the plan: the clinical pathway. The clinical pathway (also known as the health care map) covers only the key events that must occur for the patient to be discharged by the target date. Such events include consultations, diagnostic tests, physical activities the patient must perform, treatments, diet, medications, discharge planning, and patient teaching. (For more details and a completed sample of a clinical pathway, see chapter 5, Documentation in Acute Care.)

Once you've established a pathway, you must note any variances from it, grouping them by cause. Variances may result from the system, the caregivers, or a problem the patient develops, and they can be justifiable or not. For instance, you may have a patient who doesn't walk in the hall as scheduled. If he has a secondary infection that prevents him from walking, you'll list the variance as justifiable. But if the patient simply prefers to stay in bed watching television, you'll need to list the variance as unjustifiable and take steps to correct the problem.

At shift report each day, you should review the clinical pathways with the other nurses. Before you go off duty, note any changes in the expected length of stay and point out critical events scheduled for the next shift to the nurses coming on duty. Also, discuss any variances that may have occurred during your shift.

Drawbacks of case management

The case management system usually works well for a patient with one primary diagnosis, no secondary diagnoses, and few complications. But for some patients, you'll have trouble even establishing a time line. For example, you can't easily predict when treatment will succeed for a patient with a seizure disorder. For a patient with several variances, the expected course of treatment and length of stay will likely change, and documentation can become lengthy and complicated.

Nursing interventions

Documenting nursing interventions has long been standard practice. But documentation methods have changed dramatically over the years, mainly because of frustration with tedious traditional methods and the urgent economic need to streamline hospital operations. No longer must you always write lengthy narrative notes. In many cases, you can use flow sheets or refer to practice guidelines instead.

This section will help you keep pace with these changes by explaining how to perform and document your interventions, including patient teaching and the discharge summary.

Performing interventions

Nursing intervention represents a crucial step in the nursing process. When you carry out your interventions, you're putting your carefully constructed plan of care into action.

Once you've established and recorded your plan of care, you'll begin to implement it. You'll find that your interventions fall into two general categories: interdependent and independent. Before performing either type, you'll need to make a brief reassessment.

Need for reassessment

Just before performing a particular intervention, quickly reassess the patient to ensure that your plan of care remains appropriate. For example, what if the plan calls for helping the patient walk every 2 hours throughout the day, but your reassessment reveals that he recently returned from a physical therapy session and feels fatigued? In this case, making the patient walk would be inappropriate — despite the plan of care.

Types of interventions

Interdependent interventions include those you perform in collaboration with other health care professionals to help achieve a patient outcome. For example, if the outcome calls for the patient to walk independently on level surfaces, you'd support the physical therapist's regimen by reinforcing positioning and ambulation techniques between therapy sessions.

Interdependent interventions also include activities you perform at a doctor's request to help implement the medical regimen. These activities include administering medications and performing invasive procedures, such as indwelling urinary catheter insertion and venipuncture.

Independent interventions are measures you take at your own discretion, independent of other health care team members. Such interventions include instituting common comfort measures and teaching routine self-care techniques.

Documenting interventions

You need to record the fact that you performed an intervention, the time you performed it, the patient's response to it, and any additional interventions that you took based on his response (including your reasons for these additional interventions). Recording all this information makes your documentation outcome-oriented.

You can document interventions on graphic records, a patient care flow sheet that integrates all nurses' notes for a 1-day period, integrated or separate nurses' progress notes, and other specialized documentation forms, such as the medication administration record (MAR). Your facility's policies will dictate the exact style, format, and location of your documentation. You'll record interventions when you give routine care, observe changes in the patient's condition, provide emergency care, and administer medications. (See chapter 9, Documentation of Everyday Events, and chapter 10, Legally Perilous Charting Practices, for more information on charting specific interventions.)

Routine care

For years, JCAHO has encouraged health care facilities to use flow sheets for documenting routine care measures. In response, many facilities have developed these forms for such measures as making basic assessments, giving wound care, and providing hygiene. In many facilities, you may also use flow sheets to document vital signs checks, I.V. monitoring, equipment checks, patient education, and discharge summaries. Some flow sheets are simple patient care checklists; others provide space for you to record specific care given. (See chapter 4, Documentation Systems, for more information on flow sheets and samples of different types.)

Because of their brevity, flow sheets make documenting and reviewing documented material quick and easy. Specifically, they allow you to evaluate patient trends at a glance. But keep in mind that overusing flow sheets can lead to fragmented documentation that may obscure the patient's clinical picture.

Changes in condition

In your progress notes, you'll need to document any changes in your patient's condition. Suppose, for instance, that you observe a sudden increase in your patient's wound drainage. In a narrative format, your progress note describing this observation should look something like the sample note on the next page.

This example refers to a practice guideline or standard of care for patients with a nursing diagnosis of impaired skin integrity. Because this protocol mandates cleaning with 0.9% sodium chloride solution and culture and sensitivity testing for a patient with purulent wound drainage, no further orders or clarification are required.

2/5/99	1100	Left arm wound drainage has saturated six 4" x 4" gauze pads and one 4" x 8" dressing since last dressing check at 1000. Wound dimensions remain as on 2/4/99 note, but drainage now dark yellow and foul-smelling. Obtained specimens for culture and sensitivity testing and sent to the lab per impaired skin integrity practice guidelines. Cleaned wound with 0.9% sodium chloride solution. (See plan of care for dressing change orders.) Pt. states, "My arm is really throbbing." Administered Darvocet-N and repositioned patient to semi-Fowler's position with left arm supported on pillow.
		Louise Davis, RN

The note also directs the reader to the patient's plan of care for specific dressing change methods. The reader would also know to check the MAR for specific information about the pain medication given.

The note goes on to specify information about the other pain-relief measure implemented as well as the patient's comments about the pain's characteristics. It doesn't repeat information recorded elsewhere in the chart, so it's concise yet informative.

Patient teaching

With each patient, you'll need to implement the teaching plan you've created and evaluate its effectiveness. Of course, you'll also need to clearly and completely document your teaching sessions and the results. Doing so provides a permanent legal record of the extent and success of teaching. Thus, your documentation may serve as your defense against charges of insufficient patient care — even years later. Clear documentation also helps administrators gauge the overall worth of a specific patient-education program as well as helping you support your requests for improving patient care.

Direct benefits

Documenting exactly what you've taught the patient also saves time by preventing duplication of patient-teaching efforts by other staff members. By checking your notes, another nurse can determine precisely what's been covered and what she should teach next, without skipping essential information. This is important for patients with complicated needs who may receive care from several nurses.

Take the case of a hypertensive patient who requires instruction in several areas, including diet, medication, exercise, and self-care. Successful teaching hinges on a clear record of what's been taught by everyone involved in his care. When staff members communicate by documenting what they've taught and how well the patient has learned, the teaching plan can be evaluated and revised as needed and the patient will get the care he needs.

You can also use your documentation to help motivate your patient. As appropriate, show him your record of his learning successes and encourage him to continue. Moreover, by recording the patient's response to your teaching and your assessment of his progress, you're gathering some of the data necessary to evaluate the effectiveness of your teaching, the patient's degree of knowledge or competency, and the appropriateness of his learning outcomes.

Documentation tools
In many facilities, you'll document patient teaching on preprinted forms that become part of the clinical record. Using these forms not only makes documentation quicker, but also ensures that it's complete. If your facility doesn't have a preprinted form, you might talk to your supervisor about developing one. In the meantime, write accurate, detailed narrative notes to document your patient teaching.

Whether you use a preprinted form or narrative notes, keep these tips in mind:

- Check your facility's policies and procedures regarding when, where, and how to document your teaching.
- Each shift, ask yourself these questions: "What part of the teaching plan did I complete?" and "What other teaching have I given this patient or his family members?" Then document your answers.
- Make sure that your documentation indicates that the patient's ongoing educational needs are being met.
- Before discharge, document the patient's remaining learning needs.

Patient discharge

JCAHO requirements specify that when preparing a patient for discharge, you must document your assessment of his continuing care needs as well as referrals for such care. To facilitate this documentation (and to save charting time), many facilities have developed forms that combine discharge summaries and patient instructions. (See *Discharge summaries,* page 262.)

This documentation tool combines all the essential information required on a discharge summary as well as the instructions given to the patient. Typically, you'll keep one copy of the form in the medical record and give one copy to the patient. The copy you keep can then provide useful information for further teaching and evaluation.

Of course, not all facilities use these forms; some still require a narrative discharge summary. If you must use this type of documentation, be sure to include the following information:

- patient's status on admission and discharge
- significant highlights of the hospitalization
- outcomes of your interventions
- resolved and unresolved patient problems, continuing care needs for unresolved problems, and specific referrals for continuing care
- instructions given to the patient or family member about medications, treatments, activity, diet, referrals, and follow-up appointments, as well as any other special instructions.

Evaluation

The current emphasis on evaluating your interventions has changed documentation. Traditional documentation methods didn't always reflect the end results of nursing care. Today, however, your progress notes must include an assessment of your patient's progress toward the expected outcomes you established in the plan of care.

This new method, called *outcomes and evaluation documentation,* focuses on the patient's response to nursing care and thus enables the

BETTER CHARTING

Discharge summaries

By combining the patient's discharge summary with instructions for care after discharge, you can fulfill two requirements with a single form. When using this documentation method, be sure to give one copy to the patient and keep one for the record.

DISCHARGE INSTRUCTIONS

1. **Summary** Tara Nicholas is a 55-year-old woman admitted with complaints of severe headache and hypertensive crisis.
   Treatment: Nipride gtt for 24 hours
   Started Lopressor for hypertension
   Recommendation: Lose 10-15 lbs
   Follow low-sodium, low-cholesterol diet
2. **Allergies** penicillin
3. **Medications (drug, dose time)** Lopressor 25 mg at 6am and 6pm
   temazepam 15 mg at 10pm
4. **Diet** Low-sodium, low-cholesterol
5. **Activity** As tolerated
6. **Discharged to** Home
7. **If questions arise, contact Dr.** James Pritchett **Telephone No.** 525-1448
8. **Special instructions**
9. **Return visit Dr.** Pritchett **Place** Health Care Clinic
   On Date 12/15/99 **Time** 8:45 am

Tara Nicholas — **Signature of patient for receipt of instructions from doctors**

JE PRITCHETT MD — **Signature of doctor giving instructions**

nurse to provide high-quality, cost-effective care. It's now replacing narrative charting and lengthy, handwritten plans of care. (See *Writing clear evaluation statements.*)

The belief that hands-on care is more important than documentation is one reason why nurses often focus more on nursing interventions than on documenting patient responses. Outcomes and evaluation documentation forces nurses to focus on patient responses. When you evaluate the results of

Writing clear evaluation statements

Below you'll find examples of clear evaluation statements describing common outcomes. Note that they include specific details of care provided and objective evidence of the patient's response to care.

Response to p.r.n. medication within 1 hour of administration

- "Pt. states pain decreased from 8 to 4 (on a scale of 1 to 10) 10 minutes after receiving I.V. morphine."
- "Vomiting subsided 1 hr after 25 mg P.O. of prochlorperazine."

Response to patient education

- "Able to describe the signs and symptoms of a postoperative wound infection."'
- "Despite repeated attempts, pt. couldn't identify signs of hypoglycemia."

Tolerance of change or increase in activity

- "Able to walk across the room, approximately 15 feet, without dyspnea."
- "Became fatigued after 5 minutes of assisted ambulation."

Ability to perform activities of daily living, particularly those that may influence discharge planning

- "Unable to wash self independently because of left-sided weakness."
- "Requires a walker to ambulate to bathroom."

Tolerance of treatments

- "Consumed full liquid lunch; pt. stated she was hungry and wanted solid food."
- "Skin became pink and less dusky 15 minutes after nasal O_2 was administered at 4 L/min."
- "Unable to tolerate having head of bed lowered from 90 degrees to 45 degrees; became dyspneic."

your interventions, you help ensure that your plan is working.

Evaluation of care gives the nurse a chance to:

- determine if her original assessment findings still apply
- uncover complications
- analyze patterns or trends in the patient's care and his responses to it
- assess the patient's response to all aspects of care, including medications, changes in diet or activity, procedures, unusual incidents or problems, and teaching
- determine how closely care conforms with established standards
- measure how well she has cared for the patient
- assess the performance of other members of the health care team
- identify opportunities to improve the quality of care.

When to perform evaluation

Although evaluation is an ongoing process that takes place whenever you see your patient, how often you're required to make evaluations will be influenced by several factors, including where you work. If you work in an acute care setting, your facility's policy may require you to review plans of care every 24 hours. If you work in a long-term care facility, the required interval between evaluations may be up to 30 days. In either case, this doesn't mean that you shouldn't evaluate and revise the plan of care more often, if warranted.

Evaluating expected outcomes

Evaluation includes gathering reassessment data, comparing findings with the outcome criteria, determining the extent of outcome achievement (outcome met, partially met, or not met), writing evaluation statements, and revising the plan of care.

Revision starts with determining whether the patient has achieved the expected outcomes. If they have been fully met, and you decide that the problem is resolved, the plan can be discontinued. If the problem persists, the plan continues—with new target dates—until the desired status is achieved.

If outcomes have been partially met or unmet, you must identify interfering factors, such as misinterpreted information, and revise the plan accordingly. This may involve the following:

- clarifying or amending the database to reflect newly discovered information
- reexamining and correcting nursing diagnoses
- establishing outcome criteria that reflect new information and new or amended nursing strategies
- adding the revised nursing plan of care to the original document
- recording the rationale for the revisions in the nurse's progress notes.

Documenting evaluation

Evaluation statements should indicate whether expected outcomes were achieved and should list evidence supporting this conclusion. Base these statements on outcome criteria from the plan of care, and use active verbs, such as "demonstrate" or "ambulate." Include the patient's response to specific treatments (such as medication administration or physical therapy), and describe the conditions under which the response occurred or failed to occur. Document patient teaching and palliative or preventive care as well.

After evaluating the outcome, be sure to record it in the patient's chart with clear statements that demonstrate the patient's progress toward meeting the expected outcomes.

Selected references

Barnes, L.P. "Patient Teaching: Documentation of Patient Teaching," *American Journal of Maternal-Child Nursing* 21(2):111, March-April 1996.

"Charting Tips: How to Document Objectively," *Nursing97* 27(7):17, July 1997.

Chase, S.K. "Charting Critical Thinking: Nursing Judgments and Patient Outcomes," *Dimensions of Critical Care Nursing* 16(2):102-11, March-April 1997.

Godchaux, C.W., et al. "A Continuum of Care Model," *Nursing Management* 28(11):73-76, November 1997.

McCloskey, J.C., and Bulechek, G.M. "Discharge Planning," in *Nursing Interventions Classifications,* 2nd ed. St. Louis: Mosby–Year Book, Inc., 1996.

Mefford, J. "Order in a New Era: Outcome Documentation," *Caring* 15(6):18, 20, 23, June 1996.

North, S.D., and Serkes, P.C., "Improved Documentation of Initial Nursing Assessment," *Nursing Management* 27(4):30, 33, April 1996.

9

Documentation of Everyday Events

Your patient's chart communicates important information about his condition and course of treatment to other nurses and members of the health care team. Without this record, neither you nor other caregivers can do the job effectively. That's why incomplete or improper charting has enormous implications.

Poor charting poses a threat to your patient's health and to your career as well. To avert serious problems, take the time to document not only accurately, objectively, and thoroughly but also consistently and legibly—in both routine and exceptional situations.

In this chapter, you'll read about specific situations that you may encounter in your practice. Each situation is followed by a documentation example. Among the situations discussed are routine nursing procedures, common charting flaws, patient noncompliance, interdisciplinary communication, doctors' orders, and incidents.

Routine nursing procedures

Your notes about routine nursing procedures should appear in the patient's chart. Include information about the procedure, who performed it, how it was performed, how the patient tolerated it (if applicable), and any subsequent adverse effects (if applicable). Also include any patient teaching that was provided before and after the procedure.

Typically, your documentation will include drug administration, I.V. therapy, supportive care, assistive procedures, infection control, diagnostic tests, pain control, codes, change in patient's condition, intake and output monitoring, skin and wound care, patient's personal property, shift reports, and patient teaching. Some facilities use flow sheets to document repetitive procedures, such as wound care and I.V. therapy.

Drug administration

Your employer probably includes a medication administration record (MAR) in your documentation system. Commonly included in a card file (a medication Kardex) or on a separate medication administration sheet, the MAR serves as the central record of medication orders and their execution and part of the patient's permanent record.

When using the MAR, follow these guidelines:

- Know and follow your facility's policies and procedures for recording drug orders and charting drug administration.
- Make sure that all drug orders include the patient's full name, the date, the drug's name, dose, administration route or method, and frequency. When appropriate, include the specific number of doses given or the stop date. When administering a drug dose immediately—or stat—be sure to record the time. Also be certain to include drug allergy information.
- Write legibly.
- Use only standard abbreviations approved by your facility. When doubtful about an abbreviation, write out the word or phrase.
- After administering the first dose, sign your full name, licensure status, and initials in the appropriate space on the MAR.
- When transcribing a one-time order to be given on another shift, be sure to communicate information to the next shift during report, or use a medication alert sticker to flag the order.

- Record drugs immediately after administration so that another nurse doesn't give the drug again. (See *The medication Kardex,* pages 268 and 269.)

If you document medication administration by computer, chart your information for each drug right after you give it. This is particularly important if you don't use printouts as a backup. By keying in information immediately, you ensure that all health care team members have access to the latest drug administration data for the patient.

If you can't administer a prescribed drug as scheduled, document the reason (for example, the patient is having a test, which requires him not to take the drug). Many nurses omit this important step.

Occasionally, you may suspect a connection between a patient's medication and an adverse event, such as illness, injury, or even death. In such a case, follow your facility's policy on reporting adverse drug events. This information should be reported to the Food and Drug Administration (FDA) on a MedWatch form issued by the FDA. (See *Reporting adverse events and product problems to the FDA,* pages 270 and 271.)

Drugs given p.r.n.

Chart all drugs administered as needed (p.r.n.). For eye, ear, or nose drops, chart the number of drops and where they were inserted. For suppositories, chart the type of suppository (rectal, vaginal, or urethral) and how the patient tolerated it. For dermal drugs, chart the size and location of the area to which you applied the drug, and describe the condition of the skin or wound. For dermal patches, chart the location of the patch.

If you administer all drugs according to the accepted standards, you don't need to include more specific information in the chart. However, if the MAR doesn't include space to document exceptional data (such as the patient's response to drugs given p.r.n. or deviations from the drug order, such as patient refusal), document the information as narrative in the chart.

2/8/99	0900	Pt. refused KCL elixir, stating
		that it makes her feel nauseat-
		ed and that she can't stand
		the taste. Dr. Miller notified.
		K-Dur tabs ordered and given.
		Pt. tolerated K-Dur well. ———
		——————— Betty Griffin, RN

Single-dose medications

Single-dose medications, which can include a supplemental dose or a stat dose, should be documented not only in the MAR, but also in the progress notes. Your documentation should include who gave the order, why the order was given, and the patient's response to the medication. For example, if you gave a one-time order of I.V. Lasix, you would write:

2/3/99	0900	Lasix 40 mg given as per Dr.
		Singh's order. Pt. with SOB,
		crackles bilaterally, and O_2
		saturation decreased to 89%
		on room air.
2/3/99	1000	Pt. responded with urine out-
		put of 1500 ml, decreased SOB,
		and O_2 saturation increased to
		97% on room air. ———
		——————— Ann Barrow, RN.

Narcotic drugs

When you administer a narcotic, you must give the drug and document administration

(Text continues on page 272.)

BETTER CHARTING

The medication Kardex

One type of Kardex is the medication Kardex. It contains a permanent record of the patient's medications. The medication Kardex may also include the patient's diagnosis and information about allergies and diet. A sample form is shown below.

NURSE'S FULL SIGNATURE, STATUS AND INITIALS

	INIT.		INIT.		INIT.
Roy Charles, RN	RC				
Theresa Hopkins, RN	TH				

DIAGNOSIS: Heart failure, Atrial flutter

ALLERGIES: ASA DIET: Cardiac

ROUTINE/DAILY ORDERS/FINGERSTICKS/ INSULIN COVERAGE			DATE: 1/24		DATE: 1/25		DATE: 1/26		DATE:		DATE:		DATE:		DATE:		DATE:		DATE:		DATE:	
ORDER DATE	MEDICATIONS DOSE, ROUTE, FREQUENCY	TIME	SITE	INT.	SITE	INT.	SITE	INT.	SITE	INT.	SITE	INT.	SITE	INT.	SITE	INT.	SITE	INT.	SITE	INT.	SITE	INT.
1/24/99	digoxin 0.125 mg	0900	Ⓡ S.C.	RC																		
RC	I.V. q.d.	HR	68																			
1/24/99	furosemide 40 mg	0900	Ⓡ S.C.	RC																		
RC	I.V. q12h	2100	Ⓡ S.C.	TH																		
1/24/99	enalapril 1.25 mg	0511	Ⓡ S.C.	TH																		
RC	I.V. q6h	1100	Ⓡ S.C.	RC																		
		1700	Ⓡ S.C.	RC																		
1/24/99	vancomycin 1 g I.V. q.d.	2100	Ⓡ S.C.	TH																		
TH																						

The medication Kardex *(continued)*

Addressograph

PRN MEDICATION

ALLERGIES:

INITIAL	SIGNATURE & STATUS	INITIAL	SIGNATURE & STATUS	INITIAL	SIGNATURE & STATUS	INITIAL	SIGNATURE & STATUS
RC	Roy Charles, RN						
TH	Theresa Hopkins, RN						

YEAR 19 99 — P.R.N. MEDICATIONS

ORDER DATE	RENEWAL DATE	DISCONTINUED DATE	MEDICATION	DOSE	DIRECTION	ROUTE												
1/24	/	/	acetaminophen	650 mg	p.r.n. mild pain	P.O.	DATE	1/24										
							TIME GIVEN	0930										
							SITE	P.O.										
							INIT.	RC										
1/24	/	/	MSO4	2 mg	15 minutes prior to changing Ⓡ heel dressing	I.V.	DATE	1/24										
							TIME GIVEN	0930										
							SITE	Ⓡ s.c.										
							INIT.	RC										
1/24	/	/	Milk of Magnesia	30ml	q6h p.r.n.	P.O.	DATE	1/24										
							TIME GIVEN	2115										
							SITE	P.O.										
							INIT.	TH										
1/25	/	1/25	prochlorperazine	5 mg	q8h p.r.n. prn nausea and vomiting	p.O.	DATE	1/25										
							TIME GIVEN	1100	2230									
							SITE	Ⓡglut.	Ⓛglut.									
							INIT.	RC	TH									
/	/	/					DATE											
							TIME GIVEN											
							SITE											
							INIT.											
/	/	/					DATE											
							TIME GIVEN											
							SITE											
							INIT.											
/	/	/					DATE											
							TIME GIVEN											
							SITE											
							INIT.											

BETTER CHARTING

Reporting adverse events and product problems to the FDA

Even large, well-designed clinical trials can't guarantee that adverse reactions will never arise after a drug or medical device is approved for use. An adverse reaction that occurs in only 1 in 5,000 patients could easily be missed in clinical trials. The drug could also interact with other drugs in ways unrevealed during clinical trials.

As a nurse, you play a key role in reporting adverse events and product problems. Reporting such problems helps ensure the safety of products that the Food and Drug Administration (FDA) regulates. The FDA's Medical Products Reporting Program supplies health care professionals with MedWatch forms on which they can report adverse events and product problems.

What to report

Complete a MedWatch form when you suspect that a drug, a medical device, a special nutritional product, or other products regulated by the FDA are responsible for:

- death
- life-threatening illness
- initial or prolonged hospitalization
- disability
- congenital anomaly
- the need for any medical or surgical intervention to prevent a permanent impairment or an injury.

Also, promptly inform the FDA of product quality problems, such as:

- defective devices
- inaccurate or unreadable product labels
- packaging or product mixups
- intrinsic or extrinsic contamination or stability problems
- particulates in injectable drugs
- product damage.

Your responsibility in reporting

When filing a MedWatch form, keep in mind that you're not expected to establish a connection between the product and the problem. You don't have to include a lot of details; you only have to report the adverse event or the problem with the drug or the product.

What's more, you don't even have to wait until the evidence seems compelling. FDA regulations protect your identity and the identities of your patient and employer.

Further guidelines

The MedWatch form merges the individual forms used in the past to report adverse drug reactions, drug quality product problems, device quality product problems, and adverse reactions to medical devices. Send completed forms to the FDA by using the fax number or mailing address on the form.

File a separate MedWatch form for each patient, and attach additional pages if needed. If appropriate, report product problems to the manufacturer as well as to the FDA. Also remember to comply with your health care facility's protocols for reporting adverse events associated with drugs and medical devices.

Product lot numbers are used in product identification, tracking, and product recall; therefore, the lot number should be retained and a copy of the report should be kept on file by your supervisor.

FDA response

The FDA will report back to you on the actions it takes and will continue to work to instruct health care professionals about adverse events.

MEDWATCH

THE FDA MEDICAL PRODUCTS REPORTING PROGRAM

For VOLUNTARY reporting by health professionals of adverse events and product problems

Page 1 of 1

Form Approved: OMB No. 0910-0291 Expires: 4/30/96
See OMB statement on reverse

FDA Use Only

Triage unit sequence #

A. Patient information

1. **Patient identifier** In confidence
2. **Age at time of event:** or **Date of birth:**
3. **Sex** ☑ female ☐ male
4. **Weight** ___ lbs or 59 kgs

B. Adverse event or product problem

1. ☐ **Adverse event** and/or ☐ **Product problem** (e.g., defects/malfunctions)
2. **Outcomes attributed to adverse event** (check all that apply)
   - ☐ death ______ (mo/day/yr)
   - ☐ life-threatening
   - ☐ hospitalization – initial or prolonged
   - ☐ disability
   - ☐ congenital anomaly
   - ☐ required intervention to prevent permanent impairment/damage
   - ☐ other: ______
3. **Date of event** (mo/day/yr) 3/8/99
4. **Date of this report** (mo/day/yr) 3/8/99
5. **Describe event or problem**

   After Reconstituting 100 mg Vial with 10 ml. of bacteriostatic water, the drug crystallized and turned yellow.

   Drug was not given.
6. **Relevant tests/laboratory data,** including dates
7. **Other relevant history, including preexisting medical conditions** (e.g., allergies, race, pregnancy, smoking and alcohol use, hepatic/renal dysfunction, etc.)

PLEASE TYPE OR USE BLACK INK

C. Suspect medication(s)

1. **Name** (give labeled strength & mfr/labeler, if known)
   #1 Leucovorin Calcium for
   #2 Injection — 100 mg. vil
2. **Dose, frequency & route used**
   #1 100 mg. IV X 1
   #2
3. **Therapy dates** (if unknown, give duration) from/to (or best estimate)
   #1 3/8/99
   #2
4. **Diagnosis for use** (indication)
   #1 Megaloblastic Anemia
   #2
5. **Event abated after use stopped or dose reduced**
   #1 ☐ yes ☐ no ☐ doesn't apply
   #2 ☐ yes ☐ no ☐ doesn't apply
6. **Lot #** (if known)
   #1 #891
   #2
7. **Exp. date** (if known)
   #1
   #2
8. **Event reappeared after reintroduction**
   #1 ☐ yes ☐ no ☐ doesn't apply
   #2 ☐ yes ☐ no ☐ doesn't apply
9. **NDC #** (for product problems only)
   – –
10. **Concomitant medical products** and therapy dates (exclude treatment of event)

D. Suspect medical device

1. **Brand name**
2. **Type of device**
3. **Manufacturer name & address**
4. **Operator of device**
   - ☐ health professional
   - ☐ lay user/patient
   - ☐ other: ______
5. **Expiration date** (mo/day/yr)
6. model # ______
   catalog # ______
   serial # ______
   lot # ______
   other # ______
7. **If implanted, give date** (mo/day/yr)
8. **If explanted, give date** (mo/day/yr)
9. **Device available for evaluation?** (Do not send to FDA)
   ☑ yes ☐ no ☐ returned to manufacturer on ______ (mo/day/yr)
10. **Concomitant medical products** and therapy dates (exclude treatment of event)

E. Reporter (see confidentiality section on back)

1. **Name & address**
   Patricia Cohen
   987 Elm Ave
   Cincinatti, Ohio

   phone #
2. **Health professional?** ☑ yes ☐ no
3. **Occupation** RN
4. **Also reported to**
   - ☐ manufacturer
   - ☐ user facility
   - ☑ distributor
5. **If you do NOT want your identity disclosed to the manufacturer, place an " X " in this box.** ☐

FDA

Mail to: MEDWATCH
5600 Fishers Lane
Rockville, MD 20852-9787

or **FAX to:**
1-800-FDA-0178

FDA Form 3500 1/96)

Submission of a report does not constitute an admission that medical personnel or the product caused or contributed to the event.

according to federal, state, and institutional regulations. These regulations require narcotic drugs to be counted after each nursing shift to ensure an accurate drug count. Before administering a narcotic, verify the amount of drug in the container, and sign out the medication on the appropriate form.

Many facilities now use an automated storage system for narcotics that eliminates the need for counting the narcotics at end of shift. This system allows the nurse easy access (via an ID and password) to medications (including other drugs and floor stocks for nursing units). Nurses may remove one or more medications by selecting the patient, medication, and amount needed on the keypad. The nurse must then count the amount of the drug remaining in the system and enter it. Each transaction is recorded and copies are sent to the pharmacy and billing department.

Many facilities still require that a second nurse document your activity and observe you if a narcotic or part of a dose must be wasted.

If you discover a discrepancy in the narcotic count, follow your employer's policy for reporting this and file an incident report. An investigation will follow.

I.V. THERAPY

Currently, more than 80% of hospitalized patients receive some form of I.V. therapy. Whether providing fluid or electrolyte replacement, total parenteral nutrition (TPN), drugs, or blood products, you'll need to carefully document all facets of I.V. therapy — including not only administration but also subsequent complications of I.V. therapy.

Keep in mind that an accurate description of your care provides a clear record of treatments and drugs received by your patient. This record provides legal protection for you and your employer and furnishes health care insurers with the data they need to approve and provide reimbursement for equipment and supplies.

Depending on your facility's policy, you'll document I.V. therapy on a special I.V. therapy sheet or nursing flow sheet or in another format. (See *Using a flow sheet to document I.V. therapy.*)

If venipuncture requires more than one attempt, document the number of attempts made and the type of assistance required. Be sure to follow your facility's policy regarding this.

When you establish an I.V. route, remember to document the date, time, and venipuncture site together with the equipment used, such as the type and gauge of catheter or needle. You'll need to update your records each time you change the insertion site and change the venipuncture device or the I.V. tubing. Also document any reason for changing the I.V. site, such as extravasation, phlebitis, occlusion, patient removal, or a routine change according to facility policy.

1/16/99	0200	Pt. complained of pain in Ⓛ
		hand at I.V. site. Hand red-
		dened from I.V. insertion site
		to 2" above site, tender and
		warm to touch. Slight swelling
		noted. I.V. discontinued and a
		warm, moist towel applied to
		left hand. I.V. started in right
		forearm. ————
		———— Kathy Costello, RN

On each shift, be sure to document the type, amount, and flow rate of I.V. fluid, along with the condition of the I.V. site. Document each time that you flush the I.V. line, and identify any medication used to flush the line as well.

BETTER CHARTING

Using a flow sheet to document I.V. therapy

This sample shows the typical features of an I.V. therapy flow sheet.

I.V. THERAPY FLOW SHEET

Diagnosis: ® mastectomy
Venipuncture limitations: Ⓛ arm only
Permanent access: None

Date and time	1/14/99 1400	1/15/99 0800						
Patient visit	2	1						
Site status	1	1						
Procedure	R	C						
Gauge I.V. device	20	✓						
Catheter type	J	J						
Location	LPF	LPF						
Date of insertion	1/14	1/15						
Routine site rotation	—	—						
Phlebitis	1 +	1						
Infiltration	1	0						
Other	1	—						
No. of failed attempts	0	—						
Lock status	—	—						
Flush	—	—						
Tubing: Macrodrip	✓	✓						
Minidrip								
Valleylab								
Filter								
Extension	✓	✓						
Dressing change	✓	—						
Blood sample drawn	—	—						
Subcutaneous access port	—	—						
Patient response	1	1						
Patient teaching	1	1						
Nurse's initials	BG	KC						

Initials	**Signature**	**Initials**	**Signature**
BG	Betty Griffin, RN		
KC	Kathy Collins, RN		

(continued)

DOCUMENTATION OF EVERYDAY EVENTS

Using a flow sheet to document I.V. therapy *(continued)*

Date	Time	Patient care notes
1/14/99	400	I.V. D5-½NSS c̄ 40 mEq KCL infusing @ 125 ml/hr. ———— Patricia Quinn, LPN

KEY

Patient visit
- 1 Routine rounds
- 2 Unit request
- 3 Patient not available for rounds

Site status
- 1 Within normal limits
- 2 Dressing intact

Procedure
- S Start
- R Restart
- C Check
- D Discontinue
- CD Cutdown

Catheter type
- GR Groshong catheter
- PICC Peripherally inserted central catheter
- TL Triple-lumen catheter
- HI Hickman catheter
- SC Subclavian catheter
- SG Swan-Ganz catheter
- TE Tenckhoff catheter
- BR Broviac catheter

Location
- RH Right hand
- RW Right wrist
- RA Right arm
- RPF Right posterior forearm
- RC Right cubital
- RU Right upper arm
- LH Left hand
- LW Left wrist
- LA Left arm
- LPF Left posterior forearm
- LC Left cubital
- LU Left upper arm
- RF Right foot
- LF Left foot
- RJ Right jugular
- LJ Left jugular
- AB Abdomen

Phlebitis
- 1 No pain to slight pain at site; erythema and no edema; no streak; no palpable cord
- 1+ Pain at site; erythema and/or edema; no streak, no palpable cord
- 2+ Pain at site; erythema and/or edema; streak formation; nonpalpable cord
- 3+ Pain at site; erythema and/or edema; streak formation; palpable cord

Infiltration
- 0+ Slight edema — no infiltration
- 1+ Slight puffiness at site
- 2+ Swelling above or below site
- 3+ Skin cool and pale; large area of swelling above or below site

Other
- 1 Leaking
- 2 Occluded
- 3 Patient removed catheter
- 4 Other (see patient care notes)

Lock status
- 1 Site locked
- 2 Site unlocked
- 3 Caps changed

Heparin flush
- 1 Heparin
- 2 Saline

Patient response
- 1 Patient tolerated
- 2 Unresponsive
- 3 Patient agitated/combative
- 4 Other (see patient care notes)

Patient teaching
- 1 Patient/family member indicates understanding procedure
- 2 Instructed to call nurse for signs of redness, swelling, leaking, pain, or problem
- 3 Patient unable to comprehend

Take the time to document any complication precisely. For example, if extravasation occurs, stop the I.V. Then assess the amount of fluid infiltrated, provide appropriate nursing intervention, and notify the doctor. Be sure to document all pertinent information.

If a chemotherapeutic drug extravasates, follow the procedure specified by your facility. In the chart, document the appearance of the I.V. site, the type of treatment given (especially any drug used as an antidote), the kind of dressing applied to the site, and that the doctor was notified. Also be sure to record every time that you flush this kind of I.V. line and the type and amount of fluid used.

If an allergic reaction occurs while the patient is receiving I.V. therapy, notify the doctor immediately and complete an adverse reaction form. Document all pertinent information about the reaction, such as the type of reaction, when the reaction was identified, the extent of the reaction, and that it was reported to the doctor. In addition, you must document treatments and the patient's response to them.

Record any patient teaching that you perform with the patient and his family, such as explaining the purpose of I.V. therapy, describing the procedure itself, and discussing any possible complications.

Total parenteral nutrition

If a patient is receiving TPN, document the type and location of the central line, the condition of the insertion site, and the volume and rate of the solution infused. Monitor any patient receiving TPN for adverse reactions and document your observations and interventions.

When you discontinue a central or peripheral I.V. line for TPN, record the date and time and the type of dressing applied. Also describe the appearance of the administration site.

Blood transfusions

Whether you administer blood or blood components, such as packed cells, plasma, platelets, or cryoprecipitates, you must use proper identification and cross-matching procedures to ensure that the patient receives the correct blood product for transfusion. After matching the patient's name, medical record number, blood group (or type) and Rh factor (both the patient's and the donor's), the cross-match data, and the blood bank identification number with the label on the blood bag, clearly document that you did so. The blood or blood component must be identified and documented properly by two health care professionals as well.

Once you have determined that all the information is correct and matches, the consent form has been signed, and the patient's vital signs are within acceptable parameters per your facility's policy, you may administer the transfusion. On the transfusion record, document the date and time the transfusion was started and completed, the name of the health care professional that verified the information, the type and gauge of the catheter, and the total amount of the transfusion. Also record the patient's vital signs before, during, and after the transfusion as well as any infusion device used, the flow rate, and any blood warming unit that was used.

If the patient receives his own blood, document the amount of autologous blood retrieved and reinfused in the intake and output records. Also monitor and document laboratory data during and after the autotransfusion as well as the patient's pre- and posttransfusion vital signs.

Pay particular attention to the patient's coagulation profile, hemoglobin and hematocrit values, and arterial blood gas (ABG) and calcium levels.

Transfusion reaction

During a blood transfusion, the patient is at risk for developing a transfusion reaction. If he develops a reaction, stop the transfusion immediately, take down the blood tubing, and hang new tubing with normal saline solution running to maintain vein patency. Notify the doctor and the laboratory.

Date	Time	Note
2/13/99	1400	Pt. reports chills. Cyanosis of the lips noted at 1350 hours, with PRBCs transfusing. Infusion stopped. Tubing changed. I.V. of 1,000 ml D_5NSS infusing at KVO rate in Ⓡ arm. Notified Dr. Cahill. BP, 168/88; P, 104; R, 25; T, 97.6° R. Blood sample taken from PRBCs. Two red-top tubes of blood drawn from pt. and sent to the laboratory. Urine specimen obtained from catheter. Urine specimen sent to lab for UA. Gave pt. diphenhydramine 50 mg I.M. Two blankets placed on pt.
	1415	Pt. reports he's getting warmer. BP 148/80; P, 96; R, 20; T, 97.6° R.
	1430	Pt. no longer complaining of chills. I.V. of 1,000 ml D_5NSS infusing at 125 ml/hr in Ⓡ arm. BP, 138/76; P, 80; R, 18; T, 98.4° R.
		Maryann Belinsky, RN

Be sure to document the time and date of the reaction, the type and amount of infused blood or blood products, the time you started the transfusion, and the time you stopped it.

Also record the clinical signs of the reaction in order of occurrence, the patient's vital signs, any urine specimen or blood sample sent to the laboratory for analysis, any treatment given, and the patient's response to the treatment.

Some health care facilities require the completion of a transfusion reaction report that must be sent to the blood bank. (See *Transfusion reaction report.*)

Supportive care procedures

Your daily nursing interventions constitute supportive care measures. Many of these can be documented on graphic forms and flow charts; others must be described in progress notes or other forms. Among the most commonly documented nursing interventions are those that are provided before and after a surgical procedure (for example, pacemaker insertion, paracentesis, peritoneal dialysis, peritoneal lavage, or thoracic drainage) and those provided to support the patient throughout treatment (for example, cardiac monitoring, chest physiotherapy, mechanical ventilation, nasogastric [NG] tube insertion and removal, seizure management, tube feedings, and withdrawing arterial blood for analysis).

Preoperative documentation

Effective nursing documentation during the preoperative period focuses on two primary elements — the baseline preoperative assessment and patient teaching. Documenting both of these elements encourages accurate communication among caregivers. Most facilities use a preoperative checklist to verify that required data have been collected, that preoperative teaching has occurred, and that prescribed procedures and safety precautions have been executed. (See *Preoperative checklist and surgical identification form,* page 280.)

BETTER CHARTING

Transfusion reaction report

If your facility requires a transfusion reaction report, you'll include the following types of information.

TRANSFUSION REACTION REPORT

Nursing report

1. Stop transfusion immediately. Keep I.V. line open with saline infusion.
2. Notify responsible physician.
3. Check all identifying names and numbers on the patient's wristband, unit, and paperwork for discrepancies.
4. Record patient's post-transfusion vital signs.
5. Draw posttransfusion blood samples (clotted and anticoagulated) avoiding mechanical hemolysis.
6. Collect posttransfusion urine specimen from patient.
7. Record information as indicated below.
8. Send discontinued bag of blood, administration set, attached I.V. solutions, and all related forms and labels to the Blood Bank with this form completed.

Clerical errors

☑ None detected
☐ Detected

Vital signs

	Pre-TXN	Post-TXN
Temp.	98.4°	98°
B.P.	120/60	134/80
Pulse	88	80

☑ Urticaria
☐ Fever
☐ Chills
☐ Chest pain
☐ Hypotension
☐ Nausea
☑ Flushing
☐ Dyspnea
☐ Headache
☐ Perspiration
☐ Shock
☐ Oozing
☐ Back pain
☐ Infusion site pain
☐ Hemoglobinuria
☐ Oliguria or anuria

Reaction occurred

During administration? yes
After administration?
How long?
Medications added?
Previous I.V. fluids? 1 unit FFP
Blood warmed? No

Specimen collection

Blood: Difficulty collecting?
Urine: Voided Yes – Sent lab Catheterized

Comments:

Signature Jacqueline Brown, RN **Date** 2/10/99

BLOOD BANK REPORT

Unit # 22FM80507

Component Returned Yes

Volume Returned 185 ml

1. Clerical errors

☑ None detected
☐ Detected

Comments:

2. Hemolysis:

Note: If hemolysis is present in the posttransfusion sample, a posttransfusion urine sample must be tested for free hemoglobin immediately.

Patient pre-TXN sample	☑ None	☐ Slight	☐ Moderate	☐ Marked
Patient post-TXN sample	☑ None	☐ Slight	☐ Moderate	☐ Marked
Blood Bag	☑ None	☐ Slight	☐ Moderate	☐ Marked
Urine HGB (centrifuged)	☐ None	☐ Slight	☑ Moderate	☐ Marked

(continued)

DOCUMENTATION OF EVERYDAY EVENTS

Transfusion reaction report *(continued)*

BLOOD BANK REPORT *(continued)*

3. Direct antiglobulin test

Pretransfusion ______ Posttransfusion ______

If No. 2 and No. 3 are negative, steps 4 through 6 are not required. Report results to the blood bank physician. Steps 7 and 8 or further testing will be done as ordered by blood bank physician.

4. ABO and Rh Groups

Repeat testing	Cell reaction with								Serum reaction with		ABO/Rh
	Anti-A	Anti-B	Anti-A,B	Anti-D	Cont.	Du	Cont.	CCC	A_1 cells	B cells	
Pretransfusion											
Posttransfusion											
Unit #											
Unit #											

5. Red cell antibody screen

		Saline/AB				INT
Pretransfusion	**Cell**	**RT**	**37°C**	**AHG**	**CCC**	
Date of sample	I					
	II					
By:	Auto					

		Saline/AB				INT
Posttransfusion	**Cell**	**RT**	**37°C**	**AHG**	**CCC**	
Date of sample	I					
	II					
By:	Auto					

Specificity of antibody detected:

6. Crossmatch compatibility testing

Use patient pre- and post-TXN serum and the suspected unit red cells obtained from inside the container or from a segment still attached to bag. Observe appearance of blood in bag and administration tubing.

	Albumin				INT
Pretransfusion	**RT**	**37°C**	**AHG**	**CCC**	
Unit #					
Unit #					

	Albumin				INT
Posttransfusion	**RT**	**37°C**	**AHG**	**CCC**	
Unit #					
Unit #					

All units on hold for future transfusion must be recrossmatched with the posttransfusion sample.

7. Bacteriologic testing

Pretransfusion ______ Posttransfusion ______

8. Other testing results

Total bilirubin

Patient pre-TXN ______ mg/dl

Patient 6 hrs. post-TXN ___ mg/dl

Coagulation studies

Urine output studies

Pathologist's conclusions:

Signature ______ **Date** ______

Be sure to document the name of the person you notified of any abnormalities that could affect the patient's response to the surgical procedure, or any deviations from facility standards. For example, if you find there is no completed history or physical, your note might read as follows:

3/14/99	0800	No completed history and physical found in pt's medical record. O.R. charge nurse, Margaret Little, notified. Also called Dr. Steven Adler's answering service. Message given to Operator 34. ——— Susan Altman, RN

Surgical incision care

Besides documenting vital signs and level of consciousness (LOC) when the patient returns from surgery, pay particular attention to maintaining records pertaining to the surgical incision and drains and the care you provide.

Also read the records that travel with the patient from the postanesthesia care unit. (See *Documenting postsurgical status,* page 281.) Look for a doctor's order directing whether you or the doctor will perform the first dressing change. The following features of documenting surgical wound care are important:

- the date, time, and type of wound care performed
- the wound's appearance (size, condition of margins, necrotic tissue if any), odor (if any), location of any drains, and drainage characteristics (type, color, consistency, and amount)
- dressing information, such as type and amount of new dressing or pouch applied
- additional wound care procedures provided, such as drain management, irrigation, packing, or application of a topical medication
- the patient's tolerance of the procedure.

Record special or detailed wound care instructions and pain management measures on the nursing plan of care. Document the color and amount of measurable drainage on the intake and output form.

2/10/99	0830	Dressing removed from midline abd. incision; no drainage noted on dressing. Incision well approximated and intact with staples. Margins ecchymotic; small amt. of serosanguineous drainage noted from distal portion of wound. Dry 4" x 4" sterile gauze pad applied. JP in LLQ draining serosanguineous fluid. Emptied 40 ml. JP drain intact. Insertion site without redness or drainage. Split 4" x 4" gauze applied to site and taped securely. ——— Grace Fedor, RN

If the patient will need wound care after discharge, provide and document appropriate instruction. The record should show that you explained aseptic technique, described how to examine the wound for signs of infection and other complications, demonstrated how to change the dressing, and provided written instructions for home care.

Pacemaker care

Record the type of pacemaker used, the date and time of pacemaker placement, the doctor who inserted it, the reason for placement, the pacemaker settings, and the patient's response.

Preoperative checklist and surgical identification form

To document preoperative procedures, data collection, and teaching, most facilities use a checklist like the one below.

Woodview
Hospital

Pre-Operative Checklist and Surgical Identification Form

Instructions: All items checked "No" requires follow up. Follow up is to be documented. In "Additional Information / Comment" section until resolved.

Pre-Op Checklist	Yes	No	Resolved	Initials
ID Band On	✔			NRC
Allergies Noted / Bracelet	✔			NRC
History & Physical (Present & Reviewed)	✔			NRC
Surgical Informed Consent Signed	✔			NRC
Anesthesia Informed Consent	✔			NRC
Pre-Op Teaching	✔			NRC
Prep. as Ordered	N/A			
NPO After Midnight	✔			NRC
Dentures, Capped Teeth, Cosmetics,		✔		
Glasses, Contact Lenses, Wig Removed	N/A			
Voided/Catheter Inserted	✔			NRC
Medical Clearance/Physician's Name	✔			NRC
TEDS, as Ordered	N/A			
SCD, as Ordered	N/A			
PCA Teaching, as Ordered	✔			NRC
Type & Cross/Screen Drawn (If Ordered Must Have Blood Informed Consent Signed) **Blood Informed Consent Signed	N/A			
*Lab Results on Chart	✔			NRC
*EKG on Chart	✔			NRC
*Chest X-ray on Chart	✔			NRC

*Abnormal Results Results Reported To H&H Dr. Schoblitz
Time & Date 4/28/99 0800
Reported By NRC

Temp. 98.6 Pulse 84 Resp. 18 B/P 132/82

Valuables
Destination: ❑ To Safe ❑ To Family, Name ______

✘ Norma R. Clay, RN NRC
Signature of Nurse Initials

✘ ______
Signature of Transferring RN Date Time

Additional Information /Comments

Surgical Patient Identification Form

Nursing Floor RN Patient Identification

- ☑ Patient I.D. Bracelet Personally Observed
- ☑ Patient Questioned Verbally Regarding I.D., Procedure & Site
- ❑ Patient's Chart Reviewed to Verify I.D., Procedure & Site

✘ Norma R. Clay, RN 4/28/99 0800
R.N.'s Signature Date Time

Pre-Op Anesthesia Patient Identification

- ❑ Patient's I.D. Bracelet Personally Observed
- ❑ Patient Questioned Verbally Regarding I.D., Procedure & Site
- ❑ Patient's Chart Reviewed to Verify I.D., Procedure & Site

✘ ______
Anesthesiologist/Anesthetist's Signature Date Time

Operating Room and Anesthesia Personnel Patient Identification

Operative Procedure & Site: ______

ANES	CIRC Nurse	
❑	❑	Patient I.D. Bracelet Personally Observed
❑	❑	Patient Questioned Verbally Regarding I.D., Procedure & Site
❑	❑	Patient's Chart Reviewed to Verify I.D., Procedure & Site
❑	❑	Surgical Site Confirmed

✘ ______
Anesthesiologist/Anesthetist's Signature Time

✘ ______
CIRC Nurse's Signature Time

Surgeon's Patient Identification Statement

- ❑ Patient I.D. Bracelet Personally Observed
- ❑ Patient Questioned Verbally Regarding I.D., Procedure & Site
- ❑ Surgical Site Marked

✘ ______
Surgeon's Signature Time

CHARTING GUIDELINES

Documenting postsurgical status

When your patient recovers sufficiently from the effects of anesthesia, he can be transferred from the operating room–postanesthesia care unit (OR–PACU) to his assigned unit for ongoing recovery and care. As the nurse on this service, you're responsible for the four-part documentation that travels with the patient. Here are some tips for making sure that all parts of the record are present and complete.

Part 1: History

Make sure that this section of the OR–PACU report includes the patient's pertinent medical and surgical history (information that might affect the patient's response to anesthesia and his postoperative course).

Include drug allergies, medication history, chronic illnesses (coronary artery disease or chronic obstructive pulmonary disease, for example), significant surgical history and hospitalizations, and smoking history.

Part 2: Operation

Check that the following information is recorded in this section of the report, describing the surgery itself:

- the procedure performed
- the type and dosage of anesthetics administered
- the length of time the patient was anesthetized
- the patient's vital signs throughout surgery
- the volume of fluid lost and replaced
- drugs administered
- surgical complications
- tourniquet time
- any drains, tubes, implants, or dressings used in surgery and removed or still in place.

Part 3: Postanesthesia period

Be certain that this part of the record includes information about:

- pain medications and pain control devices that the patient received and how he responded to them
- interventions that should continue on the unit. For example, if the patient underwent leg surgery and had a tourniquet on for a long time, he will need more frequent circulatory, motor, and neurologic checks. Or, if the anesthesiologist inserted an epidural catheter, the record should note any doctor's orders regarding medication administration or special care procedures.
- a flow sheet showing the patient's postanesthesia recovery scores on arrival and discharge in these areas: activity level, respiration, circulation, level of consciousness (LOC), and color
- an account of unusual events or complications that occurred on the PACU — for instance, nausea or vomiting, shivering, hypothermia, arrhythmias, central anticholinergic syndrome, sore throat, back or neck pain, corneal abrasion, tooth loss during intubation, swollen lips or tongue, pharyngeal or laryngeal abrasion, and postspinal headache.

Part 4: Current status

Expect this section to describe the patient's status at the time of transfer. Information should include patient's vital signs, LOC, and sensorium.

Document the patient's LOC and vital signs, noting which arm you used to obtain the blood pressure reading. Also note any complications (such as infection, chest pain, pacemaker malfunction, or arrhythmias) and interventions taken (such as X-ray studies to verify correct electrode placement).

Document the information obtained from a 12-lead electrocardiogram (ECG). Obtain and include rhythm strips in the medical record at these times: before, during, and after pacemaker placement; anytime pacemaker settings change; and anytime the patient receives treatment resulting from a pacemaker complication.

1/9/99	0920	Pt. c̄ temporary transvenous pacemaker in Ⓛ subclavian vein. Rate 70, mA2, mV full demand. 100% ventricular paced rhythm noted on monitor. ECG obtained. Pacer sensing & capturing correctly. Site w/o redness or swelling. Dressing D & I. ——— John Mora, RN

As ECG monitoring continues, note capture, sensing rate, intrinsic beats, and competition of paced and intrinsic rhythms.

If the patient has a transcutaneous pacemaker, document the reason for this kind of pacing, the time pacing started, and the locations of the electrodes.

Paracentesis

When caring for a patient during and after paracentesis, be sure to document the date and time of the procedure and the puncture site. Also record the amount, color, viscosity, and odor of the initially aspirated fluid in your notes and in the fluid intake and output record.

If you're responsible for ongoing patient care, be sure to keep a running record of the patient's vital signs and nursing activities related to drainage and to dressing changes. The record should indicate the frequency of drainage checks (typically, every 15 minutes for the first hour, every 30 minutes for the next 2 hours, every hour for the next 4 hours, then every 4 hours for the next 24 hours) and the patient's response to the procedure. Continue to document drainage characteristics, including color, amount, odor, and viscosity.

If peritoneal fluid leakage occurs, notify the doctor and document that you did so. Be sure to include the time and the date.

Also document daily patient weight and abdominal girth measurements before and after the procedure, the number of fluid specimens sent to the laboratory for analysis, and the total volume of fluid removed.

2/12/99	1100	After procedure explained to pt. and consent obtained, Dr. Novello performed paracentesis in RLQ as per protocol. 1,500 ml cloudy, pale-yellow fluid drained and sent to lab as ordered. Site sutured with one 3-0 silk suture. Sterile 4" x 4" gauze pad applied. No leakage noted at site. Abd. girth 44" preprocedure and 42 3/4" postprocedure. Pt. tolerated procedure w/o difficulty. VSS before and after procedure as per flow sheet. Emotional support given to pt. ——— Carol Barsky, RN

Peritoneal dialysis

During and after dialysis, monitor and document the patient's response to treatment. Record his vital signs every 10 to 15 minutes for the first 1 to 2 hours of exchanges, then every 2 to 4 hours or as often as necessary. If you detect any abrupt changes in the patient's condition, document them, notify the doctor, and document your notification.

Document the amount of dialysate infused and drained and any medications added. Be sure to complete a peritoneal dialysis flowchart every 24 hours. Keep a record of the effluent's characteristics and the assessed negative or positive fluid balance at the end of each infusion-dwell-drain cycle. Also record each time that you notify the doctor of an abnormality.

Chart the patient's daily weight (immediately after the drain phase) and abdominal girth. Note the time of day and any variations in the weighing-measuring technique. Also document physical assessment findings and fluid status daily.

Keep a record of equipment problems, such as kinked tubing or mechanical malfunction, and your interventions. Also note the condition of the patient's skin at the dialysis catheter site, the patient's reports of unusual discomfort or pain, and your interventions.

1/15/99	0700	Pt. receiving exchanges q 2 hr of 1,500 cc 4.25 dialysate with 500 units heparin and 2 mEq KCL. Dialysate infused over 15 min. Dwell time 75 min. Drain time 30 min. Drainage clear, pale-yellow fluid. (See flow sheet for fluid balance.) VSS. Pt. tolerates procedure. No cramping or discomfort. Skin warm, dry at RLQ catheter site and no redness. Dry split 4" x 4" dressing applied p̄ site cleaned per protocol. ——— Liz Schaeffer, RN

Peritoneal lavage

Frequently monitor and document the patient's vital signs and any signs or symptoms of shock — for example, tachycardia, decreased blood pressure, diaphoresis, dyspnea, or vertigo.

Keep a record of the incision site's condition and document the type and size of peritoneal dialysis catheter used, the type and amount of solution instilled and withdrawn from the peritoneal cavity, and the amount and color of fluid returned. Note whether the fluid flowed freely into and out of the abdomen. Record which specimens were obtained and sent to the laboratory.

Also note any complications that occurred and the nursing actions you took to manage them.

1/2/99	1500	NG tube inserted via Ⓛ nostril, to low Gomco suction. #16 Fr. Foley catheter inserted to straight drainage. Dr. Fisher inserted #15 Fr. peritoneal catheter below umbilicus via trocar. Clear fluid withdrawn. 700 ml warm NSS instilled as ordered and clamped. Pt. turned from side to side. NSS dwell time of 10 min. Then NSS drained freely from abdomen. Fluid samples sent to lab as ordered. Peritoneal catheter removed and incision closed by Dr. Fisher. 4" x 4" gauze pad c̄ povidone-iodine ointment applied to site. Pt. tolerated procedure well VSS pre- and postprocedure. ——— Angela Novack, RN

Thoracic drainage

Record the date and time thoracic drainage began, the type of system used, the amount of suction applied to the system, and the initial presence or absence of bubbling or fluctuation in the water-seal chamber. (Bubbling in the water-seal chamber may indicate an air leak.)

Also record the initial amount and type of drainage and the patient's respiratory status.

Document how frequently you inspected the drainage system. Again, note the presence or absence of bubbling or fluctuation in the water-seal chamber, and enter the patient's respiratory status.

3/11/99	0900	Ⓛ anterior CT intact to Pleur-evac suction system to 20 cm of suction. All connections intact. 50 ml BRB drainage noted since 0800. No air leak noted + fluctuation. CT site dressing D&I, no crepitus palpated. Lungs clear bilaterally. Chest expansion equal bilaterally. No SOB noted. RR 18-20 nonlabored. O_2 @ 2 L/min via NC. ——— Andrew Ortiz, RN

Also record the condition of the chest dressings; the name, amount, and route of any pain medication you gave; complications that developed; and any subsequent interventions that you performed.

When documenting ongoing drainage characteristics, describe the color, consistency, and amount of thoracic drainage in the collection chamber. Be sure to include the time and date of each instance that you make such observations.

Keep a record of patient-teaching sessions and subsequent activities that the patient will perform, such as coughing and deep-breathing exercises, sitting upright, and splinting the insertion site to minimize pain.

Record the results of your respiratory assessments, including the rate and quality of the patient's respirations and auscultation findings. Also document the time and date when you notify the doctor of serious patient conditions, such as cyanosis, rapid or shallow breathing, subcutaneous emphysema, chest pain, or excessive bleeding.

Be sure to document each chest tube dressing change and findings related to the patient's skin condition at the chest tube site.

Cardiac monitoring

In your notes, document the date and time that monitoring began and the monitoring leads used. Commit all rhythm strip readings to the record. Be sure to label the rhythm strip with the patient's name, his room number, and the date and time. Also document any changes in the patient's condition.

1/8/99	0720	Pt. on 5-lead electrode system. ECG strip shows NSR @ a rate of 80 c̄ occasional PACs PR .16, QRS .08; 6-sec. episode of PAT - rate 160 noted @ 0710 hr. Dr. Durkin notified. Pt. asymptomatic. Peripheral pulses normal; no edema noted. Heart c̄ RRR. No murmurs, gallops or rubs. Pt. denies chest pain/discomfort. ——— Diane Goldman, RN

If cardiac monitoring will continue after the patient's discharge, document which caregivers can interpret dangerous rhythms and can perform cardiopulmonary resuscitation. Also teach troubleshooting techniques to use if the monitor malfunctions, and document your teaching efforts or referrals (for example, to equipment suppliers).

Chest physiotherapy

Whenever you perform chest physiotherapy, document the date and time of your interventions, the patient's positions for secretion drainage and length of time the patient remains in each position, the chest segments percussed or vibrated, and the characteristics of the secretion expelled (including color, amount, odor, viscosity, and the presence of blood). Also record indications of complications, the nursing actions taken, and the patient's tolerance of the treatment.

2/20/99	1415	Pt. placed on Ⓛ side c̄ foot of
		bed elevated. Chest PT and
		postural drainage performed
		for 10 min. from lower to
		middle then upper lobes, as
		ordered. Pt. had productive
		cough and expelled large amt.
		of thick yellow sputum. Lungs
		clear p̄ chest PT. Procedure
		tolerated w/o difficulty. ———
		——— Jane Goddard, RN

Mechanical ventilation

Document the date and time that mechanical ventilation began. Note the type of ventilator used for the patient and its settings. Describe the patient's subjective and objective responses to mechanical ventilation (including vital signs, breath sounds, use of accessory muscles, comfort level, and physical appearance).

Throughout mechanical ventilation, list any complications and subsequent interventions. Record all pertinent laboratory data, including results of any ABG analyses and oxygen saturation findings (as shown at top of next column).

3/16/99	1015	Pt. on Servo ventilator set at
		TV 750; FIO_2, 45%; 5 cm PEEP;
		AC of 12. RR 20 nonlabored. #8
		ETT in Ⓡ corner of mouth,
		taped securely at 22-cm mark.
		Suctioned via ETT for large
		amt. of thick white secretions.
		Pulse oximeter reading 98%. Ⓛ
		lung clear. R lung with basilar
		crackles and expiratory wheezes.
		No SOB noted. ———
		——— Janice Del Vecchio, RN

If the patient is receiving pressure support ventilation or using a T-piece or tracheostomy collar, note the duration of spontaneous breathing and the patient's ability to maintain the weaning schedule. If the patient is receiving intermittent mandatory ventilation, with or without pressure-support ventilation, record the control breath rate, the time of each breath reduction, and the rate of spontaneous respirations.

Record any adjustments made in ventilator settings as a result of ABG levels, and document any adjustments of ventilator components, such as draining condensate into a collection trap and changing, cleaning, or discarding the tubing.

Note interventions implemented to promote mobility, to protect skin integrity, or to enhance ventilation. For example, record when and how you perform active or passive range-of-motion exercises, turn the patient, or position him upright for lung expansion. Also record any tracheal suctioning done and the character of secretions.

Document assessment findings related to peripheral circulation, urine output, decreased cardiac output, fluid volume excess, or dehydration. When possible, document sleep and wake periods, noting significant trends as appropriate.

Record any teaching efforts (involving the patient and appropriate caregivers) that you carried out in preparation for the patient's discharge. Take special care to record teaching associated with ventilator care and settings, artificial airway care, communication, nutrition, and therapeutic exercise.

Also indicate teaching discussions and demonstrations related to signs and symptoms of infection and equipment functioning. List any referrals you made to equipment vendors, home health agencies, and other community resources.

NG tube insertion and removal

Record the type and size of NG tube inserted; the date, time, and route of insertion; the reason for the insertion; and confirmation of proper placement. Describe the type and amount of suction (if used); drainage characteristics, such as amount, color, consistency, and odor; and the patient's tolerance of the insertion procedure. Record when the NG tube was irrigated, along with the amount of solution used.

1/15/99	1605	# 12 Fr. NG tube placed in Ⓛ
		nostril. Placement verified and
		attached to low intermittent
		suction as ordered. Drainage
		pale green; heme −. Irrigated
		with 30 ml NSS q 2 hr. Pt.
		tolerated procedure. Hypoac-
		tive B.S. in all 4 quadrants.
		——— Vijay Rao, RN

Include in your notes any signs and symptoms signaling complications, such as nausea, vomiting, and abdominal distention. Document any subsequent irrigation procedures and continuing problems after irrigation.

Record the date and time of NG tube clamping or removal, the patient's tolerance of the procedure, and any unusual events accompanying NG tube removal, such as nausea, vomiting, abdominal distention, and food intolerance.

Seizure management

Note in the medical record that the patient requires seizure precautions, and record all precautions taken. Record the date and time that a seizure began as well as its duration and any precipitating factors. Identify any sensation that may be considered an aura. Describe any involuntary behavior occurring at onset, such as lip smacking, chewing movements, or hand and eye movements. Record any incontinence occurring during the seizure.

Document the patient's response to the seizure, the medications given, any complications resulting from the medications or the seizure, and any interventions performed. Finally, record your assessment of the patient's postictal mental and physical status.

1/19/99	1712	Pt. observed with generalized
		seizure activity lasting 2 1/2
		min. Pt. sleeping at time of
		onset. Urinary incontinence
		during seizure. Seizure pads in
		place on bed before seizure.
		Pt. placed on Ⓛ side, airway
		patent, no N/V. Dr. Gordon
		notified of seizure. Diazepam
		10 mg given I.V. as ordered.
		VS taken q 15 min. and p.r.n.
		(see flow sheet). Pt. currently
		obtunded (see neurologic flow
		sheet). No further seizure ac-
		tivity noted. ———
		——— Gale Hartman, RN

Tube feedings

Besides frequently assessing and documenting the patient's tolerance of the procedure and the feeding formula, keep careful records of the kind of tube feeding the patient is receiving (for example, duodenal or jejunal feedings or continuous drip or bolus) as well as the amount, rate, route, and method of feeding.

If you need to dilute a feeding formula, note the dilution strength for the record (for example, half- or three-quarters strength).

When you flush the feeding tube to maintain patency, be sure to document the time and the flushing solution (such as water or cranberry juice) as intake amounts. If you must replace the feeding tube, document this activity as well.

Regularly assess and document the patient's gastric function and note any prescribed medications or treatments to relieve constipation or diarrhea.

2/25/99	0700	Full-strength Pulmocare infusing via Flexiflow pump thru Dobhoff tube in Ⓡ nostril at 50 ml/hr. Tube placement checked and pt. maintained with HOB raised about 45°. 5 ml residual obtained. Pt. denies any N/V. Normal active bowel sounds auscultated x 4 quad. Diphenoxylate elixir 2.5 mg given via f.t. for continuous diarrhea. Tubed flushed with 30 ml H_2O this shift as ordered. Pt. instructed to tell nurse of discomfort. ——— Sandra Mann, RN

When administering continuous feedings, check and document the infusion rate hourly. When administering bolus feedings, document the residual contents and amount as well as placement and patency of the tube prior to feeding.

Regularly record such laboratory test findings as the patient's urine and serum glucose, serum electrolyte, and blood urea nitrogen levels as well as serum osmolality. Be sure to document any feeding complications, such as hyperglycemia, glycosuria, and diarrhea.

If the patient will continue receiving tube feedings after discharge, document any instructions you give to the patient and appropriate caregivers and any referrals you make to suppliers or support agencies.

Withdrawal of arterial blood

When you must obtain blood for ABG analysis, keep careful records of the patient's vital signs and temperature, the arterial puncture site, and the results of Allen's test. Also document any indications of circulatory impairment, such as bleeding at the puncture site and swelling, discoloration, pain, numbness, or tingling in the bandaged arm or leg.

Document the time that the blood sample was drawn, the length of time pressure was applied to the site to control bleeding and, if appropriate, the type and amount of oxygen therapy that the patient was receiving.

3/12/99	1010	Blood drawn from Ⓡ radial artery p̄ + Allen's test c̄ brisk capillary refill. Pressure applied to site for 5 min. and pressure drsg. applied. No bleeding, hematoma, or swelling noted. Hand pink, warm c̄ 2-sec. capillary refill. Sample for ABGs placed on ice and taken to lab. Pt. on 40% CAM. T 99.2Ⓛ F; Hgb 10.2. ——— Pat Toricelli, RN

When filling out a laboratory request form for ABG analysis, be sure to include the following information for laboratory records: the patient's current temperature and respiratory rate, his most recent hemoglobin level and, if he's on mechanical ventilation, the fraction of inspired oxygen, tidal volume, and control rate. In many facilities, this is entered as a computerized order.

Assistive procedures

When you assist a doctor in such procedures as bone marrow aspiration, esophageal tube insertion, insertion or removal of arterial or central venous lines, lumbar puncture, suture removal, or thoracentesis, your role also involves patient support, patient teaching, and evaluation of the patient's response.

Careful charting of these procedures is your responsibility. Document the name of the doctor performing the procedure, the equipment used, the patient's response to the procedure, the patient teaching provided, and any other pertinent information.

Bone marrow aspiration

When assisting the doctor with a bone marrow aspiration, document the date and time and the name of the doctor performing the procedure. Also describe the appearance of the specimen aspirated, the patient's response to the procedure, and the appearance of the aspiration site. Monitor the patient's vital signs after the procedure, and observe the aspiration site for bleeding. Document any pertinent information about the specimen sent to the laboratory.

1/30/99	1000	Assisted Dr. Shelbourne while he performed a bone marrow aspiration at 0915 hr. Pt. tolerated the procedure well with little discomfort. Specimens sent to lab, as ordered. The procedure was performed on the Ⓡ anterior iliac crest. No bleeding at site. VS: BP, 142/82; P, 88; R, 22. Pt. afebrile. Bed rest being maintained.
		Margaret Little, RN

Esophageal tube insertion and removal

Make sure that your documentation includes the date and time that you assisted with insertion and removal of the esophageal tube and the name of the doctor who performed the procedure.

As applicable, record the type of sedation administered, the intragastric balloon pressure, the amount of air injected into the gastric balloon port, the amount of fluid used for gastric irrigation, and the color, consistency, and amount of gastric return both before and after lavage.

Because intraesophageal balloon pressure varies with respirations and esophageal contractions, be sure to record the baseline pressure, which is the most important pressure.

Document the patient's tolerance of both the insertion and removal procedures, as shown at the top of the next page.

2/11/99	1210	Sengstaken-Blakemore tube placed w/o difficulty by Dr. Fisher via Ⓡ nostril. 50 cc air injected into gastric balloon. Abdominal X-ray obtained to confirm placement. Gastric balloon inflated c̄ 500 cc air. Tube secured to football helmet traction. Large amt. BRB drainage noted. Tube irrigated c̄ 1,800 ml of iced NSS until clear. NG tube placed in Ⓛ nostril and attached to 8 mm Ohio wall suction. Esophageal balloon inflated to 30 mm Hg and clamped. Equal BS bilat. No SOB, VSS. Pt. tolerated procedure. Emotional support given. ——— Evelyn Sutcliffe, RN

Insertion and removal of an arterial line

When assisting with insertion of an arterial line, record the doctor's name; the time and date; the insertion site; the type, gauge, and length of the catheter; and whether the catheter is sutured in place.

3/5/99	0625	#20G arterial catheter placed in Ⓡ radial artery by anesthes. Dr. Mayer on 2nd attempt after + Allen's test. Transducer leveled and zeroed. Readings accurate to cuff pressures. Site w/o redness or swelling. 4" x 4" gauze pad c̄ povidone-iodine ointment applied. Ⓡ hand and wrist taped and secured to arm board. Line flushes easily. Good waveform on monitor. Pt.'s hand pink and warm c̄ 2-sec. capillary refill. ——— Lisa Chang, RN

At removal, record the time and date, doctor's name, length of the catheter, and condition of the insertion site. If any catheter specimens were obtained for culture, be sure to document that too.

Insertion and removal of a central venous line

Typically when you assist the doctor who inserts a central venous (CV) line, you'll need to document the time and date of insertion; the type, length, and location of the catheter; the solution infused; the doctor's name; and the patient's response to the procedure. Other measures that need to be noted include the time of the X-ray study performed to confirm the line's safe and correct placement, the X-ray results, and your notification of the doctor of the results.

2/24/99	1100	Procedure explained to pt. and consent obtained by Dr. Chavez. Pt. in Trendelenburg position and TLC placed by Dr. Chavez on 1st attempt in Ⓡ SC. Cath. sutured in place c̄ 3-0 silk and sterile dressing applied per protocol. All lines flushed c̄ 100 units heparin and PC X-ray obtained to confirm line placement. VSS. Pt. tolerated procedure well. ——— Louise Flynn, RN

After assisting with a CV line's removal, record the time and date of removal and the type of dressing applied. Note the length of the catheter and the condition of the insertion site. Also document collecting any catheter specimens for culture or other analysis.

Lumbar puncture

During lumbar puncture, observe the patient closely for such signs and symptoms as a change in LOC, dizziness, or changes in vital signs. Report these observations to the doctor and document them carefully.

Also record the initiation and completion time of the procedure and the number of test tube specimens of cerebrospinal fluid (CSF) as they are obtained. Document the patient's tolerance of the procedure and any pertinent information about the specimens in the chart.

Monitor the patient's condition, and keep him in a flat supine position for 6 to 12 hours. Encourage fluid intake, assess him for headache, and check the puncture site for leaking CSF. Document all of your observations and interventions.

2/8/99	9:00am	Procedure explained to patient.
		Pt. positioned, side lying for
		lumber puncture. Procedure
		began at 9am and ended at
		9:35am. Pt. draped and prepped
		by MD. Specimen obtained on 1st
		attempt by MD. Clear straw
		colored CSF noted. Pt. toler-
		ated procedure without diffi-
		culty. Vitals signs stable during
		procedure. Pt. maintained in
		supine position as instructed.
		Due to flat positioning, and
		NPO status, NSS infusion
		started at 100 ml/hr. Puncture
		site dressed by MD. Site clear
		dry and intact. No leakage. Pt.
		without complaints of headache
		or dizziness. ———
		——— Jeanette Kane, RN

Suture removal

Although suture removal is primarily a doctor's responsibility, this procedure may be delegated to a skilled nurse with a written medical order. When documenting this procedure, note the appearance of the suture line, the date and time the sutures were removed, and whether the wound site contained purulent drainage. If you suspect infection at the site, notify the doctor, collect a specimen, and send it to the laboratory for analysis.

2/14/99	10:30am	Order obtained from MD to
		remove sutures from index
		finger. Suture line well approx-
		imated and healed. No drainage
		present upon assessment. Site
		clean and dry. No redness.
		Patient complaining of "a numb
		feeling" when the finger is
		touched. All three sutures
		removed without difficulty. Dry
		Bandaid applied to the finger.
		——— Pauline Primas, RN

Thoracentesis

When assisting with thoracentesis, assess the patient for any sudden or unusual pain, faintness, dizziness, or vital sign changes. Report these observations to the doctor immediately, and record them as soon as possible. Document the date and time, the name of the doctor performing the procedure, the amount and quality of fluid aspirated, and the patient's response to the procedure.

If later symptoms of pneumothorax, hemothorax, subcutaneous emphysema, or infection occur, notify the doctor immediately and document your observations and interventions on the chart. Also note whether you sent a fluid specimen to the laboratory for analysis.

3/10/99	11:00am	Procedure explained to patient
		and consent obtained by Dr.
		McCall. Pt. positioned over
		secured bedside table. RLL
		thoracentesis performed by MD
		without incident. Sterile 4" x 4"
		dressing applied to site. Site
		clean and dry, no redness or
		drainage present. 900ml of
		blood-tinged serosanguineous
		fluid aspirated. Specimen sent
		to lab as ordered. Vital signs
		stable. Pt. denies SOB or
		dyspnea. Bilateral breath sounds
		auscultated. Chest X-ray pending.
		——— Ellen Pritchett, RN

Infection control

Meticulous record keeping is an important contributor to effective infection control. Various federal agencies require documentation of infections so that the data can be assessed and used to help prevent and control future infections. In addition, the data you record help your health care facility meet national and local accreditation standards.

Typically, you must report to your facility's infection control department any culture result that shows a positive infection and any surgery, drug, elevated temperature, X-ray finding, or specific treatment related to infection. (See *Reporting diseases and infections,* page 292.)

Document to whom you reported the signs and symptoms of suspected infection, instructions received, and treatments initiated. Always follow standard precautions against direct contact with blood and body fluids, and be sure to document that you've done so, as shown at the top of the next column.

Teach the patient and his family about these precautions, and document this also. Record the dates and times of your interventions both in the patient's chart and on the Kardex. Document any breach in an isolation technique and file an incident report should this occur. If the doctor prescribes a drug to treat the infection, record this as well.

1/28/99	1300	Wound and skin precautions
		maintained. Pt. temperature
		remains elevated at 102.3° R.
		Amount of purulent drainage
		from the incision has increased
		since yesterday. Dr. Levick
		notified. Repeat C&S ordered.
		Specimen obtained and sent to
		the lab. ———
		——— Lynne Kasoff, RN

Be sure to communicate the results of any culture and sensitivity studies to the doctor so that he may prescribe the appropriate drug to treat the infection. Also inform the infection control practitioner. Record the patient's response to this drug.

Diagnostic tests

Before receiving a diagnosis, most patients undergo testing—as simple as a blood test or as complicated as magnetic resonance imaging.

Begin documenting diagnostic testing with any preliminary assessments you make of a patient's condition. For example, if your patient is pregnant or has certain allergies, record this information because it might affect the test or the test result. If the patient's age, illness, or disability requires special preparation for the test, enter this information in his chart as well.

Always prepare the patient for the test, and document any teaching you've done about the test itself and any follow-up care associated with it. Be sure to document the administration or withholding of drugs and prepara-

Reporting diseases and infections

The Centers for Disease Control and Prevention, the Occupational Safety and Health Administration, the Joint Committee on Accreditation of Health Care Organizations, and the American Hospital Association all require health care facilities to document and report certain diseases acquired in the community or in hospitals and other health care facilities.

Generally, the health care facility reports diseases to the appropriate local authorities. These authorities notify the state health department, which in turn reports the diseases to the appropriate federal agency or national organization.

Because regulations vary from community to community and state to state and because different agencies focus on different data, the list of reportable diseases that appears below isn't conclusive and may change periodically.

- Acquired immunodeficiency syndrome (AIDS)
- Amebiasis
- Animal bites
- Anthrax (cutaneous or pulmonary)
- Arbovirus
- Botulism (food-borne, infant)
- Brucellosis
- Campylobacteriosis
- Chancroid
- Chlamydial infections
- Cholera
- Diarrhea of the newborn, epidemic
- Diphtheria (cutaneous or pharyngeal)
- Encephalitis (postinfectious or primary)
- Food poisoning
- Gastroenteritis (institutional outbreaks)
- Giardiasis
- Gonococcal infections
- Gonorrhea
- Group A beta-hemolytic streptococcal infections (including scarlet fever)
- Guillain-Barré syndrome
- Haemophilus influenza Type B
- Hepatitis A, infectious (include suspected source)
- Hepatitis B, serum (include suspected source)
- Hepatitis C (include suspected source)
- Hepatitis, unspecified (include suspected source)
- Histoplasmosis
- Kawasaki disease
- Lead poisoning
- *Legionella* infections (Legionnaires' disease)
- Leprosy
- Leptospirosis
- Listeriosis
- Lyme disease
- Lymphogranuloma venereum
- Malaria
- Measles (rubeola)
- Meningitis (all types)
- Meningococcal disease
- Mumps
- Neonatal hypothyroidism
- Pertussis
- Phenylketonuria
- Plague (bubonic or pneumonic)
- Poliomyelitis (spinal paralytic)
- Psittacosis (ornithosis)
- Rabies
- Reye's syndrome
- Rickettsial diseases (including Rocky Mountain spotted fever)
- Rubella (German measles) and congenital syndrome
- Salmonellosis
- Shigellosis
- Syphilis (congenital < 1 year)
- Syphilis (primary or secondary)
- Tetanus
- Toxic shock syndrome
- Toxoplasmosis
- Trichinosis
- Tuberculosis
- Tularemia
- Typhoid and paratyphoid fever
- Yellow fever

tions, special diets, food or fluid restrictions, enemas, and specimen collection.

3/18/99	0700	24-hour urine test for creatinine clearance started. Pt. taught purpose of this test and how to collect urine. Sign placed on pt.'s door and in bathroom. Urine placed on ice in bathroom. ——— Paul Steadman, RN

Pain control

Your primary goal is to eliminate or minimize your patient's pain. Determining its severity can be difficult, however, because pain is subjective. You can use a number of tools to assess pain; when you use them, always document the results. (See *Assessing and documenting pain,* page 294.)

When charting pain levels and characteristics, first determine where the patient feels the pain and whether it's internal, external, localized, or diffuse. Also find out whether the pain interferes with the patient's sleep or other activities of daily living. Describe the pain in the patient's own words and enter them in the chart.

Be aware of the patient's body language and behaviors associated with pain. Does he wince or grimace? Does he move or squirm in bed? What positions seem to relieve or worsen the pain? What other measures (heat, cold, massage, drugs) relieve or heighten the pain? All of this information is important in assessing your patient's pain and should be documented.

Enter into the chart whichever interventions you take to alleviate your patient's pain, and document the patient's responses to your interventions.

3/19/99	1600	Pt. admitted to room 304 with diagnosis of pancreatic cancer and severe pain in LLQ. Pt. taking Percocet 2 tabs q 4 hr. at home without relief at present. Dr. Martin notified. Dilaudid 2 mg. ordered and given I.V. @ 1600 hrs. VS stable. Pt. resting at present ——— K. Comerford, RN

Patient-controlled analgesia

Some patients may be receiving narcotics via a patient-controlled analgesia (PCA) infusion pump. These pumps allow patients to self-administer boluses of a narcotic analgesic I.V., subcutaneously, or epidurally within limits prescribed by the doctor. To avoid overmedication, an adjustable lockout interval inhibits delivery of additional boluses until the appropriate time has elapsed. PCA increases the patient's sense of control and reduces anxiety, reduces drug use over the postoperative course, and gives enhanced pain control.

Be sure to document the amount of narcotics used during your shift, and document the patient's response to the treatment and any patient teaching done. (See *PCA flow sheet,* page 295.)

Codes

Guidelines established by the American Heart Association (AHA) direct you to keep a written, chronological account of a patient's condition throughout resuscitative efforts. If you're a designated recorder for a patient's cardiopulmonary arrest record, document therapeutic interventions and the patient's responses to these as they occur. Don't rely on

(Text continues on page 297.)

BETTER CHARTING

Assessing and documenting pain

Used appropriately, standard assessment tools, such as the McGill-Melzack Pain Questionnaire and the Initial Pain Assessment Tool (developed by McCaffery and Beebe), provide a solid foundation for your nursing diagnoses and plans of care. If your health care facility doesn't use standardized pain questionnaires, you can devise other pain measurement tools, such as the pain flow sheet or the visual and graphic rating scales that appear below. Whichever pain assessment tool you choose, remember to document its use and include the graphic record in your patient's chart.

Pain flow sheet

Possibly the most convenient tool for pain assessment, a flow sheet provides a standard for reevaluating the patient's pain at ongoing and regular intervals. It's also beneficial for patients and families, who may feel too overwhelmed by the pain experience to answer a long, detailed questionnaire.

If possible, incorporate pain assessment into the flow sheet you're already using. Generally, the easier the flow sheet is to use, the more likely you and your patient will be to use it.

PAIN FLOW SHEET

Date and time	Pain rating (0 to 10)	Patient behaviors	Vital signs	Pain rating after intervention	Comments
1/16/99 0800	*7*	*Wincing, holding head*	*186/88 98-22*	*5*	*Dilaudid 2 mg I.M. given*
1/16/99 1200	*3*	*Relaxing, reading*	*160/80 84-18*	*2*	*Tylox ī P.O. given*

Visual analog pain scale

In a visual analog pain scale, the patient marks a linear scale containing words or numbers that correspond to his perceived degree of pain. Draw a scale to represent a continuum of pain intensity. Verbal anchors describe the pain's intensity; for example, "no pain" begins the scale and "pain as bad as it could be" ends it. Ask the patient to mark the point on the continuum that best describes his pain.

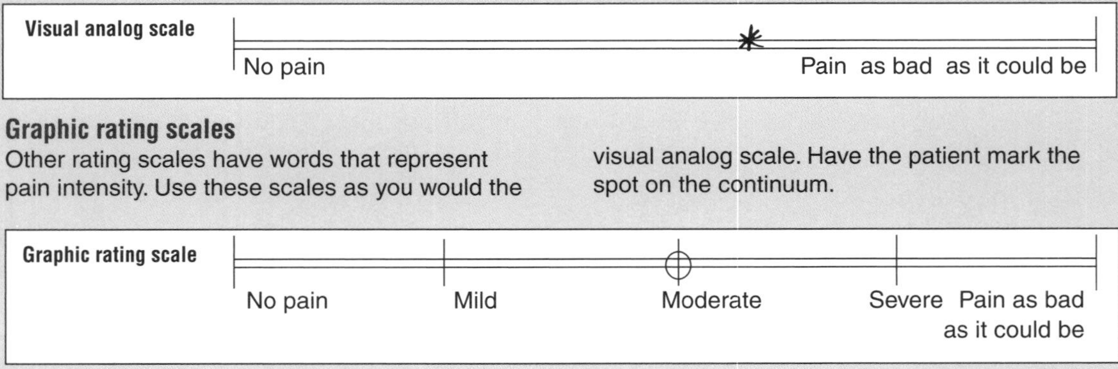

Graphic rating scales

Other rating scales have words that represent pain intensity. Use these scales as you would the visual analog scale. Have the patient mark the spot on the continuum.

BETTER CHARTING

PCA flow sheet

The form shown below is used to document the use of patient-controlled analgesia (PCA). PCA allows the patient to self-administer a narcotic analgesic as needed yet within limits prescribed by the doctor.

Date 3/22/99

Medication (Circle one) Meperidine 300 mg in 30 cc (10mg/1ml)
Morphine 30 mg in 30 cc (1 mg/ml) (circled)

	7–3 Shift				3–11 Shift				11–7 Shift			
Time (enter in box)	1200	1400			1600							
New cartridge inserted	OR											
PCA settings Lockout interval 7 (minutes)		7			7							
Dose volume 1 (ml/dose)												
Four-hour limit 30												
Continuous settings 1 (mg/hr)												
Respiratory rate	18	20			20							
Blood pressure	150/70	130/62			128/70							
Sedation rating 1. Wide awake 2. Drowsy 3. Dozing, intermittent 4. Mostly sleeping 5. Only awakens when stimulated	1	2			3							
Analgesia rts (1—10) Minimal Pain – 1 Maximum Pain – 10	7	8			6							
Additional doses given (optional doses)	3ml/OR											
Total ml's delivered (total from ampule)	3	6			15							
ml's remaining	27	24			15							

RN SIGNATURE (7–3 SHIFT) Janet Green, RN **Date** 3/22/99

RN SIGNATURE (3–11 SHIFT) Karen Singleton, RN **Date** 3/22/99

RN SIGNATURE (11–7 SHIFT) ______ **Date** ______

BETTER CHARTING

Keeping a resuscitation record

Here's an example of the completed resuscitation record for inclusion in your patient's chart.

CODE RECORD

Pg. _1_ of _1_

Arrest Date: _5/9/99_
Arrest Time: _0600_
Rm/Location: _431-2_
Discovered by: _C. Brown_
☑ RN ☐ MD
☐ Other

Methods of alert:
☑ Witnessed, monitored: rhythm _V fib_
☐ Witnessed, unmonitored
☐ Unwitnessed, unmonitored
☐ Unwitnessed, monitored; rhythm ______
Diagnosis: _Post anterior wall MI_

Condition when needed:
☑ Unresponsive
☐ Apneic
☐ Pulseless
☐ Hemorrhage
☐ Seizure

Ventilation management:
Time: _0635_
Method: _oral ET tube_
Precordial thump: _0631_
CPR initiated at: _0631_

Previous airway:
☐ ET tube
☐ Trach
☑ Natural

Addressograph

CPR PROGRESS NOTES

VITAL SIGNS						I.V. PUSH					INFUSIONS				ACTIONS/PATIENT RESPONSE
Time	Pulse CPR	Resp. rate Spont; bag	Blood pressure	Rhythm	Defib (joules)	Atropine	Epinephrine	Lidocaine	NA bicarb	Bretylium	Lidocaine	Procain.	Isuprel	Dopamine	Responses to therapy, procedures, labs drawn/results
0631	CPR	Bag	0	V fib			1 mg								No change.
0632		Bag	0	V fib	200										ABGs drawn. Ⓡ fem pressure applied.
0633	CPR	Bag	0	Asystole	300		1 mg								No change
0639	40	Bag	60 palp	SB PVCs				75			✔				Oral intubation by Dr. Hart
0645	60	Bag	80/40	SB PVCs							✔				CCU ready for patient

ABGs & Lab Data

Time Spec Sent	pH	PCO	Po_2	HCO_3	Sat%	Fio_2	Other
0633	7.1	76	43	14	80%		

Resuscitation outcome

☑ Successful ☑ Transferred to _CCU_ at _0648_
☐ Unsuccessful — Expired at ______
Pronounced by: ______ MD
Family notified by: _S. Quinn, RN_
Time: _0645_
Attending notified by: _S. Quinn, RN_ Time _0645_
Code Recorder _S. Quinn, RN_
Code Team Nurse _B. Mullen, RN_
Anesthesia Rep. _J. Hanna, RN_
Other Personnel _Dr. Hart_
B. Russo, RT

your memory to record the sequence of events. (See *Keeping a resuscitation record.*)

If a code is called, you'll complete a *code record,* a form that incorporates detailed information about the code (including observations, interventions, and any drugs given to the patient).

1/24/99	2100	Summoned to the pt.'s room @ 2020 hr. by a shout from roommate. Found pt. unresponsive without respirations or pulse. Roommate stated, "He was talking to me; then all of a sudden he started gasping and holding his chest." Code called. Initiated CPR with Ann Barrow, RN. Code team arrived @ 2023 hr. and continued resuscitative efforts. (See code record.) Pt. groaned and opened eyes @ approx. 2030 hr. (see neurologic flow sheet). Notified Dr. Cooper @ home @ 2040 hr. and explained situation—will be in immediately. Pt. transferred to ICU @ 2035 hr. Family notified of pt.'s condition and transfer. ——— Delia Landers, RN

Some health care facilities use a resuscitation critique form to identify actual or potential problems with the resuscitation process. This form tracks personnel responses and response times as well as the availability of appropriate drugs and functioning equipment.

Change in patient's condition

One of your major documentation responsibilities is documenting any change in a patient's condition. Your note should include the patient's complaint, your assessment and interventions, whom you notified, what you reported, and what instructions you received. When documenting your observations, avoid using vague words such as "appears." For example, instead of merely writing "stools appear bloody," describe the stool's characteristics, such as color, amount, frequency, and consistency.

3/28/99	1500	Pt. had moderate sized, soft, dark brown stools positive for blood c̄ a guaiac test. ——— Jackie Paterno, RN.

Intake and output monitoring

Many patients require 24-hour intake and output monitoring. They include surgical patients, patients on I.V. therapy, patients with fluid and electrolyte imbalances, and patients with burns, hemorrhage, or edema.

You'll keep most intake and output sheets at the patient's bedside or by the bathroom door to remind you to measure and document his intake and output. If the patient is incontinent, document this as well as tube drainage and irrigation volumes.

For easy reference, list the volumes of specific containers. Infusion devices make documenting enteral and I.V. intake more accurate. But keeping track of intake that isn't premeasured — for example, food such as gelatin that is normally fluid at room temperature — requires the cooperation of the patient, family members (who may bring him snacks and soft drinks or help him to eat at the health care facility), and other caregivers. So make sure that everyone understands how to record or report all foods and fluids that the patient consumes orally.

BETTER CHARTING

Charting intake and output

As this sample shows, you can monitor your patient's fluid balance by using an intake and output record.

Name: Josephine Klein
Medical record #: 49731
Admission date: 2/13/99

INTAKE AND OUTPUT RECORD

	INTAKE						OUTPUT				
	Oral	Tube feeding	Instilled	I.V. and IVPB	TPN	Total	Urine	Emesis Tubes	NG	Other	Total
Date 2/15/99											
0700–1500	250	320	H_2O 50	1100		1720	1355				1355
1500–2300	200	320	H_2O 50	1100		1670	1200				1200
2300–0700	0	320	H_2O 50	1100		1470	1500				1500
24hr total	450	960	H_2O 150	3300		4860	4055				4055
Date											
24hr total											
Date											
24hr total											
Date											
24hr total											

Key: IVPB = I.V. piggyback TPN = total parenteral nutrition NG = nasogastric

Standard measures

Styrofoam cup	240 ml	Water (large)	600 ml	Milk (large)	600 ml	Ice cream, sherbet, or gelatin	120 ml
Juice	120 ml	Water pitcher	750 ml	Coffee	240 ml		
Water (small)	120 ml	Milk (small)	120 ml	Soup	180 ml		

Don't forget to count I.V. piggyback infusions, drugs given by I.V. push, patient-controlled analgesics, and any irrigation solutions that aren't withdrawn. You'll also need to know whether the patient receives any fluids orally or I.V. while he's off of your unit.

Recording fluid output accurately requires the cooperation of the patient and staff members in any other departments your patient goes to. If he's ambulatory, remind him to use a urinal or a commode.

The amount of fluid lost through the GI tract is normally 100 ml or less daily. However, if the patient's stools become excessive or watery, they must be counted as output. Vomiting, drainage from suction devices and wound drains, and bleeding are other measurable sources of fluid loss. (See *Charting intake and output.*)

Skin and wound care

The skin is the largest organ. Along with the hair, nails, and glands, it protects the body from microorganisms, ultraviolet light radiation, fluid loss, and the stress of mechanical forces. Most cuts, scrapes, and other minor wounds heal in a few days. When more serious wounds, such as pressure ulcers, fail to heal quickly and require long-term care and special assessments, careful documentation is essential.

Pressure ulcers

The National Pressure Ulcer Advisory Panel defines a pressure ulcer as "any lesion caused by unrelieved pressure resulting in damage to underlying tissue." When assessing your patient for the potential to develop a pressure ulcer you need to consider pressure, friction, shearing, and moisture as potential risk factors.

Because many patients are liable to develop pressure ulcers, always document findings related to the patient's skin condition. Clearly note in the record whether a patient had a pressure ulcer upon admission or whether the ulcer developed in the health care facility. Be sure to follow your facility's policy when documenting your findings. Failure to document an existing wound on admission can result in legal action.

Many facilities now use assessment tools, such as the Braden scale, to assess all patients at admission for the presence or risk of developing pressure ulcers.

When a chronically ill or immobile patient enters your unit with a pressure ulcer, record its location, appearance, size, depth, and color and the appearance of exudate from that ulcer.

2/10/99	1400	Pt. admitted by stretcher to
		room 418B. Pt. lethargic, skin
		dry. Incontinent of urine. 1"
		wide black pressure ulcer noted
		on Ⓡ heel. Purulent, yellow
		drainage noted on ulcer's
		dressing. Dr. Kelly notified.
		Surgical consult ordered for
		debridement of ulcer. Ⓡ foot
		elevated on 2 pillows. Heel and
		elbow protectors applied. Skin
		lotion applied. Incontinent
		care given hourly. No other
		skin breakdown noted. Buttocks
		reddened but epidermis intact.
		——— Rachel Moreau, RN

Flow sheets that have defined cues can make your documentation easier. Even if you use a flow sheet, it's a good idea to write a note in the medical record if and when you notify a doctor about any changes in the wound or surrounding tissue.

If the patient's skin condition worsens during hospitalization, his stay may be extended, in which case you'll need a clear record of skin care and related factors. This is especially important because family members typically think that pressure ulcers stem from poor nursing care, although certain risk factors—such as obesity, poor nutritional status, decreased hemoglobin level, immobility, infection, incontinence, and fractures—are equally responsible.

If your health care facility requires you to photograph pressure ulcers found at the time of admission, always date the photographs. You can then evaluate changes in a patient's skin condition by comparing his current skin integrity with previous photographs.

Wound care

Wound assessment and care has changed dramatically in the past 10 years and is continually evolving. One major change has been the shift from dry dressings to moisture-retentive dressings. However, one thing that hasn't changed is the need for good documentation. Be sure to include all of these points when documenting a wound assessment:

- wound size, including length, width, and depth in centimeters
- wound shape
- wound site, drawn on a body plan to document the exact location
- wound stage
- characteristics of drainage, if any, including amount, color, and presence of odor
- characteristics of the wound bed, including description of tissue type, such as granulation tissue, slough, or epithelial tissue, and percentage of each tissue type
- character of the surrounding tissue
- presence or absence of eschar
- presence or absence of pain
- presence or absence of undermining or tunneling (in centimeters)

Shift reports

Your facility may require an end-of-shift report (sometimes called a *unit report* or *24-hour report*). These documents, which track both conditions and activities on the unit, provide a running record of the patient census, staff-to-patient ratio, bed utilization, patient emergencies or acute changes, patient or family problems, incidents, equipment and supply problems, number of high-risk procedures, and other important data.

These reports are typically reviewed by nursing administrators charged with solving the day-to-day problems of a unit. (See *Documenting the events of your shift.*)

Personal property

Encourage patients to send home their money, jewelry, and other valuable belongings. If a patient refuses to do so, make a list of his possessions and store them according to your facility's policy.

The list of the patient's valuables should include a description of each one. To protect yourself and your employer, ask the patient (or a responsible family member) to sign, or witness, the list that you compile so that you

BETTER CHARTING

Documenting the events of your shift

Most health care facilities require the charge nurse to complete an end-of-shift report. The form below is an example of the information most facilities need to know.

Date: 2/26/99 **Charge nurse:** Donna Moriarty, RN

Patient census: Start of shift 38 End of shift: 37

Number of admissions 2 Number of transfers 2 in, 3 out

Deaths 0 Codes 0

Comments

One patient transferred to SICU postop

Staff profile: Start of shift: 9 End of shift: 7

RNs 4 Orientees 0 LPNs 3

Students 0 Nursing assistants 2

Agency 0 Other 0

Called in sick Unit clerk — not replaced

Late 0 Floated One aide, 1 LPN floated out halfway through shift

Unit workload during shift

Quiet ____ Busy but steady ____ Very busy X Understaffed X

Equipment and supply problems

I.V. pumps not available. No sterile drsg. kits in supply cart. Not enough linen.

High-risk procedures performed

CVP line insertion, wound debridement, chest tube insertion

Assignment, personnel, or performance problems

Staff floated out 4 hr. into shift to cover sick calls on another unit—increased pt. ratio for rest of staff.

Patient or family problems

Mr. Hale in room 516-B — his condition deteriorated rapidly—developed acute abdomen and required emergency surgery. Family distraught — need time and privacy to speak with doctor and clergy. Conference room is too small to accommodate more than 10 people (18 family members present). Because room doubles as staff lounge, privacy is difficult to maintain.

Number of incident reports filed: None **Number of problem logs completed:** None

both understand which items you're responsible for.

Use objective language to describe each item, noting its color, approximate size, style, type, and serial number or other distinguishing feature. Don't assess the item's value or authenticity. For example, you might describe a diamond ring as a "clear, round stone set in a yellow metal band."

Besides jewelry and money, include dentures, eyeglasses or contact lenses, hearing aids, prostheses, and clothing on the list. If your patient is homeless, he may have all of his personal belongings with him. You'll need to identify and tag each item.

3/18/99	1300	Pt. admitted to room 318 with
		one pair of brown glasses, upper
		and lower dentures, a yellow
		metal ring with a red stone, a
		pink bathrobe, and a black radio.
		Paul Cullen, RN

Place valuable items in an envelope and other personal belongings in approved containers; then label them with the patient's identification number. Never use garbage containers, laundry bags, or any other unauthorized receptacle for valuables; they could be discarded accidentally.

If the patient refuses to remove a ring, explain that it may have to be cut off if it compromises his circulation. If he decides to leave it on anyway, tape it in place. Be sure to document your conversation and actions.

COMMON CHARTING FLAWS

Ideally, every chart you receive from the nurses on the previous shift will be complete and accurate. Unfortunately, this is not always the case. Although you can't necessarily affect what other nurses do, you can try to make your own charting flawless so it doesn't mislead other caregivers.

BLANK SPACES IN CHART OR FLOW SHEET

Follow your facility's policy regarding blank spaces on forms. A blank space may imply that you failed to give complete care or assess the patient fully.

Because flow sheets have increased in size (sometimes to four to six pages), nurses may be required to fill in only those fields or prompts that apply to their patient. It is now common for health care facilities to have a written policy on how to complete such forms correctly. For example, if information requested on a form doesn't apply to a particular patient, your facility's policy may require you to write "N/A" (not applicable) or draw a line through empty spaces.

3/19/98	1500	20 y/o male admitted to room
		418B by wheelchair. #20 angio-
		cath inserted in Ⓛ antecubital
		vein with I.V. of 1,000 ml D5-
		½NSS infusing at 125 ml/hr.
		O_2 at 2 L/min. via NC. Demerol
		50 mg given I.M. for abdominal
		pain. Relief reported.
		David Dunn, RN

This leaves no doubt that you addressed every part of the record. It also prevents others from inserting information that could change the meaning of your original documentation.

Care given by someone else

Unless you document otherwise, anyone reading your notes assumes that they are a firsthand account of care provided. In some settings, nursing assistants and technicians aren't allowed to make formal charting entries. If this is the case in your facility, determine what care was provided, assess the patient and the task performed (for example a dressing change), and document your findings. Be sure to record the full names and titles of unlicensed personnel who provided care; don't just record their initials.

1/23/99	0600	Morning care provided by Kevin Lawson, NA, who stated that patient moaned when being turned.
		Camille Dunn, RN

If your facility allows unlicensed personnel to chart, you may have to countersign their notes. If your facility's policy states that the unlicensed person must provide care in your presence, don't countersign unless you actually witness her actions. If the policy says that you don't have to be there, your countersigning indicates that the note describes care that other person had the authority and competence to perform and that you verified that the procedure was performed.

You can specifically document that you reviewed the notes and consulted with the technician or assistant on certain aspects of care. Of course, you must document any follow-up care you provide. (For more information on countersigning, see chapter 10, Legally Perilous Charting Practices.)

Late entries

Late entries are appropriate in several situations:

- if the chart was unavailable when you needed it (as shown below) — for example, when the patient was away from the unit (in X-ray or physical therapy)

2/14/99	0900	(Chart not available 2/13/99 1500 hr.)
		On 2/13 @ 1300 hr., pt. stated she felt faint when getting OOB on 2/13 @ 1200 hr and fell to the floor. States she did not hurt herself and did not think she had to tell anyone about this until her husband encouraged her to report it. No bruises or lacerations noted. Pt. denies pain. Dr. Muir examined pt. at 1320 hr on 2/13.
		Elaine Kasmer, RN

- if you need to add important information after completing your notes
- if you forgot to write notes on a particular chart.

Keep in mind, however, that a late or altered chart entry can arouse suspicions and can be a significant problem in the event of a malpractice lawsuit. (See *Avoid late additions,* page 304.)

ON TRIAL

Avoid late additions

If the court uncovers alterations in a patient's chart during the course of a trial, suspicions may be aroused. The court may logically infer that additional alterations were made. In such situations, the value of the entire medical record may be brought into question.

That's what happened to the nurse involved in one case. She failed to chart her observations of a postoperative patient for 7 hours, during which time the patient died. The patient's family later sued the hospital, charging the nurse with malpractice. The nurse insisted that she had observed the patient, but because her particular unit was understaffed and overpopulated, she wasn't able to record her observations. She explained that the assistant director of nursing later instructed her about the hospital's policy on charting late additions. The nurse subsequently added her observations to the patient's medical record.

However, the court wasn't convinced that the nurse had indeed observed the patient during the postoperative period. Suspicious of the altered record, it ruled that the nurse's failure to chart her observations at the proper time supported the plaintiff's claim that she'd made no such observations.

If you must make a late entry or alter an earlier entry, find out if your health care facility has a protocol for doing so. Many do. If not, the best approach is to add the entry to the first available line, and label it "late entry" to indicate that it's out of sequence. Then record the time and date of the entry and, in the body of the entry, record the time and date it should have been made.

Corrections

When you make a mistake on a chart, correct it promptly. Never erase, cover, completely scratch out, or otherwise obscure an erroneous entry because this may imply a cover-up. If the chart ends up in court, the plaintiff's attorney will be looking for anything that may cast doubt on the chart's accuracy. Erasures or the use of correction fluid or heavy black ink to obliterate an error are red flags. (See *Correcting a charting error.*)

Patient noncompliance

Suppose a patient won't comply with nursing or medical interventions—for example, such common instructions as "Follow your diet," "Don't get out of bed without assistance," "Take your medicine as directed," or "Keep your doctor's appointment for a checkup." Beyond explaining the importance of following such instructions, you may be able to do little. But you must chart the noncompliance.

In the chart, describe any patient behavior that goes against your instructions; then report the problem to the appropriate person. Note any attempts to encourage the patient's compliance, even if unsuccessful. If the patient's care is questioned later, the record will be an important factor in your defense. Below you'll find examples of specific types of noncompliance.

Dietary restrictions

If your patient is on dietary restrictions and you discover unauthorized food or beverages at his bedside, point out to him the need to follow his prescribed dietary plan. Document

BETTER CHARTING

Correcting a charting error

When you make a mistake documenting on the medical record, correct it by drawing a single line through it and writing the words "mistaken entry" above or beside it. Follow these words with your initials and the date. If appropriate, briefly explain the necessity for the correction.

Make sure that the mistaken entry is still readable. This indicates that you're only trying to correct a mistake, not cover it up.

Date	Time	Progress notes
1/19/99	0900	Mistaken entry J.M. 1/19/99 ~~Pt. walked to bathroom.~~
		~~States he experienced no~~
		~~difficulty urinating.~~
		~~John Moda, RN~~

the noncompliance and your patient teaching, and notify the patient's doctor.

2/17/99	1400	Pt. found with milkshake and
		cookies at bedside. Discussed
		with pt. his need to maintain
		1,800-calorie ADA diet. Pt. re-
		fused to remove these foods,
		stating, "I'll eat what I want."
		Dr. Mayer notified that pt. is
		not complying with prescribed
		diabetic diet. Dietitian called to
		meet with pt. and wife.
		Claire Bowen, RN

Out of bed against advice

Even after you've told a patient that he must not get out of bed alone and that he must call you for help, you may go to his room and find him climbing over the bed rails or discover relatives helping him to the bathroom because they don't want to disturb you.

Either scenario puts the patient at risk for a fall and you at risk for a lawsuit. What can you do? You can clearly document your instructions and anything that the patient does in spite of them (as shown in the example below). Be sure to include any devices being used to ensure patient safety, such as bed alarms or leg alarms. This shows that you recognized the potential for a fall and that you tried to prevent it.

2/10/99	0300	Assisted pt. to bathroom. Weak,
		unsteady on feet. States she
		gets dizzy when she stands. In-
		structed pt. to call for assis-
		tance to get OOB. Side rails up.
		Call button within reach.
		Joseph Romano, RN
2/10/99	0430	Found pt. walking to bathroom.
		Stated she got OOB by herself.
		Reminded her to call for assis-
		tance. Said she understood.
		Joseph Romano, RN

Medication abuse or refusal

If the patient refuses or abuses prescribed medication, describe the event in his chart.

Here are some examples of situations that need careful documentation:

- You discover unprescribed drugs at the patient's bedside. Document the type of medication (pills or powders), the amount, and its appearance (color and shape).
- You find a supply of his prescribed drugs in his bedside table, indicating that he is hoarding his medication instead of swallowing each dose. Record the type of medication that you found and the amount.
- You try to give the patient prescribed medications and he refuses. Document his refusal and the reason for it, assuming he tells you. Also be sure to name the medications. Taking these steps will ensure that the patient's refusal isn't misinterpreted as an omission or a medication error on your part.
- You observe that the patient's behavior suddenly changes after he has visitors (see the example below), and you suspect the visitors of providing him with contraband (narcotics or other drugs, for example). Document how the patient appeared before and after the visitors came to see him.

1/2/99	1100	Visitor present at bedside. Pt.
		alert, oriented. I.V. $D_5$1/2NSS
		infusing at 125 ml/hr.
		Eileen Sullivan, RN
1/2/99	1125	Upon entering room, I found
		pt. lethargic. Pupils were con-
		stricted, speech was slurred. Pt.
		stated, "My friend gave me
		something to help with the
		pain." Dr. Ettingoff notified
		and told of lethargy, slurred
		speech, and pinpoint pupils.
		Eileen Sullivan, RN
1/2/99	1130	Dr. Ettingoff in to see pt. Nar-
		can administered as ordered.
		Eileen Sullivan, RN

Discharge instructions

At discharge, review the discharge instructions and discuss the date on which the patient will have a follow-up evaluation. If the patient will make the appointment himself, encourage him to do so, explaining the need for ongoing medical care.

Document the date on which the patient is expected to return for a follow-up visit and the date on which you discussed the appointment with him. This protects you from claims that you neglected to inform him of the need to return for medical care.

Also document any related patient teaching that you performed and any written instructions that you provided. If feasible, mail a reminder letter with a return receipt requested. If you should be accused of negligence related to follow-up care, you can then point to tangible evidence of your attempt to encourage the patient's compliance.

1/12/99	1300	Pt. notified to return to see
		Dr. Bonn on 1/26/99 at 0900.
		Discussed this with pt. and his
		wife.
		Laura E. Cray, RN

Refusing treatment

Infinitely more serious than minor instances of noncompliance, refusing treatment is not just an important patient care and safety issue—it's a critical documentation concern as well.

Any mentally competent adult can refuse treatment. And in most cases, the health care personnel who are responsible for the patient's care can remain free of legal jeopardy as long as they fully inform the patient about his medical condition and the likely consequences of refusing treatment. The courts recognize a competent adult's right to refuse medical treatment, even when that refusal will clearly result in his death.

When your patient refuses treatment, inform him of the risks involved in making such a decision. If possible, inform him in writing. If he continues to refuse, notify the doctor, who will then decide on the most appropriate plan of action.

2/8/99	2000	Pt. refusing to have I.V. inserted, stating that he's "sick and tired of being stuck." Explained to pt. the need for I.V. fluids and antibiotics and likely result of refusing treatment. Dr. Eisenberg notified. Dr. Eisenberg spent time with pt. Pt. still refusing I.V. Orders written to force fluids, repeat electrolytes in morning, and give amoxicillin P.O. —— Barbara Tyson, RN

Make sure that you document the patient's exact words in the chart. To protect yourself legally, document that you didn't provide the prescribed treatment because the patient refused it. Then ask the patient to sign a refusal-of-treatment release form.

If the patient refuses to sign the release form, document this refusal in the progress notes. For additional protection, your facility's policy may require you to ask the patient's spouse or closest relative to sign another refusal-of-treatment release form. Document whether the spouse or another relative does this. (See chapter 2, Legal and Ethical Implications of Documentation.)

Interdisciplinary communication

Because health care involves teamwork, all interdepartmental and interdisciplinary communication about the patient must be documented. This includes calls from the laboratory informing you of a patient's test results, calls you make to the doctor about the patient's condition, and calls from patients requesting advice. In addition, you may on occasion have to give a patient's family bad news over the telephone, and this too must be noted in the chart.

Information from other departments

When a department, such as the laboratory or X-ray department, notifies your unit of a patient's test results, you need to notify the doctor of any abnormal results and then document your notification, including the doctor's name and the time he was notified.

1/4/99	1400	Laboratory technician Donald Boyle called floor to report pt.'s random blood glucose level of 486. Dr. Somers notified. Stat blood glucose ordered. Pt. being monitored until results available. —— Peggy Irwin, RN

Reports to doctors

You've just phoned the doctor to tell him about his patient's deteriorating condition. He listens as you give laboratory test results and the patient's signs and symptoms, thanks you for the information, and hangs up —without giving you an order. Unless you properly docu-

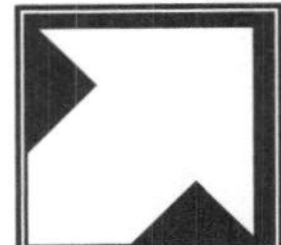

CHARTING GUIDELINES

Ensuring clear communication

To ensure clear communication when discussing a patient's care with a doctor on the phone, remember to keep the following points in mind:

- If you don't know the doctor, ask him to state and spell his full name.
- Include the exact time you contacted the doctor. To establish proof, you could have the hospital operator dial the number for you, or have another nurse listen in and then cosign the time of notification. If you don't note the time you called, allegations may later be made that you failed to obtain timely medical treatment for the patient.
- Always note in the chart the specific change, problem, or result you reported to the doctor, along with the doctor's orders or response. Use his own words, if possible.
- If you're reporting a critical laboratory test result (for example, a low serum potassium level of 3.2 mEq/L) but don't receive an order for intervention (such as potassium replacement therapy), be sure to verify with the doctor that he doesn't want to give an order. Then document this fact in the progress notes. For example, you'd write: "Dr. Jones informed of potassium of 3.2 mEq/L. No orders received."
- If you think a doctor's failure to order an intervention puts your patient's health at risk, follow the chain of command and notify your supervisor. Then be sure to document your action.

ment your conversation with him, the doctor could claim he wasn't notified should this patient's care subsequently come into question. (See *Ensuring clear communication.*)

Nurses often write "Notified doctor of patient's condition." This statement is too vague. In the event of a malpractice suit, it allows the plaintiff's lawyer (and the doctor) to imply that you didn't communicate the essential data. The chart should include exactly what you told the doctor.

2/15/99	2215	Called Dr. Spencer regarding
		increased serous drainage
		from pt.'s (L) chest tube. Dr.
		Spencer's order was to ob-
		serve the drainage for 1 more
		hr and then call him.
		Danielle Bergeron, RN

Telephone advice to patients

Nurses, especially those working in hospital emergency departments (ED), frequently get requests to give advice to patients by telephone. A hospital has no legal duty to provide a telephone-advice service, and you have no legal duty to give advice to anyone who calls.

The best response to a telephone request for medical advice is to tell the caller to come to the hospital because you can't assess his condition or treat him over the phone. Like all rules, however, this one has its exceptions — for example, a life-threatening situation when someone needs immediate care, treatment, or referral.

Accepting responsibility

If you do dispense advice over the phone, keep in mind that a legal duty arises the minute you say, "Okay, let me tell you what to do." You now have a nurse-patient relationship, and you're responsible for any advice you give. Once you start to give advice by telephone, you can't decide midway through that you're in over your head and simply hang up; that could be considered abandonment. You must give appropriate advice or a referral—for example, "After listening to you, I strongly suggest that you come to the ED or call your doctor."

If the caller is a patient you cared for recently, you may choose to give him advice. For example, if the doctor prescribed medication and gave him an instruction sheet, you probably told him to call if he had any questions. Obviously, you wouldn't refuse to answer his questions if he called.

If the question is elementary, such as "Can I take this diuretic with orange juice?," you're probably safe answering. However, direct any questions that are more specific to the doctor, especially if the patient's symptoms have changed.

If you do decide to give telephone advice, establish a system of documenting such calls—with a telephone log, for example. The log should include the date and time of the call, the name of the caller (if he'll give it), the address of the caller, the caller's request or chief complaint, the disposition of the call, and the name of the person who made that disposition.

The disposition will depend on the request. For example, you may give the caller a poison-control number or suggest that he come to the ED for evaluation. Document whatever information you give, as shown at the top of the next column.

Some nurses hesitate to use a telephone log because they assume that if they don't document, they won't be responsible for the

11/6/99	1615	Louis Chapman phoned asking
		how big a cut has to be to re-
		quire stitches. I asked him to
		describe the injury. He describ-
		ed a 4" gash in his Ⓛ leg from
		a fall. I recommended that he
		apply pressure to the cut and
		come into the ED to be assessed.
		——— Claire Bowen, RN

advice they give. This assumption is faulty. A patient may make only one call to the hospital, usually about something important to him. He'll remember that; you may not.

The telephone log can provide evidence and refresh your recollection of the event. It may remind you that you didn't tell the patient to take two acetaminophen tablets to lower his fever of 105° F (40.6° C). Instead you told him to come to the ED. Or maybe you told a young athlete to come to the ED for an X-ray of his injured ankle.

When you log such information, the law presumes that it is true because you wrote it in the course of ordinary business.

Giving bad news by phone

Sometimes you may have the unpleasant task of telephoning a patient's family member with news of a patient's deteriorating condition or death. Be sure to chart the date, the time, and the name of the family member notified.

Doctor's orders

Because most patient treatments require doctor's orders, careful and accurate documentation of these orders is crucial.

Written orders

No matter who transcribes a doctor's orders—an RN, LPN, or unit secretary —a second person needs to double-check the transcription for accuracy. Your unit should also have some method of checking for transcription errors, such as performing 8-hour or 24-hour chart checks.

Night-shift nurses usually do the 24-hour check by placing a line across the order sheet to indicate that all orders above the line have been checked. They also sign and date the sheet to verify that they've done the 24-hour medication check. The nurse caring for the patient will perform the 8-hour check.

When checking a patient's order sheet, always make sure that the orders were written for the intended patient. Occasionally, an order sheet stamped with one patient's ID plate will inadvertently be placed in another patient's chart. By double-checking, you'll avert potential mistakes.

If an order is unclear, ask the doctor who wrote it to clarify it. Don't waste time asking other people for their interpretation; they'd be guessing too. If a doctor is known to have poor handwriting, ask him to read his orders to you before he leaves the unit.

Preprinted orders

Many health care facilities use preprinted order forms to make doctor's orders easier to read and interpret. If this is the case in your facility, don't automatically assume that a preprinted order is a flawless document in the medical record; it isn't. You may still need to clarify its meaning with the doctor who filled it out. (See *Avoiding pitfalls of preprinted order forms.*)

Verbal orders

Errors made interpreting or documenting verbal orders can lead to mistakes in patient care and liability problems for you. Clearly, verbal orders can be a necessity—especially if you're providing home health care. But in a health care facility, try to take verbal orders only in an emergency when the doctor can't immediately attend to the patient.

In most cases, verbal orders should not include do-not-resuscitate (DNR) or no-code orders.

Carefully follow your facility's policy for documenting a verbal order, and use a special form if one exists. Usually, you'll follow this procedure:

- If time and circumstances allow, have another nurse read the order back to the doctor.
- Record the order on the doctor's order sheet as soon as possible. Note the date and time, and then record the order verbatim.
- On the following line, write "VO" for verbal order. Then write the doctor's name and the name of the nurse who read the order back to the doctor.
- Sign your name and draw a line for the doctor to sign.
- Draw lines through any spaces between the order and your verification of the order.
- Record in ink the type of drug, the dosage, the time you administered it, and any other information your facility's policy requires.

3/23/99	1500	Digoxin 0.125 mg P.O. now
		and daily in a.m. Furosemide
		40 mg P.O. now and daily star-
		ting in a.m. V.O. Dr. Blackstone
		taken by ————————
		———— Judith Schilling, RN, &
		———————— Carla Roy, RN

CHARTING GUIDELINES

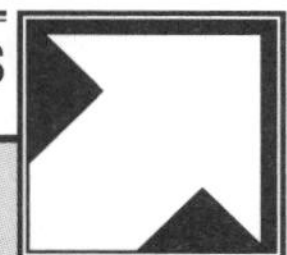

Avoiding pitfalls of preprinted order forms

When documenting the execution of a doctor's preprinted order, make sure that you've interpreted and carried out the order correctly. Even though these forms aim to prevent problems (caused by illegible handwriting, for example), they may still be misread. Here are some considerations for using preprinted forms.

Insist on approved forms
Use only preprinted order forms that have your health care facility's approval and the seal of approval of the medical records committee. Most facilities stamp or print an identification number or code on the form. When in doubt, call the medical records department — the doctor may be using a form he developed or one provided by a drug manufacturer.

Require compliance with policies
To enhance communication and continuity, a preprinted order form needs to comply with facility policies and other regulations. For example, a postoperative preprinted order form shouldn't say "Renew all previous orders" if facility policy requires specific orders. It also shouldn't allow you to select a drug dose from a range ("meperidine 50 to 100 mg I.M. q 4 h," for example) if that's prohibited in your state. Alert your nurse-manager if any order form requires you to perform duties that are outside your scope of practice.

Make sure the form is completed correctly
Many preprinted order forms list more orders than the doctor wants you to follow, so he'll need to indicate which specific interventions he's ordering. For example, he may check the appropriate orders, put his initials next to them, or cross out the ones he doesn't want.

Ask for clarity and precision
Make sure that the doctor orders drug doses in the unit of measure in which they're dispensed. For example, make sure that the form uses the metric system instead of the error-prone apothecary system. Report any errors to your nurse-manager.

Promote proper nomenclature
Ask doctors to use generic drug names, especially when more than one brand of a generic drug is available (for example, "acetaminophen" instead of "Tylenol"). If only one brand of a drug is available, its name can be included in parentheses after the generic name — for example, "dobutamine (Dobutrex)."

Take steps to avoid misinterpretation
Unapproved, potentially dangerous abbreviations and symbols — such as q.d., U, and q.o.d. — don't belong on preprinted order forms. Improper spacing between a drug name and its dosage can also contribute to medication errors. For example, a 20-mg dose of Inderal written as "Inderal20 mg" could be misinterpreted as 120 mg.

Ensure that the copy is readable
If your facility uses a no-carbon-required form, make sure that the bottom copy contains an identical set of preprinted orders; this is the copy that goes to the pharmacy. All lines on the bottom copy should also appear on the top copy — extra lines on the pharmacy copy can hide decimal points (making 1.5 look like 15, for example) and the tops of numbers (making 7 look like 1 and 5 look like 3).

Make sure that the doctor countersigns the order within the time limits set by your facility's policy. Without this countersignature, you may be held liable for practicing medicine without a license.

Telephone orders

Your patient is having trouble breathing. Your assessment findings include bilateral crackles on auscultation and dependent edema. The doctor, who's busy in an emergency, gives you a telephone order for oxygen.

Normally, you should accept only written orders from a doctor. But in a situation such as this, when the patient needs immediate treatment and the doctor isn't available to write an order, telephone orders are acceptable.

Telephone orders may also be taken to expedite care when new information is available that doesn't require a physical examination (such as laboratory data). Keep in mind that telephone orders are for the patient's well-being and not strictly for convenience. They should be given directly to you, rather than through a third party.

Carefully follow your facility's policy for documenting a telephone order. Generally, you'll follow this procedure:

- Record the order on the doctor's order sheet as soon as possible. Note the date and time; then write the order verbatim. On the next line, write "T.O." for telephone order. (Don't use "P.O." for phone order; that abbreviation could be misinterpreted to mean "by mouth.") Then write the doctor's name and sign your name. If another nurse listened to the order with you, have her sign the order too.

2/4/99	1100	M.S. Contin 30 mg P.O. now
		and q 12 hr for pain. Bisacodyl
		suppos. ī PR now. May repeat
		x 1 if no results. ————
		— T.O. Dr. Kaufman/Jane Goddard, RN,
		———— & Carol Barsky, RN

- Draw lines through any blank spaces in the order.
- Make sure that the doctor countersigns the order within the set time limits. Without his signature, you may be held liable for practicing medicine without a license.

To save time and avoid errors, consider asking the doctor to send a copy of the order by fax machine. (See *Advantages of faxing orders.*)

Clarifying doctor's orders

Although unit secretaries may transcribe orders, the nurse is ultimately responsible for the accuracy of the transcription. Only you have the authority and knowledge to question the validity of orders and to spot errors.

Follow your health care facility's policy for clarifying orders that are vague or possibly erroneous. If you don't have a policy to cover a particular situation, contact the prescribing doctor, and always document your actions. Then ask your nursing administrator for a step-by-step policy to follow so you'll know what do if the situation ever recurs.

An order may be correct when issued but improper later because of changes in the patient's status. When this occurs, delay the treatment until you've contacted the doctor and clarified the situation. Follow your facility's policy for clarifying an order. (See *When in doubt, question orders,* page 314.)

Clarify ambiguous orders with the doctor. Document your efforts to clarify the order, and document whether the order was carried out. If you believe a doctor's order is in error, you must refuse to carry it out until you receive clarification. Keep a record of your refusal together with the reasons and an account of all communication with the doctor. Inform your immediate supervisor. If the order is correct as written, initial and check off each line. Below the doctor's signature, sign your name, the date, and the time.

DNR orders

When a patient is terminally ill and his death is expected, his doctor and family (and the patient if appropriate) may agree that a DNR (do not resuscitate), or no-code, order is appropriate. The doctor writes the order, and the staff carries it out when the patient goes into cardiac or respiratory arrest.

1/19/99	1900	DO NOT RESUSCITATE THIS
		PATIENT. — Deepak Patel, MD

Because DNR orders are recognized legally, you'll incur no liability when a patient you don't try to resuscitate later dies. You may, however, incur liability if you initiate resuscitation counter to the DNR order.

Every patient with a DNR code should have a written order on file. The order should be consistent with the facility's policy, which often requires that such orders be reviewed every 48 to 72 hours.

If a terminally ill patient without a DNR order tells you orally that he doesn't want to be resuscitated in a crisis, document his statement as well as his degree of awareness and orientation. Then contact the patient's doctor and your nurse-manager, and ask for assistance from administration, legal services, or social services.

Increasingly, patients are deciding in advance of a crisis whether or not they want to be resuscitated. Health care facilities must

CHARTING TIMESAVER

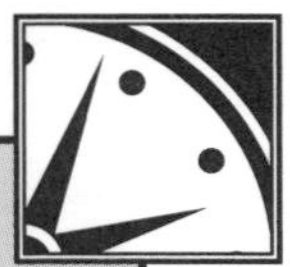

Advantages of faxing orders

The facsimile, or fax, network in most hospitals now includes the clinical laboratory, pharmacy, and radiology and cardiology departments. Faxing has two main advantages: It speeds transmittal of doctor's orders and test results to different departments, and it reduces the likelihood of errors.

Speeds communication

Faxing allows doctors to back up phone orders in writing for the patient's chart. Orders can be faxed not only to you on the unit but also to the pharmacy, radiology department, and other relevant departments. The results: no more time wasted calling the department and waiting to get through and no more time spent waiting for orders to be picked up.

In return, the receiving department gets a copy of the original order (needed for filling the order and for department files). If an order can't be filled, the receiving department can contact the doctor for clarification or for a new order, again reducing delays in filling orders and wasting your time as a go-between. An additional advantage comes from the fax machine itself, which prints the date and time the order was sent and the department it came from.

Faxing also allows staff members to transmit exact copies of X-rays, laboratory test results, and electrocardiogram strips in as little as 15 seconds.

Reduces errors

Using a fax network helps you and other staff members prevent errors by checking one another's work and consulting the doctor directly about unresolved problems. What's more, faxing provides printed accounts, promoting accurate documentation.

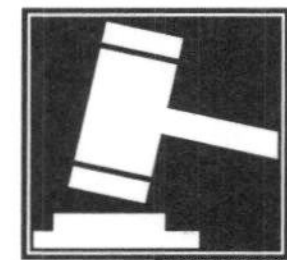

ON TRIAL

When in doubt, question orders

Always question a doctor's order if it seems strange or "not right."

In *Poor Sisters of Saint Francis Seraph of the Perpetual Adoration, et al. v. Catron* (1982), a hospital was held liable for negligence because a nurse failed to question a doctor's order about an endotracheal tube.

The doctor ordered that the tube be left in the patient's trachea for an excessively long period: 5 days instead of the standard 2 to 3 days. The nurse knew that 5 days was exceptionally long, but instead of clarifying the doctor's order and documenting her actions, she followed the order.

As a result, the patient's voice box was irreparably damaged, and the court ruled the hospital negligent.

provide written information to patients concerning their rights under state law to make decisions regarding their care, including the right to refuse medical treatment and the right to formulate an advance directive. (See chapter 2, Legal and Ethical Implications of Documentation.)

This information must be provided to all patients, usually upon admission. You must also document that the patient received this information and whether he brought a written advance directive with him. (See *Documenting advance directives.*) In some instances, you can file a photocopy of the directive in the patient's record.

As a nurse, you have a responsibility to help the patient make an informed decision about continuing treatment. If the patient's wishes differ from those of his family or doctor, make sure that the discrepancies are thoroughly documented in the chart.

INCIDENTS

A patient injury — typically referred to as an *incident* — is a serious situation. It may be the result of patient action, staff action, or equipment failure. Chart all patient injuries caused by falls, restraints, burns, or other factors. Then file an incident report in compliance with your health care facility's procedure. Also file an incident report whenever a patient insists on being discharged against medical advice.

An incident report serves two functions. First, it informs the administration of the incident, allowing the risk management team to consider changes that might prevent similar incidents in the future. Second, it alerts the administration and the health care facility's insurance company to a potential claim and the need for further investigation.

Only a person with firsthand knowledge of an incident should file a report, and only the person making the report should sign it. Never sign a report describing circumstances or events that you didn't witness. Each person with firsthand knowledge should fill out and sign a *separate* report. Your report should:

- identify the person involved in the incident
- document accurately and objectively any unusual occurrences that you witnessed
- record details of what happened and the consequences for the persons involved; include sufficient information so that admin-

CHARTING GUIDELINES

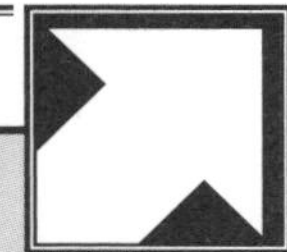

Documenting advance directives

Spurred by patients' requests and the passage of self-determination laws in many states, more and more health care facilities are requiring documentation of advance directives or lack of same.

An advance directive is a legal document by which a person tells his medical caregivers how he prefers to be treated in an illness from which he can't reasonably expect to recover. Advance directives also include living wills (which instruct the doctor to administer no life-sustaining treatment) and durable powers of attorney (which name another person to act in the patient's behalf for medical decisions in the event that the patient can't act for himself).

Because these laws vary from state to state, be sure to find out how your state's law applies to your practice and to the medical record.

Previously executed directive

If a patient has previously executed an advance directive, request a copy of it for his chart and make sure that his doctor is aware of it. Some health care facilities routinely make this request a part of admission or preadmission procedures.

Also be sure to document the name, address, and phone number of the person entrusted with decision-making power.

Presently executed directive

If a patient wants to execute an advance directive during his stay in your facility, he can do so as long as he's a competent adult. In such a case, the record should include documented proof of competence (usually the responsibility of the medical, legal, social services, or risk management department) along with the signed and witnessed, newly executed advance directive.

Directives about nutrition and hydration

If you practice in an area with laws related to artificial nutrition and hydration (nourishment provided by invasive tubes and I.V. lines), record the patient's wishes if these issues are not addressed in his advance directive.

Revocation of the directive

Legally, the patient can revoke an advance directive at any time either orally or in writing. In such a case, include a copy of the written revocation in the record, or sign and date a statement in the patient's medical record explaining that the patient made the request orally. Consult your facility's policy and state laws pertaining to living wills and advance directives; revocation statements may need to be countersigned.

istrators can decide whether the matter requires further investigation

- avoid opinions, judgments, conclusions, or assumptions about who or what caused the incident
- avoid making suggestions about how to prevent the incident from happening again.

Detailed statements from witnesses and descriptions of remedial action are normally part of an investigative follow-up; don't include them in the incident report itself. Although the incident report isn't part of the patient's chart, it may be used later in litigation. Don't note in the chart that you filed an incident report, but do include the clinical details of the incident in the chart. Make sure that the descriptions in the incident report are consistent with those in the chart. (See chapter 2, Legal and Ethical Implications of Documentation.)

After it's filed, the incident report may be reviewed by the nursing supervisor, the doc-

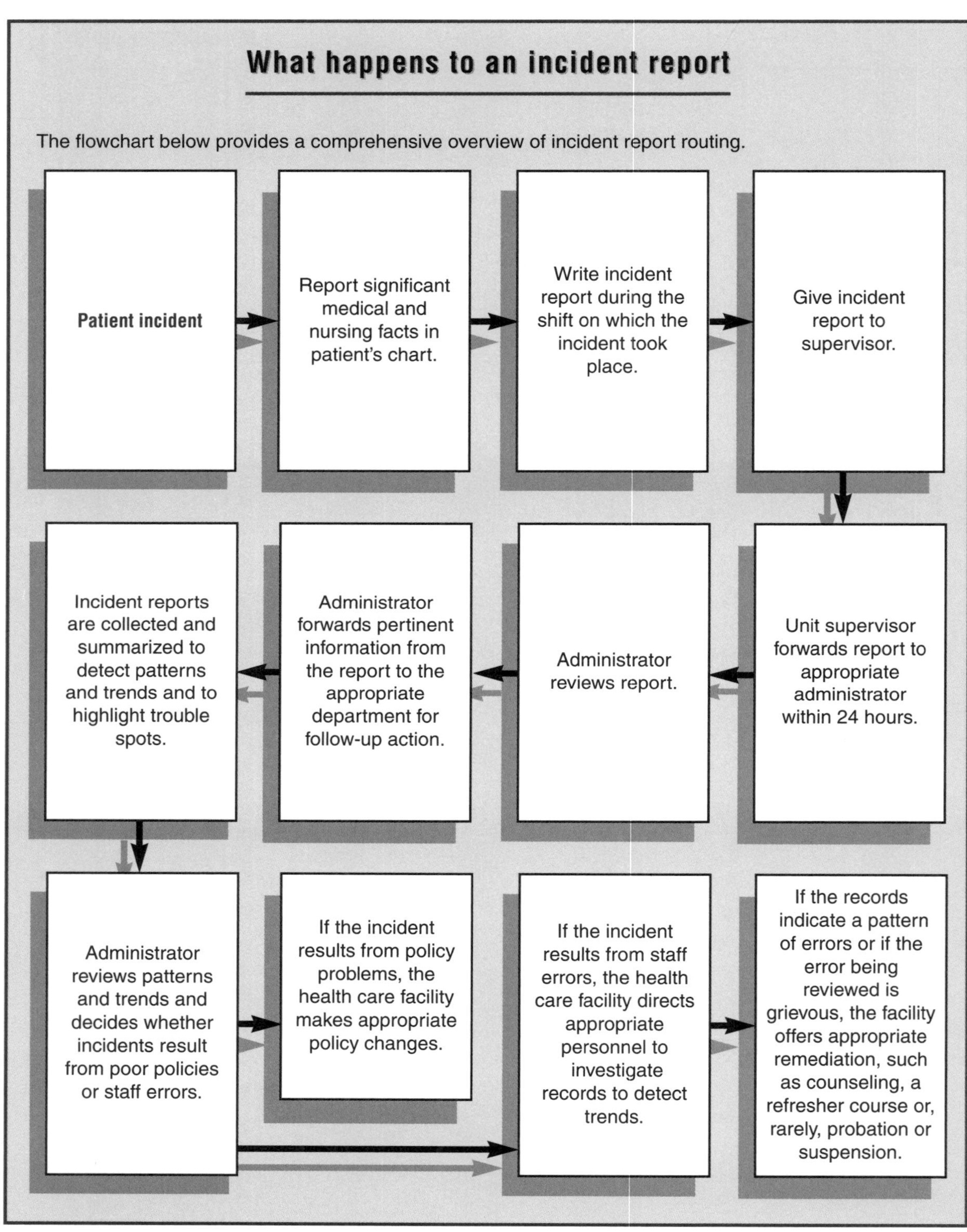
What happens to an incident report
The flowchart below provides a comprehensive overview of incident report routing.
Patient incident
Report significant medical and nursing facts in patient's chart.
Write incident report during the shift on which the incident took place.
Give incident report to supervisor.
Unit supervisor forwards report to appropriate administrator within 24 hours.
Administrator reviews report.
Administrator forwards pertinent information from the report to the appropriate department for follow-up action.
Incident reports are collected and summarized to detect patterns and trends and to highlight trouble spots.
Administrator reviews patterns and trends and decides whether incidents result from poor policies or staff errors.
If the incident results from policy problems, the health care facility makes appropriate policy changes.
If the incident results from staff errors, the health care facility directs appropriate personnel to investigate records to detect trends.
If the records indicate a pattern of errors or if the error being reviewed is grievous, the facility offers appropriate remediation, such as counseling, a refresher course or, rarely, probation or suspension.

tor called to examine the patient, appropriate department heads and administrators, the health care facility's attorney, and the insurance company. (See *What happens to an incident report.*)

Falls

Current research shows that falls — involving patients, visitors, and staff — constitute most of the incidents reported on clinical units. Among the events qualifying as falls are slips, slides, knees giving way, faints, or tripping over equipment.

Consequences of falls include prolonged hospitalization, increased hospital costs, and liability problems.

Risk assessment and prevention

Because falls raise so many problems, your health care facility may require an all-out risk assessment and prevention effort. If so, you'll need to document your role in this activity. For example, if your facility requires a risk assessment form for patients, complete it and keep it in the patient's chart. (See *Determining a patient's risk of falling,* page 318.)

Avoiding falls

There are no foolproof ways to prevent every patient from falling, but the following strategies may help. As required by your health care facility, document the following safety interventions:

- Keep the bed's side rails raised or lowered, when indicated, and include your decision to do so in the chart as part of your interventions for addressing the nursing diagnosis of "Risk for trauma."
- Monitor the patient regularly — continuously, if his condition requires it — and document your findings.
- Offer a bedpan or commode regularly, and chart this care measure.
- Provide an adequately lighted, clean, and clutter-free environment.
- Make sure that someone helps and supports the patient whenever he gets out of bed and that he has proper footwear for walking safely.
- Make sure that adequate staff are available to transfer him, if necessary.
- Apply restraints or mechanical devices as ordered that provide a warning signal when a patient tries to climb out of bed.
- Suggest that a relative or friend stay with the patient.
- Patients taking medications that cause orthostatic hypotension, central nervous system depression, or vestibular toxicity need special nursing care when a doctor's orders require them to be in a chair for meals. If you can't supervise such a patient while he's sitting, make sure that another member of the health care team does.

Charting falls

If a patient falls despite precautions, be sure to chart the event and file an incident report. Check the patient for bruises, lacerations, or abrasions. Note any pain or deformity in the extremities, particularly the hip, arm, leg, or lumbar spine. Assess blood pressure while the patient is lying down and sitting up. Look for a drop of 20 to 30 mm Hg in the systolic reading, which may indicate orthostatic hypotension. Perform a neurologic assessment. Check for slurred speech, weakness in the extremi-

BETTER CHARTING

Determining a patient's risk of falling

Certain patients have a greater risk of falling than others. Using a chart such as the one below, which was developed for use with older patients, can help you determine the extent of the risk. To use the chart, check each applicable item and total the number of points. A score of 10 or more indicates a risk of falling.

POINTS	PATIENT CATEGORY
	Age
1 ___	80 or older
2 ✔	70 to 79 years old
	Mental state
0 ___	Oriented at all times or comatose
2 ___	Confused at all times
4 ✔	Confused periodically
	Duration of hospitalization
0 ✔	Over 3 days
2 ___	0 to 3 days
	Falls within the past 6 months
0 ___	None
2 ✔	1 or 2
5 ___	3 or more
	Elimination
0 ✔	Independent and continent
1 ___	Uses catheter, ostomy, or both
3 ___	Needs help with elimination
5 ___	Independent and incontinent
1 ✔	**Visual impairment**
3 ___	**Confinement to chair**
2 ___	**Blood pressure** Drop in systolic pressure of 20 mm Hg or more between lying and standing positions

POINTS	PATIENT CATEGORY
	Gait and balance Assess gait by having the patient stand in one spot with both feet on the ground for 30 seconds without holding onto something. Then have him walk straight ahead and through a doorway. Next, have him turn while walking.
1 ___	Wide base of support
1 ✔	Loss of balance while standing
1 ___	Balance problems when walking
1 ___	Diminished muscle coordination
1 ___	Lurching or swaying
1 ___	Holds on or changes gait when walking through a doorway
1 ___	Jerking or instability when turning
1 ___	Needs an assistive device, such as a walker
	Medications How many different drugs is the patient taking?
0 ___	None
1 ___	1
2 ✔	2 or more

___	Alcohol	___	Cathartics
___	Anesthetics	___	Diuretics
___	Antihistamines	___	Narcotics
✔	Antihypertensives	___	Psychotropics
___	Antiseizure drugs	___	Sedative hypnotics
✔	Antidiabetics	___	Other drugs (specify)
___	Benzodiazepines		

POINTS	PATIENT CATEGORY
1 ✔	Check if the patient has changed drugs, dosage, or both in the past 5 days.
13	**TOTAL**

ties, or a change in mental status. Notify the patient's doctor, who should assess the patient.

3/6/99	1400	Pt. found on floor beside her
		bed and chair. Pt. c/o pain in
		her Ⓡ hip area and difficulty
		moving Ⓡ leg. No abrasions or
		lacerations noted. BP elevated
		at 158/94; P, 94; R, 22. Pt.
		states she fell trying to get to
		her chair. Mental status un-
		changed. Dr. Dayoub notified.
		Pt. returned to bed. Hip X-ray
		reveals fractured Ⓡ hip. Pt.
		medicated for hip pain. Family
		notified by Dr. Dayoub. Pt.
		assessed hourly. Discussed the
		need for side rails with pt.
		Instructed her in use of call
		button. Side rails up at pres-
		ent. ———— Beverly Kotsur, RN

Restraints

Restraints are defined as any method of physically restricting a person's freedom of movement, physical activity, or normal access to his body. Restraints can cause numerous problems, including limited mobility, skin breakdown, impaired circulation, incontinence, and strangulation.

Restraints are "prescriptive devices"—you can't use them unless you have a doctor's order. (Some states may authorize other licensed health care professionals to prescribe restraints.) In most facilities, the order must be renewed by the doctor every 24 hours. (See *Physical restraint order,* page 320.) You'll need to consult your facility's policy for the correct protocol to follow in emergencies—for example, when the patient's safety is at risk and you have no time to obtain an order.

Institutional restraint policies, procedures, and protocols should be based on professional practice standards and then approved by appropriate committees. Depending on the institution involved, the committee will include members of the medical staff, nursing staff, and safety committee. Policies and protocols must specify your facility's definition of restraints, who is authorized to carry out the order, and how the order will be conveyed.

If you are ordered to use restraints on a patient, avoid causing pain or injury to the patient by applying them in a safe manner. (See *Using restraints safely,* page 321.)

The medical record of all restrained patients must show evidence of the following:

- written orders for restraint or seclusion
- name of licensed independent practitioner who ordered the restraint
- reason for the restraint
- type of restraint
- attempted alternatives to restraints, if any
- reassessment by a licensed independent practitioner for a continuation of the original order
- monitoring and reassessment of the patient in restraints. (See *Quality assurance outcome monitor for soft restraints,* page 322.)

If a competent patient makes an informed decision to refuse restraints, the facility may require the patient to sign a release that would absolve the facility of liability should injury result from the patient's refusal to be restrained.

Burns

Burns are another common cause of injury to patients. Patients are burned by spilled hot food or liquids, hot baths, and electrical equipment. Always assess the risk of burns

BETTER CHARTING

Physical restraint order

A form such as the one shown here must be in the patient's chart before physical restraints are applied.

Date: 2/12/99 **Time:** 0315

Reason for restraint use (circle all that apply):

To prevent:

1. Falls
2. (circled) Removal of indwelling lines/tubes ® subclavian CV line
3. (circled) Self-extubation
4. Other

Duration of restraint: (Not to exceed 24 hr) 24 hr

Type of restraint (circle all that apply):

Vest

(Left mitt) (Right mitt)

Left wrist Right wrist

Left ankle Right ankle

Other

Doctor's signature Colette Hendler, MD

and take appropriate precautions.

Patients who have hand tremors should be cautioned not to handle hot foods or liquids by themselves. Patients with decreased sensation in their feet or hands should be taught to test bathwater with an unaffected extremity. Explain to patients taking medication causing drowsiness that they may be more prone to burns and need to be cautious. Document these instructions and the patient's response to this information in your notes.

If a patient in your care does burn himself, always document the injury in his chart.

1/8/99	1100	Pt. dropped hot cup of tea on
		® thigh. Area slightly pink, sen-
		sitive to touch, with no edema.
		Dr. Adler notified. Cold com-
		presses ordered and applied.
		Pt. tolerates cold compress
		well. Tylenol Extra-Strength
		500 mg X 1 given with relief.
		——— Colleen Cameron, RN

Discharge AMA

Although a patient can choose to leave a health care facility against medical advice

ON TRIAL

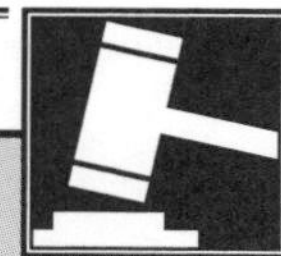

Using restraints safely

Improperly restraining a patient can leave you vulnerable to a host of legal charges, such as negligence, professional malpractice, false imprisonment, and battery. The case discussed below is about a nurse who failed to use restraints effectively.

The patient who slipped away

In *Robison v. Micheline Faine and Catalano's Nurse Registry, Inc.* (1987), the nurse, Micheline Faine, was required to restrain the patient, Ms. Robison, before leaving her hospital room. With the time for lunch break approaching, Faine tied the patient in a restraining device and left to find a relief nurse. Once the relief nurse entered the room, Faine left for lunch.

When Faine returned 20 minutes later, she found that Ms. Robison was gone, although the restraining device was still attached to the bed and the side rails were up. While Faine had been at lunch, Ms. Robison had slipped out of the restraint, left the hospital through an emergency stairway leading to the roof, and attempted to jump to a nearby tree. She fell to the ground and sustained serious injuries.

No exemption from liability

At the malpractice trial, the judge instructed the jury to exempt Ms. Faine from liability. But an appeals court disagreed. It ruled that Ms. Faine wasn't automatically exempt from liability because the patient would have been unable to free herself if the restraining device had been tied correctly. The appeals court ordered a new trial for Ms. Faine to determine whether she was negligent.

(AMA) at any time, the law requires clear evidence that he's mentally competent to make that choice. In most facilities, an AMA form serves as a legal document to protect you, the doctors, and the facility should any problems arise from a patient's unapproved discharge.

The AMA form should clearly document that the patient knows he's leaving against medical advice, that he's been advised of the risks of leaving and understands them, and that he knows he can come back. If a patient refuses to sign the AMA form, document this refusal on the form and enter it in his chart. Use the patient's own words to describe his refusal.

Include the following information on the AMA form:

- patient's reason for leaving AMA
- names of relatives or others notified of the patient's decision and the dates and times of the notifications
- explanation of the risks and consequences of the AMA discharge, as told to the patient, including the name of the person who provided the explanation
- instructions regarding alternative sources of follow-up care given to the patient
- list of those accompanying the patient at discharge and the instructions given to them
- patient's destination after discharge.

Document any statements and actions reflecting the patient's mental state at the time he chose to leave the facility. This will help

BETTER CHARTING

Quality assurance outcome monitor for soft restraints

This form lists criteria for the use of soft restraints and for ensuring that interventions are properly documented.

Date: 1/30/99 **Department:** Nursing
Room No.: 325 **Staff signature:** Pamela Petrakis, RN

Criteria: Soft restraint: Any use of soft restraints (padded mitts, cloth wrist or ankle restraints, cloth vests)	**Satisfactory**	**Unsatisfactory**
1. Is there documentation of clinical justification for restraint?	√	
2. Does the documentation show that less restrictive measures were attempted prior to restraints?	√	
3. Is a clinical assessment documented prior to the use of restraint by an RN?	√	
4. Is there a doctor's order for each incident of restraint documented within 8 hours of restraints? Signed within 24 hours?	√	
5. Is the time of going into restraint specified in the doctor's order?	√	
6. Is the doctor's order time limited? Use "Not to exceed 24 hours" instead of "up to."	√	
7. Is there an RN progress note written describing this incident? (Prior to and after D/C of restraint)	√	
8. Does the restraint documentation reflect that the patient's needs were not neglected? (Review flow sheet.)	√	
9. Does documentation reflect interventions of staff with patient after restraint?	√	
10. Is the restraint record complete?	√	
11. Does the documentation reflect the physical status of the patient prior to use of restraint and after removal of restraint?	√	
12. Is the order renewed every 24 hours?	√	

Comments:

protect you, the doctors, and the facility against a charge of negligence. The patient may later claim that his discharge occurred while he was mentally incompetent and that he was improperly supervised while he was in that state.

1/4/99	1400	Pt. found in room packing his clothes. When asked why he was dressed and packing, he stated, "I'm tired of all these tests. They keep doing tests, but they still don't know what's wrong with me. I can't take any more. I'm going home." Dr. Giordano notified and came to speak with pt. Pt.'s wife notified and she came to the hospital. She was unable to persuade husband to stay. Pt. willing to sign AMA form. AMA form signed. Pt. told of possible risks of his leaving the hospital with headaches and hypertension. Pt. agrees to see Dr. Giordano in his office in 2 days. Discussed appointment with pt. and wife. Pt. going home after discharge. Accompanied patient in wheelchair to main lobby, with wife. Pt. left at 1445 hr.
		Lynn Nakashima, RN

Also check your facility's policy regarding incident reports. If the patient leaves without anyone's knowledge or if he refuses to sign the AMA form, you'll probably be required to complete an incident report.

Missing patient

Suppose the same patient never said anything about leaving, but on rounds you discover he's missing. First, of course, try to find him in the building. Attempt to contact his home. If he's gone, notify your nurse-manager, the patient's doctor, and the police, if necessary. The police are usually called if there is a possibility of the patient hurting himself or others, especially if he has left the facility with any medical devices.

In the chart, note the time that you discovered the patient missing, your attempts to find him, and the people notified. Include any other pertinent information.

Selected references

"Charting Tips: How to Document Objectively," *Nursing97* 27(7):17, July 1997.

Cirone, N.R. "Charting Tips: Documenting Return Demonstrations," *Nursing97* 27(12):17, December 1997.

Craven, G.A., et al. "What to Do When You Note a Medication Error," *Massachusetts Nurse* 68(2): 1-2, February 1998.

Eggland, E.T. "Charting Smarter: Using New Mechanisms to Organize Your Paperwork," *Nursing95* 25(9):34-42, September 1995.

Eggland, E.T. "Charting Tips: Avoiding Incomplete Charting," *Nursing95* 25(10):73, October 1995.

Fitzpatrick, L., and Fitzpatrick, T. "Blood Transfusion: Keeping Your Patient Safe," *Nursing97* 27(8):34-41, August 1997.

Maher, V.F. "Charting Tips: Countersigning Notes By Others," *Nursing97* 27(6):17, June 1997.

Miller, B. "Meeting JCAHO Patient-Education Standards," *Nursing Management* 28(5):55-58, May 1997.

Miller, D.L. "Notes from the Field: Improving Interdisciplinary Communication," *Nursing Management* 29(4):47, 49, April 1998.

Scharf, L. "Revising Nursing Documentation to Meet Patient Outcomes," *Nursing Management* 28(4):38-39, April 1997.

Schuster, J. "Looking Out for Adverse Drug Reactions," *Nursing97* 27(11):34-39, November 1997.

Snyder, B. "An Easy Way to Document Patient Education," *RN* 59(3):43-45, March 1996.

Thorman, M. "Documenting Wound Care for Pressure Ulcers," *Topics in Geriatric Rehabilitation* 13(1):33-43, September 1997.

Tibbitts, M.G. "Patients Who Fall: How to Predict and Prevent Injury," *Geriatric Nursing* 51(9): 24-33, September 1996.

10

Legally Perilous Charting Practices

If you're ever named in a malpractice suit that proceeds to court, your documentation may be your best defense. It provides a running record of your patient care. How and what you documented—and even what you didn't document—will heavily influence the outcome of the trial.

Credible evidence

Typically, the outcome of every malpractice trial boils down to one question: Whom will the jury believe? The answer usually depends on the credibility of the evidence. In a malpractice suit, a plaintiff presents evidence designed to show that he was harmed or injured because care provided by the defendant (in this case, the nurse) failed to meet accepted standards of care. The nurse, of course, strives to present evidence demonstrating that she provided an acceptable standard of care. However, if she can't offer believable evidence, the jury may have no choice but to accept the plaintiff's evidence. Even worse, if the nurse's evidence—including the medical record—is discredited, the plaintiff's attorney may convince a jury of her negligence.

In a malpractice suit, jurors may view the medical record as the best evidence of what really happened. It may be the hinge that swings the jury's verdict.

Negligent or not

If you have actually been negligent and have truthfully documented the care given, the medical record will naturally be the plaintiff's best evidence, as it should be. In such instances, the case will probably be settled out of court.

If you haven't been negligent, the medical record should be your best defense, providing the best evidence of quality care. If the charted record makes you *seem* negligent, however, the jurors may conclude that you *were* negligent, because they base their decision on the evidence. The lesson: A "bad" medical record can be used to make a good nurse look bad. A "good" medical record should defend those who wrote it.

By knowing how to chart, what to chart, when to chart, and even who should chart, you'll create a solid record. And knowing how to handle legally sensitive situations, such as difficult and nonconforming patients; how to avoid misinterpreting written records; and how to protect yourself when charting on computer, faxing records, and giving telephone advice, will offer additional safeguards.

How to chart

You may assume that every nurse knows how to chart, but this isn't necessarily so. Charting is a craft that's refined with experience. A skilled nurse knows that she needs to document that the standard of care was delivered, keeping in mind that it's not only *what* she charts but *how* she charts that's important.

Chart objectively

The medical record should contain descriptive, objective information: what you see, hear, feel, smell, measure, and count—not what you suppose, infer, conclude, or assume. The chart may also contain subjective information, but only when it's supported by documented facts.

Stick to the facts

To make sure that you keep the medical record factual, follow these simple rules:

- *Record only what you see and hear.* For example, don't record that a patient pulled out his I.V. line if you didn't witness him doing so. Do, however, describe your findings — for example, "Found pt., arm board, and bed linens covered with blood. I.V. line and venipuncture device were untaped and hanging free."

Similarly, don't record that a patient fell out of bed if you didn't see him fall. If you saw him lying on the floor, record that. If the patient says he fell out of bed, record that. If you heard a muffled thud, went to the patient's room, and found him lying on the floor, record that. (See *Avoiding assumptions.*) An example of how to document a patient's fall appears below.

1/8/99	0600	Heard pt. scream. Found pt.
		lying beside bed. Pt. has lacer-
		ation 2 cm long on forehead.
		Side rails up. Pt. stated he
		climbed over side rails to go
		to the bathroom. BP 184/92,
		P 96, R 24. Dr. Phillips notified
		and ordered X-ray. Pt. c/o
		pain in Ⓡ hip. Pt. taken for
		X-ray of Ⓡ hip. ————
		———— Sonia Benoit, RN

- *Describe — don't label — events and behavior.* Expressions such as "appears spaced out," "flying high," "exhibiting bizarre behavior," or "using obscenities" mean different things to different people.

If a plaintiff's attorney asked you to define those terms, could you do it? Even if you could, would you be likely to gain or lose credibility in the process?

Facts, accurately reported, reflect professionalism. Subjective conclusions force you into the uncomfortable position of having to defend your own words. You will almost always lose credibility and distract the jury from the fact that you provided the standard of care to the patient.

ON TRIAL

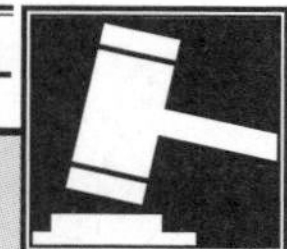

Avoiding assumptions

Always aim to record the facts about a situation — not your assumptions or conclusions. In the following example, a nurse failed to document the facts and instead charted her assumptions about a patient's fall. As a result, she had to endure this damaging cross-examination by the plaintiff's attorney.

ATTORNEY: Would you read your fifth entry for January 6th, please?
NURSE: "Patient fell out of bed. . . ."
ATTORNEY: Thank you. Did you actually see the patient fall out of bed?
NURSE: Actually, no.
ATTORNEY: Did the patient tell you he fell out of bed?
NURSE: No.
ATTORNEY: Did anyone actually see the patient fall out of bed?
NURSE: Not that I know of.
ATTORNEY: So these notes reflect nothing more than conjecture on your part. Is that correct?
NURSE: I guess so.
ATTORNEY: Is it fair to say then, that you charted something as fact even though you didn't know it was?
NURSE: I suppose so.
ATTORNEY: Thank you.

- *Be specific.* Your goal in documenting is to describe facts clearly and concisely. To do so, use only approved abbreviations and express your observations in quantifiable terms.

For example, the conclusion "output adequate" is vague. Give an exact measurement, such as "1,200 ml." Similarly, "Pt. appears to be in pain" is vague. Ask yourself why he "appears to be in pain" and document the specific findings — for example, "Pt. requested pain medication after complaining of severe but slow-onset lower back pain radiating to his right leg, 6 on a scale of 0 to 10. No numbness or tingling, no edema. Color of extremity pink, temperature warm."

Similarly, avoid catchall phrases such as "Pt. comfortable." Instead, describe his comfort. Is he resting, reading, sleeping? This type of information is more helpful and informative.

Here's an example of specific, clear documentation:

2/11/99	1400	Dressing removed from Ⓡ
		mastectomy site. Incision is
		pink. No drainage. Measures
		12.5 cm long and 2 cm wide.
		Slight bruising noted near cen-
		ter of incision. Dressing dry.
		Drain site below mastectomy
		incision measures 2 cm x 2 cm.
		Bloody, dime-sized drainage
		noted on drain dressing. No
		edema noted. Betadine dres-
		sings applied. Pt. complaining
		of mild incisional pain, 3 on a
		scale of 0 to 10. 2 Tylox P.O.
		given at 1330 hours. Pt. re-
		ports relief at 1355.
		Joan Delaney, RN

Use neutral language

Avoid including inappropriate comments or language in your notes. Not only are such comments unprofessional, but they can also trigger difficulties in legal cases.

For example, one elderly patient's family became upset after the patient developed pressure ulcers. They complained that the patient wasn't receiving adequate care. The patient later died of natural causes.

However, because the patient's family was dissatisfied with the care the patient received, they sued. In the patient's chart, under prognosis, the doctor had written "PBBB." After learning that this stood for "pine box by bedside," the insurance company was only too happy to settle for a significant sum.

Avoid bias

Don't use words that suggest a negative attitude toward the patient. For example, don't use unflattering or unprofessional adjectives, such as *obstinate, drunk, obnoxious, bizarre,* or *abusive,* to describe the patient's behavior.

Remember, the chart is a legal document. Imagine how your harsh words would sound in court. They most certainly would invite the plaintiff's attorney to attack your professionalism with an argument such as this: "Look at how this nurse felt about my client — she called him 'rude, difficult, and uncooperative.' It's right here in her own handwriting! No wonder she didn't take good care of this patient — she didn't like him."

If a patient is difficult or uncooperative, document the behavior objectively. That way, the jurors will draw their own conclusions.

1/19/99	1400	I attempted to give pt.
		medication, but he said, "I've
		had enough pills. Now leave
		me alone." Explained the
		importance of the medication
		and attempted to determine
		why he would not take it. Pt.
		refused to talk. Dr. Ellis
		notified that medication was
		refused.
		Anne Curry, RN

Keep the medical record intact

Take special care to keep the patient's chart complete and intact. Discarding pages from the medical record, even for innocent reasons, is bound to raise doubt in the jury's mind about the chart's reliability.

Suppose, for example, you spill coffee on a page, blurring several entries. You remove the original page from the chart, copy it, and place the copy in the chart. Then you discard the original. Imagine having to admit to a jury that you destroyed original evidence.

You could try to explain that you did so for an innocent reason, but the jury could be difficult to convince. Jurors are skeptical; they must be. Giving them a reason to doubt you makes the plaintiff's job a lot easier and yours much more difficult.

When something is considered part of the official record, never discard or destroy it. If you replace an original sheet with a copy, cross-reference it with lines like these: "Recopied from page 4" or "Recopied on page 6." Be sure to attach the original. If a page is damaged, note "reconstructed charting," and attach the damaged page. (See *Consequences of missing records.*)

ON TRIAL

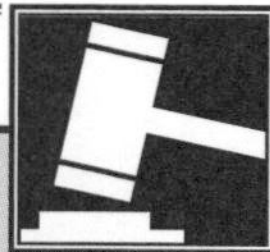

Consequences of missing records

The case of *Battocchi v. Washington Hospital Center,* 581 A.2d 759 (D.C. App. 1990) underscores the significance of keeping the medical record intact. In this case the plaintiffs brought a medical malpractice suit against the hospital and a doctor for injuries sustained by their son during forceps delivery.

The nurse in attendance documented the events and her observations of the delivery immediately after the delivery. Later, the hospital's risk management personnel obtained the chart for analysis but apparently lost the nurse's notes from the record.

The court ruled in favor of the hospital and doctor, holding that the jury couldn't presume negligence and causation against them simply because the hospital lost the attending nurse's notes.

However, on appeal, the District of Columbia Court of Appeals sent the case back to the trial court so that the lower court could rule whether the hospital's loss of the records stemmed from negligence or impropriety.

What to chart

When you're busy, getting your work done may seem more important than documenting every detail. But from a jury's viewpoint, an incomplete chart suggests incomplete nursing care. This is one of the most serious and common charting errors. It's no accident that a popular saying among malpractice attorneys is "If it wasn't charted, it wasn't done."

That's not literally true, of course, but it's an easy conclusion for a jury to draw. You may have performed a nursing procedure that you simply forgot to chart. If the chart doesn't back you up, though, you'll have a hard time convincing a jury to accept your version of events.

Ask yourself, What is your responsibility to the patient? It is to deliver the accepted standard of care and to document it in order to communicate with other health care providers and establish a permanent record of care. If this is done, you can defend yourself. Areas of documentation that are frequently

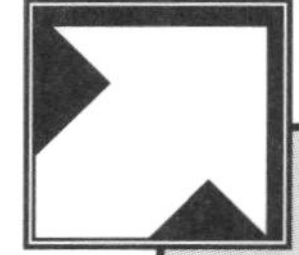

CHARTING GUIDELINES

Keeping the record clean

What you say and how you say it are of utmost importance in documentation. Keeping the patient's chart free of negative, inappropriate information—potential legal bombshells —can be quite a challenge when you're writing detailed narrative notes. Here are some guidelines to help you sidestep charting pitfalls and record an accurate account of your patient's care and status.

Avoid reporting staffing problems
Even though staff shortages may affect patient care or contribute to an incident, you should not refer to staffing problems in a patient's chart. Instead, discuss them in a forum that can help resolve the problem. In a confidential memo or an incident report, call the situation to the attention of the appropriate personnel, such as your nurse-manager. Also review your hospital's policy and procedure manuals to determine how you're expected to handle this situation.

Keep staff conflicts and rivalries out of the record
Entries about disputes with nursing colleagues (including characterization and criticism of care provided), questions about a doctor's treatment decisions, or reports of a colleague's rude or abusive behavior reflect personality clashes and don't belong in the medical record. They're not legitimate concerns about patient care.

As with staffing problems, address concerns about a colleague's judgment or competence in the appropriate setting. After making sure that you have the facts, talk with your nurse-manager. Consult with the doctor directly if an order concerns you. Share your opinions, observations, or reservations about colleagues with your nurse-manager only; avoid mentioning them in a patient's chart.

If you discover personal accusations or charges of incompetence in a chart, discuss this with your supervisor.

Handling incident reports
A confidential, administrative communication, an incident report is filed separately from the patient's chart. Some facilities require the notation, "Incident form completed," while others require you not to document in the chart that an incident report was filed. Be familiar with your facility's policy so you'll know how to accurately chart this.

You should always document the facts of an incident in the patient's chart. For example, "Found pt. lying on the floor at 1250 hours. Vital signs: BP 120/80, P 76, T 98.2°. Notified Dr. Gary Dietrich at 1253 hours, and he saw pt. at 1300 hours" is a sufficient and accurate statement of the facts.

Steer clear of words associated with errors
Terms such as by *mistake, accidentally, somehow, unintentionally, miscalculated,* and *confusing* can

reviewed in malpractice cases include timely vital signs, reporting changes in the patient's condition, medications given, patient responses, and discharge teaching.

Failure to document diminishes your ability to testify confidently and persuasively about the details—any one of which could be critical to the verdict. Of course, you should never document some things, such as conflicts among the staff. (See *Keeping the record clean.*)

Record critical and extraordinary information

When you encounter a critical or an extraordinary situation, take pains to document the details thoroughly. Failure to chart such situa-

LEGALLY PERILOUS CHARTING PRACTICES

be interpreted as admissions of wrongdoing. Instead, let the facts speak for themselves — for example, "Pt. was given Demerol 100 mg I.M. at 1300 hours for abdominal pain. Dr. was notified at 1305 and is on his way here. Pt.'s vital signs are BP 120/82, P 80, R 20, T 98.4°."

If the ordered drug dose was 50 mg, this entry will let other health care providers know that the patient was overmedicated.

Avoid naming names

Naming another patient in someone else's chart violates confidentiality. Use the word *roommate* or a room and bed number to describe the other patient.

Never chart that you informed a colleague of a situation if you only mentioned it

Telling your nurse-manager in the elevator or rest room about a patient's deteriorating condition doesn't qualify as informing her, but it *does* violate patient confidentiality. The nurse-manager is likely to forget the details. She may not even realize you expect her to intervene. You need to clearly state why you're notifying her so she can focus on the facts and take appropriate action. Otherwise, you can't say you've informed her. Chart the patient's deterioration in the record and chart the time you notified your supervisor.

tions can have serious repercussions. (See *What you don't document can hurt you,* page 332.)

Consider the case of Tommy York, who was left partially paralyzed and severely brain damaged after an accident. He was admitted to the hospital for intensive rehabilitation.

Soon after he arrived, his parents told his nurse that a support from the right side of his wheelchair was missing and that they had noticed scratches on their son's right arm. The nurse failed to record the parents' or her own observations.

Later, the patient's hip became red, swollen, and increasingly painful. Although Tommy's mother pointed this out to the nurse, she again failed to record any observations.

Finally, the patient was diagnosed with a broken hip. The parents sued and the court ruled the hospital negligent in record keeping. The plaintiff was awarded $250,000, the maximum allowable in the state where the lawsuit was filed. (See *Recording critical information: A case in point,* page 333.)

The example below shows how to document extraordinary information correctly.

2/19/99	0900	Digoxin 0.125 mg P.O. not
		given because of nausea and
		vomiting. Dr. Kelly notified
		that digoxin not given. Dr.
		Kelly gave order for digoxin
		0.125 mg I.V. Administered at
		0915 hours. ————
		———— Ruth Bullock, RN

Chart full assessment data

Failing to document an adequate physical assessment is a key factor in many malpractice suits. When initially assessing your patient, focus on his chief complaint, but also document all his concerns and your findings.

After completing the initial assessment, establish your nursing plan of care. A well-written plan of care provides a clear approach to the patient's problems and can assist in your defense — *if* it was carried out.

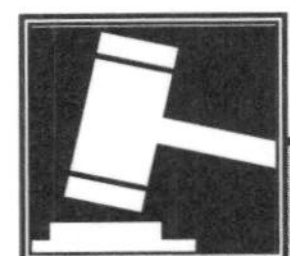

ON TRIAL

What you don't document can hurt you

Only careful documentation can substantiate your version of events. Consider the situations below.

The case of the supposed phone call

A patient was admitted to the hospital for surgery for epicondylitis (tennis elbow). After the surgery, a heavy cast was applied to his arm. The patient complained to the nurse of severe pain, for which the nurse repeatedly gave pain medication.

The next morning, when the surgeon visited, he split the patient's cast. By that time, the ulnar nerve was completely paralyzed and the patient was left with a permanently useless, clawed hand.

The patient subsequently sued the nurse for failing to notify the surgeon about his pain. At the deposition, the dialogue between the nurse and the plaintiff's attorney sounded like this:

ATTORNEY: Did you call the doctor?
NURSE: I must have called him.
ATTORNEY: Do you remember calling him?
NURSE: Not exactly, but I must have.
ATTORNEY: Do you have a record of making that call?
NURSE: No, I don't.
ATTORNEY: If you'd made such a call, shouldn't there be a record of it?
NURSE: Yes, I guess so.
ATTORNEY: "Guess" is right; you can't really say that you made that call. You can only "guess" that you "must have."

The case of the documentation deficit

In the case of *Sweeney v. Purvis,* 665 So. 2d 926 (Ala., 1995), a 42-year-old woman was transferred to a rehabilitation facility 10 days after being admitted to the hospital with a brain infarction. On her first day there, she attended therapy sessions without a problem.

The next day, after therapy, she had cramping in her left leg that wasn't relieved by analgesics. She also complained of pain in her left heel. The nursing staff called the doctor, who ordered a heating pad applied to the affected leg.

The patient reported little pain that evening, but the next day her left leg appeared swollen so she stayed in bed. When she tried to get out of bed, she again had pain. The LPN caring for her noted a positive Homans' sign, which may indicate the presence of a blood clot. The RN on duty also got a positive response and reported it to her manager. Believing that the manager would notify the doctor, the RN didn't document the positive Homans' sign or tell the next shift about it.

The next morning, a nurse practitioner and an RN examined the patient. Because her left calf appeared enlarged, the nurses were concerned about her undergoing therapy — if a clot were present, movement could cause it to move to her lung. When told about her condition, the doctor told the nurses to get her up for therapy.

That afternoon at lunch, the patient shook, turned blue, and developed pinpoint pupils. Then her breathing and pulse stopped. Paramedics transported her to the hospital, where she died.

The administrator of the patient's estate sued the doctor and his professional corporation for wrongful death. In court, the RN who noted the positive Homans' sign testified that she told her manager about it and the manager told her she would contact the doctor. But the RN didn't chart her actions or tell the next shift of her findings.

The nurse-manager testified that she didn't recall the RN telling her about the patient's condition and she didn't remember contacting the doctor. The doctor testified that he didn't recall the nurse-manager notifying him of the positive Homans' sign. What's more, no documentation in the nurses' notes, the doctor's orders, or the interdisciplinary progress notes supported the RN's claim that the doctor was notified.

The jury decided in favor of the plaintiff and awarded $500,000 in damages.

The lesson? Appropriate nursing assessments aren't enough if you don't document your findings. This patient's death might have been averted if the nurse had written "positive Homans' sign" in the chart.

ON TRIAL

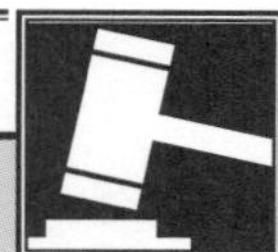

Recording critical information: A case in point

This case illustrates the significance of documenting critical information accurately as proof that you provided the accepted standard of care.

Failure to document

Patti Bailey was admitted to the hospital to deliver her third child. During her pregnancy, she'd gained 63 lb, her blood pressure had risen from 100/70 in her first trimester to 140/80 at term, and an ultrasound done at 22 weeks showed possible placenta previa.

In the 4 hours after her admission, she received 10 units of oxytocin in 500 ml of dextrose 5% in lactated Ringer's solution. Documentation during this period was scant — her blood pressure was never recorded, and there were only single notations of the fetal heart rate and how labor was progressing. The nurses failed to record the baby's reaction to the drug as well as the nature of the mother's contractions.

Suddenly, after complaining of nausea and epigastric pain, Mrs. Bailey suffered a generalized tonic-clonic seizure. Because her condition was so unstable, she couldn't undergo a cesarean section, and her baby girl was delivered by low forceps. Mrs. Bailey developed disseminated intravascular coagulation and required 20 units of whole blood, platelets, and packed red blood cells within 8 hours of delivery.

Incredibly, Mrs. Bailey's nurse had documented nothing in the labor or delivery records or the progress notes.

Deficient policy and procedure manuals

When the unit's policy and procedure manuals were reviewed, no protocol for administering oxytocin and assessing the patient was included. At the very least, the manuals should have recommended using an oxytocin flow sheet to record vital signs, labor progress, fetal status, and changes in the drug administration rate.

The result

Although Mrs. Bailey recovered, her daughter has seizures and is developmentally disabled. Now age 15, the daughter can't walk or talk and has a gastrostomy tube for nutrition. The case was settled out of court for $450,000; the nurse and hospital were held responsible for one-third of the judgment and the doctor paid the rest.

Phrase each patient problem statement clearly, and don't be afraid to modify the statement as you gather new assessment data. Also, state the plan of care for solving each problem and then identify the actions you intend to implement. (See *Using good interview techniques to improve documentation,* page 334.)

Document discharge instructions

Hospitals today commonly discharge patients earlier than in years past. As a result, the patient and his family must change dressings; assess wounds; deal with medical equipment, tube feedings, and I.V.s lines; and perform other functions that a nurse traditionally performed.

To perform these functions properly, the patient and his home caregiver must receive adequate instruction. The responsibility for these instructions is usually the nurse's. If a patient receives improper instructions and an injury results, you could be held liable.

Many hospitals distribute printed instruction sheets describing treatments and home care procedures that provide adequate in-

Using good interview techniques to improve documentation

Assessing a patient's condition adequately is part of your professional and legal responsibility. That means following up and documenting each of the patient's complaints. Documenting your data can be easier when you know how to ask questions that elicit the most information from your patient. What follows is an example of an open-ended interview with a patient being assessed for abdominal pain.

NURSE: How would you describe the pain in your abdomen?

PATIENT: It's dull but constant. Actually, it doesn't bother me as much as my blurry eyesight.

NURSE: Tell me about your blurry eyesight.

PATIENT: When I work long hours at my computer, all the words and lines seem to blend together. Sometimes it happens when I watch television too. I probably should see my eye doctor, but I haven't had the time.

NURSE: We'll be sure to follow up on your blurred vision. Now how about that abdominal pain. How does it affect your daily routine and your sleep?

A lot of things went right in this interview.

- First, the nurse didn't dismiss the patient's vision problem. If she had and it turned out to be serious, she might have been judged negligent.
- Second, she asked open-ended questions so that the patient could explain his answers rather than simply saying "yes" or "no."
- Third, she didn't put words in the patient's mouth. For example, she avoided saying, "The abdominal pain bothers you when you try to sleep, doesn't it?" That would have been a leading question. And the patient, assuming the nurse knows the right answer because she's a nurse, might have answered "yes"—even if the correct answer was "no."

struction. The chart should indicate which materials were given and to whom.

Courts typically consider these teaching materials as evidence that instruction took place. However, to support testimony that instructions were given, the materials should be tailored to each patient's specific needs and include any verbal or written instructions that were provided. If caregivers practice procedures with the patient and family in the hospital, this should be documented too, along with the results.

When to chart

Finding the time to chart can be a problem during a busy shift. But timely entries are crucial in malpractice suits.

Ideally, you'll document your nursing care and other relevant activity when you perform it, or not long after—but never before performing it. Documenting ahead of time makes your notes inaccurate and also omits information about the patient's response to intervention. Even though you may subsequently do what you charted, this practice can lead the plaintiff's attorney to pose a question such as: "Is it your regular or even occasional practice to chart something in anticipation of doing it?" If you answer "yes," the jury won't perceive the chart as a reliable indicator of what you actually did. From that point on, your credibility and that of the medical record will be compromised. (See *Understanding the importance of timely documentation,* pages 336 and 337.)

Who should chart

You, and only you, should chart your nursing care and observations. At times, because of understaffing or other circumstances, you may be tempted to ask another nurse to complete your portion of the medical record. However, doing so is illegal and is prohibited by your state's nurse practice act.

Do your own charting

Having someone else chart for you can result in disciplinary actions that range from reprimand to suspension of your nursing license. It may also cause harm to your patient if your coworker makes an error or misinterprets information.

If the patient sues you for negligence, you could be held accountable, along with your employer, because delegated documentation is illegal and may constitute fraud.

Delegating documentation duties has another consequence. It destroys the credibility and value of the medical record, leading reasonable nurses and doctors to doubt the accuracy of the chart, and it diminishes the record's value as legal evidence. A judge will give little, if any, weight to a medical record that contains secondhand observations or hearsay evidence. To avoid this unsafe practice, do your own charting and refuse to do anyone else's.

Countersign cautiously

Countersigning, or signing off on someone else's entry, requires good judgment. Although countersigning doesn't imply that you performed the procedure, it does imply that you reviewed the entry and approved the care given.

To act correctly and to protect yourself, review your employer's policy on countersigning and proceed accordingly. Does your facility interpret countersigning to mean that the licensed practical nurse (LPN), graduate nurse, or nurse's aide performed the nursing actions in the countersigning registered nurse's presence? If so, don't countersign unless you were there when the actions occurred.

On the other hand, if your facility acknowledges that you don't necessarily have time to witness your coworkers' actions, your countersignature implies that the LPN or nurse's aide had the authority and competence to perform the care described. In countersigning, you verify that all required patient care procedures were carried out.

If policy does require you to countersign a subordinate's entries, be careful. Review each entry, and make sure it clearly identifies who did the procedure. If you sign off without reviewing an entry, or if you overlook a problem the entry raises, you could share liability for any patient injury that results.

What should you do if another nurse asks you to document her care or sign her notes? In a word, don't. Unless your hospital policy authorizes or requires you to witness someone else's notes, your signature will make you responsible for anything written in the notes above it.

Charting legally sensitive situations

Among the most legally charged situations are those involving dissatisfied patients and patients who carry out "nonconforming" behavior, such as refusing treatment, leaving the

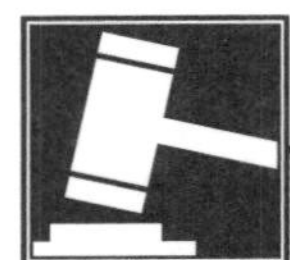

ON TRIAL

Understanding the importance of timely documentation

Although you would never document care before providing it, you may wait until the end of your shift or until your dinner break to complete your nurse's notes. That's what one nurse did. Some time later she was summoned to court as a witness in a malpractice suit. She took the witness stand, answered the attorney's questions, and regularly referred to and read from the chart while doing so. She relied heavily on it for her defense and, in the process, implicitly asked the jury to do the same.

The plaintiff's attorney began his cross-examination by asking the nurse to read from her entries. After a few minutes, here's what happened:

ATTORNEY: Excuse me, may I interrupt? As I listened to you read these entries, a question occurred to me. Maybe it occurred to the jury, too. Would you tell us whether you make the entries you are reading at the time of the events they describe?

NURSE: Well, no, I would have made them sometime later.

ATTORNEY: You're sure?

NURSE: Yes.

ATTORNEY: Thank you. Now, I'd like you to look at the chart and tell the jury whether you noted the time that you actually gave the patient his medication.

NURSE: No, I didn't.

ATTORNEY: Now, I'd like you to look at the chart again and tell the jury whether you indicated the time that you made the entry.

NURSE: No.

ATTORNEY: Given the absence of those two pieces of information, how could you so promptly and confidently respond to my original question? How can you remember so clearly now that you made the entry sometime after the event it describes? Is it because your regular practice is to wait until the end of your shift to chart each and every detail of every event that transpired over your entire shift, and that you rely solely on your memory when making all these entries?

NURSE: Well, yes, that's true.

ATTORNEY: Would you tell the jury how long a shift you worked that day?

NURSE: A 10-hour shift.

ATTORNEY: And how many patients did you see over that 10-hour period?

NURSE: About 15.

ATTORNEY: Now, each of these 15 patients was different, correct? Each had his own individualized plan of care that corresponded to his particular health problems, isn't that right?

NURSE: That's right.

ATTORNEY: And how many different times did you see each of these different patients over the 10-hour period?

NURSE: I probably saw each one, on average, about once an hour.

ATTORNEY: In other words, you probably had 150 patient contacts on that shift alone, is that correct?

NURSE: I suppose so.

ATTORNEY: Now, during the course of your shift, do unexpected events sometimes develop? Unanticipated developments that must be attended to?

NURSE: Sometimes, yes.

ATTORNEY: And when these situations occur, do they distract you from things you had planned to do?

NURSE: Sometimes.

ATTORNEY: After working such a long shift, do you sometimes feel tired?

NURSE: Yes.

ATTORNEY: And at the end of a shift, are you sometimes in a hurry? With things to do, places to go, people to see?

NURSE: Yes.

ATTORNEY: Now, would you tell the jury the purpose of the chart you keep for each patient?

NURSE: Well, we want to communicate information about the patient to others on the health care team, and we want to develop a historic account of the patient's problems, what's been done for him, and his progress.

ATTORNEY: So, other people rely on the information in this chart when they make their own decisions about the patient's care?
NURSE: Yes, that's true.
ATTORNEY: So you'd agree that the chart must be reliable?
NURSE: Yes.
ATTORNEY: And you'd agree that it must be factual and accurate in all respects?
NURSE: Yes.
ATTORNEY: And you'd agree that it needs to be comprehensive and complete, wouldn't you?
NURSE: Yes, I would.
ATTORNEY: So you're trying to develop a record that is factual, accurate, and complete at a time when you are sometimes tired, sometimes in a hurry, after working 10 consecutive hours and seeing 15 different patients 10 different times, and after having dealt with unexpected and distracting events. Is that the essence of your testimony?
NURSE: Well. . . yes.
ATTORNEY: Thank you. You may continue to read your entries to the jury.

By attacking the timeliness of charted entries, the attorney undermined their reliability, accuracy, and completeness. The jurors will now probably be skeptical of the chart and the nurse as well.

How to prevent untimely entries

So, how do you prevent this situation? By timely charting. Some nurses may carry a notepad to keep working notes of events while they are fresh in their mind. This is not recommended because during a lawsuit a plaintiff's attorney could subpoena your notes, hoping to find discrepancies between them and the chart. If he succeeds, he'll use those discrepancies to discredit the chart. This will also corroborate that timely charting does not exist.

health care facility against medical advice, or mishandling equipment.

Handle difficult patients with care

No doubt you've cared for dissatisfied patients and heard remarks like these: "I've been ringing and ringing for a nurse. I could have died before you got here!" or "This food is terrible — take it away!" or "I've never seen such filth in my life. What kind of a hospital is this, anyway?" These are the sounds of unhappy patients. If you tend to dismiss them, you may be increasing your risk of a lawsuit.

Try to put out the fire

The first step in defusing a potentially troublesome situation is to recognize that it exists. Most nurses know the signs of a difficult patient: constant grumpiness, endless complaints, no response to friendly remarks, not a trace of a smile when you try a little humor. You don't have to accept the situation; instead, try to improve it. Here are three simple strategies:

- Continue reaching out to the patient, even if he doesn't respond.
- Ask your colleagues to support and reinforce your efforts.
- Record the details of all patient contacts. (See *Documenting precisely,* page 338.)

Record significant patient communications

If a patient suggests that he's going to sue you and other caregivers, document this on the progress notes and report it to your nurse-manager or your employer's legal department or attorney. An example of an entry in the progress notes appears on the next page.

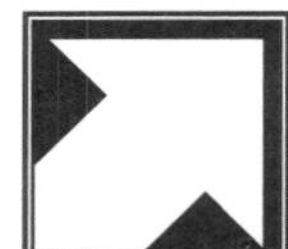

CHARTING GUIDELINES

Documenting precisely

Patients or their families may believe a bad outcome is due to poor care. As you know, this is not always the case. Here's an example of how precise documentation saved the day for one nurse.

A son wanted to sue a hospital and nurse for an incident involving his elderly father, who had been hospitalized for a cholecystectomy. Several days after surgery, his father became disoriented and disorderly, fell out of bed, and broke both hips. He never walked again.

In talking with his attorney, the son claimed, "That nurse either didn't know or didn't care that Dad was confused and agitated. She did nothing to protect him from harm. I want to sue."

The son's description of the father's care sounded like nursing negligence — until the attorney reviewed the patient's record and the nurse's notes. The nurse provided a detailed account of the events preceding the fall. Clearly, she not only knew about the patient's problem but also did everything she could to protect him. Specifically, she:

- confined him to bed with a Posey restraint in compliance with the doctor's order
- assigned an aide to stay with him when he became agitated
- made sure the side rails were always up
- notified coworkers and asked them to watch the patient (his bed was visible from the nurses' station)
- charted all times that the patient and restraint were checked.

The record established that the nurse not only acted properly but also showed concern for the patient. The patient's son was convinced that this unfortunate accident was just that — an accident.

Even if the case had gone to court, that nurse would have been well prepared to meet any challenge to her memory. The details were all there, in black and white.

1/26/99	1000	Pt. stated that he plans to file suit against this facility for causing his bed sores. ——— ——— Dave Bevins, RN

Chart patient's nonconforming behavior

Occasionally, a patient does something — or fails to do something — that may contribute to an injury or explain why he hasn't responded to nursing and medical care. Document these behaviors and the outcomes.

Although patients have the right to refuse medical and nursing care, be sure to document on the progress notes any behavior that contradicts medical instructions and the fact that you informed the patient of the possible consequences of his actions.

Failure to provide information

You may occasionally encounter a patient who refuses to provide accurate or complete information about his health history, current medications, or treatments. He may be uncooperative for various reasons: He thinks too many caregivers have asked him the same questions too many times, he doesn't understand the significance of the information, he's fearful or disoriented, or he's suspicious of why you want him to divulge personal information. Or he may have severe pain, a psychiatric problem, or a language barrier.

In such situations, try to obtain the information from other sources or forms. Clearly document any trouble you've had in communicating with the patient.

Here's an example of what to chart when a patient refuses to answer questions:

2/5/99	0830	When asked for a list of his
		current medications, the pt.
		said, "Why do you want to
		know? What business is it of
		yours? I don't know why I
		have to answer that question."
		——— Nora Martin, RN

Unusual possessions

Document any unauthorized personal belongings discovered in the patient's possession (including alcoholic beverages, tobacco, heating pads, medications, vitamins, and other items that should be checked by the biomedical department before use). Describe the object and how you disposed of it. Here's an example:

2/9/99	1100	Found 3 cans of unopened
		beer in pt.'s bedside table
		when checking his soap supply.
		Explained to pt. that beer was
		not allowed in the hospital.
		Took beer to nurse's station
		to be sent home with family.
		Dr. Kennedy notified at 1140
		hours. He stated he would
		discuss this with pt. on rounds
		later today. Pt. denied having
		drunk any alcohol during
		hospitalization. No alcohol
		odor on breath. No empty cans
		in the trash or room. ———
		——— Elaine Kasmer, RN

Misuse of equipment

At times, a patient may manipulate equipment or misuse supplies (such as pressing keys on a pump or monitor, detaching tubing, or playing with switches) without understanding the consequences. When misuse occurs, document in the progress notes what you saw the patient do (or what he told you he did) and what you did about the problem. Here's an example:

2/6/99	0930	I.V. rate set at 60 ml/hr,
		1,000 ml D_5W 1,000 ml in bag.
		——— K. Comerford, RN
		Checked I.V. 840 ml left in
		bag. Pt. stated, "I flicked the
		switch because I didn't see
		anything happening. Then I
		pressed the green button and
		the arrow." BP 110/82, P 80, T
		98.4°. No signs of fluid
		overload. Breath sounds clear
		bilaterally. Instructed pt. not
		to touch the pump or I.V.
		Repositioned pump to limit pt.
		access. Dr. Huang notified at
		1030 hours. ——— K. Comerford, RN

AMA discharges and elopements

If a patient decides to leave the hospital against medical advice (AMA), notify your nurse-manager, the patient's doctor, and possibly a member of the patient's family, who may be able to persuade the patient to stay.

Expect the patient's doctor to inform the patient of the risks posed by refusing further treatment. Then, if the patient still intends to leave, complete the paperwork required by your facility, and chart the time and the patient's condition in the chart. Chart the patient's desire for leaving AMA and any reason he gave. Also document how he left, such as by cab, with a friend or family member, or by wheelchair. (For more information on documenting AMA discharges, see chapter 9, Documentation of Everyday Events.)

If the patient elopes from the health care facility without having said anything about leaving, look for him on your unit immediately and notify security, your nurse-manager, and the patient's doctor and family. If the patient is at risk for harming himself or others, notify the police. Document the time you discovered the patient missing, your attempts to find him, and the times and people notified. The legal consequences of a patient leaving the facility without medical permission can be particularly severe if he is confused or mentally incompetent, especially if he's injured or dies of exposure as a result of his absence.

Interpreting medical record entries

Keeping your own documentation neat and legible should be a primary goal. But what about other caregivers who aren't careful about their handwriting? Misinterpreting medical record entries can lead to mistakes in care. If you can't read handwritten notes or orders, ask for clarification.

To avoid making an error, always make sure you clearly understand a written order before carrying it out. If you have questions, clarify the order with the doctor who wrote it. Don't ask other nurses or doctors on the unit—they would be guessing, too.

An assistant director of nursing at a well-known general hospital learned this lesson when she decided to help out on an understaffed pediatric unit. A doctor ordered 3 ml of a digitalis glycoside for an infant. Not realizing that he meant the pediatric elixir, she administered 3 ml of an injectable, adult-strength digitalis glycoside. This was equivalent to about five times what the doctor intended. When the infant died, her parents successfully sued the nurse and the hospital. (See chapter 9, Documentation of Everyday Events, for more on clarifying orders.)

Minimizing other legal risks

The use of computers, fax machines, and telephones poses a number of other legal risks that nurses can take steps to minimize.

Privacy and computer charting

The legal implications of computerized medical records are still evolving. In most cases, computer records serve as legitimate substitutes for handwritten ones. But some state laws require health care facilities with electronic records to maintain handwritten records as well.

The most pressing legal questions associated with computer charting concern the threat to patient privacy and confidentiality. With traditional record keeping, access to information is restricted simply by keeping the record on the unit. With a computerized system, such information can be retrieved by anyone who has the proper entry code.

Health care professionals and computer programmers have devised safeguards to protect a patient's privacy. The primary safeguard is the signature code. By developing a series of access codes, programmers can limit access

CHARTING GUIDELINES

Maintaining confidentiality with computer charting

The American Nurses Association and the American Medical Records Association offer these guidelines for maintaining the confidentiality of computerized medical records.

Never share your password or computer signature

Never give your personal password or computer signature to anyone — including another nurse in the unit, a nurse serving temporarily in the unit, or a doctor. Your health care facility can issue a short-term password authorizing access to certain records for infrequent users.

Log off if not using your terminal

Don't leave a computer terminal unattended after you've logged on. (Some computers have a timing device that shuts down a terminal after a certain period of disuse.)

Follow protocol for correcting errors

Follow your health care facility's protocol for correcting errors. Computer entries are part of the patient's permanent record and, as such, can't be deleted. In most cases, however, you can correct an entry error before storing the entry. To correct an error after storage, mark the entry "error" or "mistaken entry," add the correct information, and date and sign the entry. If you record information in the wrong chart, write "error" and "wrong chart," draw a line through the entry, and sign off. (See the example above right.)

~~2/14/99~~	~~1400~~	~~Pt. out of bed to sit in~~
		~~chair for first time. Pt.~~
		~~followed directions well,~~
		~~but needed help of 2~~
		~~nurses. BP 110/82. Pulse~~
		~~74 before transfer, BP~~
		~~118/88, P 86 after~~
		~~transfer. Stayed in chair~~
		~~1 hr. Required less~~
		~~assistance on return.~~
		Error, wrong chart.
		Beth Marshall, RN

Make backup files

Make sure that stored records have backup files — an important safety feature. If you inadvertently delete part of the permanent record (even though there are safeguards against this), type an explanation into the file along with the date, the time, and your initials. Submit an explanation in writing to your nurse-manager, and keep a copy.

Never display patient information

Don't leave information about a patient displayed on a monitor where others can see it. Also, don't leave print versions or excerpts of the patient's medical record unattended. Keep a log that accounts for every copy of a computer file that you've printed.

Remember, a diagnosis of acquired immunodeficiency syndrome or human immunodeficiency virus infection is part of the patient's confidential record. Disclosing this information to unauthorized people may have significant legal implications. For any other diagnosis, follow your health care facility's confidentiality procedures.

to the records. For example, a nurse's code would allow her to view a patient's entire record, but a lab technician's code would produce only the doctor's orders for laboratory studies. Never search for information on an unassigned patient. (See *Maintaining confidentiality with computer charting.*)

Various laws protect the privacy of a patient's medical records. The Federal Privacy Act of 1974 protects the confidential medical information of patients in federal facilities. In some states, nurse practice acts impose legal duties to safeguard patients' privacy.

Privacy and faxing

Faxing patient information is an increasingly common practice in health care facilities. A breach of patient confidentiality can occur if the information is inadvertently faxed to an incorrect destination.

The American Health Information Management Association recommends these safeguards when faxing:

- Before sending a fax, call the intended recipient to say that it is coming.
- Clearly note on the fax cover sheet that the accompanying material is confidential.
- Ask the recipient to send a return fax verifying receipt of the information.
- If you don't receive a verification receipt, check the fax machine's internal log to determine where the fax was sent. If the information went to the wrong number, send another fax to that number asking the recipient to destroy the material.
- For added safety, before sending a fax, check the number before you dial, check it on the fax machine display, and recheck it before hitting the "send" button.

Telephone advice

Nurses commonly receive phone calls from recently discharged patients or their family members who have questions about care at home. Remember that you are legally responsible for any advice you give over the phone and must document it properly.

Be sure to keep a log of the date and time of the call, the caller's name and address, the caller's request or chief complaint, whether the advice sought was for the caller or another person (such as a mother calling about her baby's temperature), the advice you gave, the protocol you followed (if any), other caregivers notified, and your name.

Selected references

Allenby, J. "Dialogue and Discussion: A Release of Patient Results—A Freedom of Information Issue?" *Clinical Laboratory Science* 10(1):1, January-February 1997.

DeMarzo, M. "Advice of Counsel: Be Careful about Giving Advice Online," *RN* 61(2):54-55, February 1998.

Elnitsky, C., et al. "Are Hospital Incidents Being Reported?" *Journal of Nursing Administration* 27(11):40-46, November 1997.

Markus, K. "Legal File: Your Legal Risk in Giving Advice or Care," *Healthweek* 2(20):15, October 6, 1997.

Perry, L. "Critical Incidents, Crucial Issues: Insights into the Working Lives of Registered Nurses," *Journal of Clinical Nursing* 6(2):131-37, March 1997.

11

Malpractice Lawsuits

Every practicing nurse is at risk for a malpractice lawsuit. However, you can substantially reduce your risk of such a lawsuit by providing the accepted standard of care to your patients. The standard of care — the minimum criteria for job proficiency — includes creating timely and accurate documentation. If you provide the standard of care but fail to document it, you leave yourself open to an indefensible lawsuit. (See *Why nurses are sued.*)

If you fail to document, chart haphazardly, or tamper with a patient's record, the jury is likely to conclude that you also failed to provide appropriate care or that you have something to hide. What kind of documentation can withstand legal scrutiny? Documentation that shows you provided care meeting standards set forth by federal regulations, state laws, hospital policies, and your profession.

Each state has laws that define malpractice. Although these laws are worded differently, they all stipulate that malpractice occurs when a patient suffers because of a health care professional's failure to meet standards of care. These standards guide others in judging the quality of care you and your colleagues provide.

In a malpractice claim, the patient's (plaintiff's) attorney tries to prove that a standard of care wasn't met. Documentation that fails to provide evidence that the standard was met makes the attorney's job that much easier. (See *Spotlight on documentation in court,* page 346.)

If you're ever involved in a malpractice lawsuit, you'll feel more secure if you know that your documentation stands on its own merit. You'll also feel more confident if you know what happens before a trial. Pretrial preparations include knowing what to do and what not to do if your patient's medical record is subpoenaed, what steps you and your attorney should take if you and your employer are sued, and how to conduct yourself during a deposition and, later, during a trial.

Your pretrial role

Your involvement in pretrial activities may begin before the patient is discharged. If a mishap has occurred or the patient is dissatisfied with the care that was delivered, your supervisor or the Quality Assurance/Risk Management Department of your facility may begin an investigation or a review of the care. This is actually an ideal time to review the care given because memories are fresh and any "evidence," such as specific equipment, is readily available. In other cases, your involvement may begin at a later date, when the patient or his attorney requests a copy of the medical records. A review may begin at that time if it has not already occurred.

If such proactive steps aren't taken, the first indication you or your facility may have of an impending lawsuit may be the receipt of a complaint filed against you. Because nurses are usually employees rather than independent contractors, the hospital or facility is typically named in the suit. If you were an employee who provided care to the patient, you will also be named in the suit. Eventually, you'll be asked to appear at a deposition. If you refuse to appear voluntarily, you'll be subpoenaed; if you still fail to appear, you'll likely be held in contempt of court. Most defendants appear without being subpoenaed.

Why nurses are sued

Malpractice charges against a nurse can result from various situations. In many of these situations, the lawsuit-triggering event may have been out of your control. What remains in your control, however, is your timely and accurate documentation of the patient's condition, your nursing interventions, and other relevant data.

If you accurately document that you provided appropriate care, the record should protect you and your employer and may go a long way toward averting a malpractice suit. The following are some common occurrences that can lead to malpractice claims.

Medication administration

- Incorrect medications
- Incorrect route of administration
- Administration to the wrong patient
- Incorrect dosage
- Incorrect time of administration
- Injury from injections

Obstetric and related care

- Nursing negligence causing injury during delivery
- Delay in notifying doctor
- Failure to monitor during labor
- Failure to monitor neonate's condition
- Failure to provide proper neonatal care

Patient falls

- Side rails left down
- Medicated patients left unattended
- Patient left unattended on stretcher or examination table
- Wheelchairs left unsecured
- Inappropriate patient transfers
- Injury caused when moving or turning patient
- Inappropriate use of physical or chemical restraints

Surgery and related care

- Foreign object left in patient
- Failure to adhere to patient's nothing-by-mouth order
- Negligent postoperative monitoring and care

Care involving I.V. lines, catheters, and tubes

- Infiltration
- Negligence causing emboli
- Incorrect placement
- Inappropriate number of insertion attempts
- Injection of improper solution
- Improper catheter size
- Failure to monitor

Failure to monitor or communicate

- Failure to record information or recording of inaccurate information
- Failure to use standard abbreviations
- Failure to notify doctor
- Failure to document doctor notification

Personal liability

- Damage to or theft of patient's property
- Malicious acts or violence
- Intentionally wrongful conduct (such as sexual abuse)
- Breach of confidentiality
- Invasion of privacy
- Slander or libel
- False imprisonment

Understanding subpoenas

You may first learn that you're involved in a lawsuit when you're served legal notification — a subpoena, or summons — that a plaintiff has filed charges against you (the defendant) and that you must appear at a certain time and place to testify and respond to these charges.

The court can subpoena not only your presence but also the medical record (which includes your nursing documentation). A *subpoena duces tecum* is a command to produce

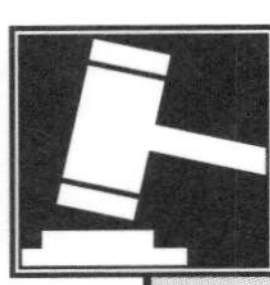

ON TRIAL

Spotlight on documentation in court

In a malpractice lawsuit, the patient's medical record testifies to the quality of care that was provided. Its importance in the courtroom cannot be exaggerated, as illustrated by the following cases.

Failure to document communication with the doctor

Many significant malpractice cases are brought against nurses who fail to notify the doctor of changes in the patient's condition. For instance, in *Cruz v. West Volusia Hospital Authority d/b/a West Volusia Memorial Hospital,* Volusia County, Florida Circuit Court No. 95-10313 (1997), a woman in labor was given Pitocin by her obstetrician. Six hours later, the fetal monitor indicated prolonged variable decelerations for 1½ hours. The nurse failed to inform the obstetrician of the fetal distress or document it. As a result, the baby suffered hypoxic ischemic encephalopathy. The parties reached an out-of-court settlement for $2,425,000.

Failure to document patient monitoring

In *Cloughly v. St. Paul Fire and Marine Insurance Company,* Washington County, Arkansas Circuit Court, Case No. C1V95-996 (1997), a 28-year-old woman who entered the hospital with an asthma attack was placed on a portable ventilator in the intensive care unit. While being transferred to radiology for a computed tomography scan, she became cyanotic twice and exhibited a low pulse rate. Although a code was called in radiology, the woman suffered hypoxia, resulting in spastic quadriparesis. Her attorney claimed the portable ventilator was not delivering enough oxygen during her trip to radiology because it had not been set up properly. Although there was no evidence that the portable ventilator was not functioning properly, neither the hospital nor the nurse documented how it was set up and there was no record that oxygen saturation readings had been taken. A $2,125,000 settlement was reached prior to trial.

In another case, *Toinkham, Administrator of Estate of Muncey, v. Mt. Carmel Health d/b/a Mt. Carmel East Hospital,* Franklin County, Ohio Court of Common Pleas, Case No. 94CVA-09-6736 (1997), a 39-year-old patient went to the emergency department with severe right flank pain that was diagnosed as a kidney stone. After receiving I.V. morphine and Dilaudid, the patient experienced an oxygen saturation drop but quickly recovered with supplemental oxygen. After being transferred to the floor, he was given additional I.M. morphine and Phenergan. He was later found in total cardiac arrest and could not be revived.

His family's attorney alleged that the nurses did not properly assess, monitor, and care for him before and after the injection of morphine because these actions were not documented in the medical record. A $433,415 verdict was returned at trial.

certain documents (such as the medical record) that may be used as evidence at trial. This type of subpoena is usually served on a hospital, a clinic, or an office, but it may be served on a nurse if she possesses the documents, as in the case of a nurse practitioner or a midwife who may maintain separate files.

The medical record is a critical legal document. It describes (or fails to describe) acts, events, conditions, diagnoses, and opinions at or near the time of the alleged malpractice event and is kept by a person with firsthand knowledge or a duty to record. It's considered trustworthy because entries are made contemporaneously and must meet established standards. Juries assume that the information in the medical record is true. Although this presumption can be challenged in court, it's hard to rebut.

Reviewing the medical record

Once you've received notice that a lawsuit has been filed, you need to familiarize yourself with the medical record. By the time the case is filed, several years may have elapsed since you cared for the patient. The medical record will refresh your memory and assist with preparation for your deposition.

Avoid tampering with the record

During this review, you may notice that certain nursing interventions that you always perform — from dates and times to such events as vital signs or changes in condition — were not recorded. *Do not* add to, delete from, or otherwise change the record. Making changes at this time would not only violate your state's nurse practice act and codes of conduct, but also be tantamount to falsification or alteration (or both). Moreover, your care may have met the accepted standard and not be the cause of the patient's injury at all. However, if the jury learns that the document was altered or falsified in any way whatsoever, there will be an appearance of impropriety. (See *Types of tampering,* page 348.)

Attorneys on both sides have document investigators who can easily analyze papers and inks and identify signs of alteration and falsification. In addition, by the time a lawsuit has been filed, the patient's attorney already has a copy of the medical record and knows the contents so well that he'll be able identify any alterations immediately.

Implications of tampering

Tampering with a patient's medical record to protect yourself can only create problems and suspicion. Even if you consider correcting an error that may have nothing to do with the focus of the lawsuit, you'll damage your credibility and that of the record — and you could end up losing a case you should have won. For example, suppose you hung the wrong I.V. solution. That fact might have no bearing on a malpractice suit brought by a patient with a postoperative wound infection unrelated to the I.V. infusion. However, if you tamper with the record to conceal your error, the entire case becomes suspect. As a result, your insurance company might have to make an expensive out-of-court settlement that would not have been necessary if you hadn't tampered with the medical record.

The case of *Pyle v. Morrison,* 716 S.W. 2d 930 (1986), illustrates this point. A malpractice suit was brought against doctors for their treatment of a child's fractured arm. The jury decided in favor of the plaintiffs — $400,000 for the child and $15,000 for the father. The deciding factor was the testimony of a nurse who said that she thought a portion of the medical record had been altered after the child's surgery. Her testimony cast doubt on the credibility of the medical record in the minds of the jurors.

Altering or falsifying the medical record also can extend the statute of limitations — the time period each state gives an injured party to file a lawsuit. Because these acts can be interpreted as a form of fraud and fraud has a longer statute of limitations than malpractice, the plaintiff's attorney would have more time to prepare a case against you — perhaps as long as 10 years.

Types of tampering

Tampering with the medical record is both unethical and illegal. But exactly what constitutes tampering?

Delayed charting

The medical records department is responsible for ensuring that the record is completed within a defined time period to comply with state statutes, third-party payer guidelines, and the guidelines of the Joint Commission on Accreditation of Healthcare Organizations. If you are asked by the department to supply a missing signature to charting that is clearly yours (for example, in your handwriting), it's permissible to sign your name. However, write the date on which you signed, rather than the date of the action that was originally charted. *Do not add* any other information. Charting must be contemporaneous, and any additions may be viewed as alterations.

Omissions

Never allow anyone—including your peers, your supervisors, hospital administrators, and the hospital attorney—to coerce you to *not* chart factual, objective, and relevant information. For example, if a patient fell but was apparently uninjured, chart the fall anyway. Days or weeks later, a fatal hematoma could be discovered, and the failure to chart the fall could be seen as an attempt to avoid responsibility. Even if an autopsy eventually reveals that the cause of death was an aneurysm rather than the fall, the fact that a fall occurred and was not charted will create the appearance that information was withheld.

Intentionally failing to chart information that is relevant to the patient may result in punitive damages, an award above and beyond the amount that would compensate the patient for his injuries. In addition, you could be liable in a civil suit that is separate and distinct from a malpractice action, and you could lose your license.

Accidental destruction of records

Never rewrite your notes and discard the original, even for an innocent reason like spilling coffee on a page. In a lawsuit, you'd have trouble convincing the plaintiff's lawyer that your actions were so innocent. Both the attorney and the jury would likely assume that the evidence in the missing document was so damaging that you had to destroy it.

If you accidentally damage or destroy a part of your nurse's notes, follow this procedure:

- If you can recall what the original notes said, create another page titled "Reconstructed notes from memory" or "Notes reconstructed from original of 3/19/99" and write down what you remember. (Do not call the new notes "copied notes;" you would not be able to copy them if they were illegible.)
- Give a reason for the rewrite, such as "Original illegible due to coffee spill." Sign and date the entry.
- Retain the original page, and place it in the record with the newly written page.

To reduce the risk of accidentally damaging or destroying the medical record, avoid eating or drinking while charting.

You could even face charges of "aggravated and outrageous conduct" if the plaintiff's attorney successfully argues that the record was intentionally altered or falsified because of conspiracy or fraud. The judge could then allow the jury to award punitive damages to the plaintiff—a penalty that's intended to punish you. Punitive damages exceed the actual damages and may not be covered by your insurance policies, so you'd end up paying out of your own pocket.

As a precaution to prevent tampering, write every entry in ink. Date each entry, record the time, and sign it. Write on consecutive lines. If there's a blank space at the end of your entry, draw a line through it so that

Settling out of court

Research indicates that only about 10% of all malpractice lawsuits actually go to trial; the rest are settled out of court. Therefore, if you're ever involved in a malpractice suit, your chances of settling out of court are good.

When you discuss an out-of-court settlement with your attorney, remember these points:

- If you're covered by professional liability insurance, the terms of your policy determine whether you, your attorney, or your insurer controls the settlement. Most policies don't permit the nurse to settle a case without the consent of the insurer. However, many policies permit the insurer to settle without the consent of the nurse being sued.
- If you do not have your own malpractice insurance separate and distinct from that of your employer, your only representation may be from your employer. The attorney who represents your facility will be meeting with you and all other involved parties during the discovery process. It will be up to that attorney and your facility's administration whether to pursue settlement options or proceed to trial.
- Once you are represented by an attorney, you are precluded from communicating with the patient and his representative or attorney, and vice versa. All communication takes place through the attorneys for each side.
- Provide your insurer's representative and your attorney with all the information you can about the case. Then they can evaluate the plaintiff's and your liabilities and determine whether settlement options are indicated.
- Remember that settling out of court does not mean that you admit any wrongdoing. The law regards settlement as a compromise between two parties to end a lawsuit and avoid further expense. You may choose to reach a settlement rather than incur greater financial and emotional expenses by defending your innocence at a trial.
- Ask your attorney about the terms of the settlement. You'll usually be expected to keep the settlement agreement confidential.

no one can insert words at the end of your entry.

Dealing with your insurer

Contact your supervisor immediately if you are served with a complaint or a subpoena or are contacted by an attorney in any way. Find out whether your employer's attorney will represent you or whether you'll need to retain your own. Be aware that if your employer's attorney represents you, he may decide to settle the case out of court. This may be in the employer's best interest, but not in yours, especially if you weren't negligent. In this situation, consider consulting your own attorney to advise you. (See *Settling out of court.*)

Many nurses believe they don't need personal medical malpractice insurance. This could not be further from the truth for a number of reasons. First, you won't be covered by your facility's insurance if you're considered an independent contractor rather than an employee. Second, even if you *are* an employee, there are situations in which your employer may refuse to defend you. For example, the employer could find that you were acting outside the scope of your employment, perhaps by not following protocol or policy.

Furthermore, your interests might diverge from those of the facility. For instance, if the facility decides to pay damages in a case in which a doctor is at fault and you are also

Choosing liability insurance

To find the professional liability coverage that fits your needs, compare the features of a number of policies. Understanding insurance policy basics will enable you to shop more intelligently for the coverage you need. If you already have professional liability insurance, the information below may help you better evaluate your coverage. Information about nursing malpractice insurance can also be found in nursing journals and on the Internet. Many insurance companies have web sites or a toll-free telephone number to call to talk to an agent.

Type of coverage

Ask your insurance agent if the policy only covers claims made before the policy expires (claims-made coverage) or if it covers any negligent act committed during the policy period (occurrence coverage). Keep in mind that an occurrence policy provides more coverage than a claims-made policy.

Coverage limits

All malpractice insurance policies cover professional liability. Some also cover personal liability, medical payments, assault-related bodily injury, all property damage, paid leave of absence while preparing your case, and attorney representation at state board disciplinary hearings.

The amount of coverage varies, as does your premium. For example, depending on your nursing specialty, a policy costing about $100 a year may provide up to $1 million for each incident (single-occurrence limit) and up to $3 million per year (the maximum annual protection).

Remember that professional liability coverage is limited to acts and practice settings specified in the policy. Make sure your policy covers your nursing role, whether you're a student, a graduate nurse, or a working nurse with advanced education and specialized skills, such as a nurse practitioner, midwife, or nurse anesthetist.

Options

Find out whether the policy limits your choice of attorney or limits the number of hours for which the attorney would be paid. Also check whether the policy would provide coverage for the following incidents:

- negligence on the part of nurses under your supervision
- accidental misuse of equipment
- negligent administration of medications
- mistakes made while providing care in an emergency outside your employment setting
- lawsuit filed against you by your employer (the hospital)
- additional coverage beyond that provided in the workplace (such as for volunteer nurse activities).

Definition of terms

Definition of terms can vary from policy to policy. If your policy includes restrictive definitions, you won't be covered for actions outside those guidelines. For the best protection, seek broad definitions and ask for examples of actions the company has not covered.

named in the case, your name would then be reported to the National Practitioner's Data Bank, which keeps a record of settled cases. However, if you had your own attorney, he could negotiate to have you dismissed from the claim and no report would be made to the data bank or the state board of nursing.

If you do have your own professional liability insurance, find your representative's name on your policy and notify him right away. If you don't do this within the time specified on your policy, your insurance company (insurer) can refuse to cover you. (See *Choosing liability insurance.*)

Duration of coverage

Insurance is an annual contract that can be renewed or canceled each year. The policy usually specifies how it can be canceled, for example, in writing by either you or the insurance company. Some contracts require 30 days' notice for cancellation. If the company cancels the policy, you'll probably be given at least 30 days' notice.

Exclusions

Ask your agent about exclusions—areas not covered by the insurance policy. Examples include "This policy does not apply to injury arising out of performance of the insured of a criminal act" or "This policy does not apply to nurse-anesthetists." Midwives, nurse practitioners, correctional system nurses, and flight nurses may also be subject to exclusions because of the increased risk and liability associated with these types of nursing. In addition, nursing faculty and student nurses may simply be overlooked by some insurers.

Other insurance clauses

All professional liability insurance policies contain "other insurance" clauses that address payment obligations when a nurse is covered by more than one insurance policy, such as the institution's policy and the nurse's personal liability:

- The *pro rata* clause states that two or more policies in effect at the same time will pay any claims in accordance with a proportion established in the individual policies.
- The *in excess* clause states that the primary policy will pay all fees and damages up to its limits, at which point the second policy will pay any additional fees or damages up to its limits.
- The *escape clause* relieves an insurance company of all liability for fees or damages if another insurance policy is in effect at the same time; in effect, the clause states that the other company is responsible for all liability.

If you are covered by more than one policy, be alert for "other insurance" clauses and avoid purchasing a policy with an escape clause for liability.

Additional tips

Here is some additional information that will guide you in the purchase of professional liability insurance:

- The insurance application is a legal document. If you provide any false information, the policy may never take effect or may become void.
- If you're involved in nursing administration, education, research, or advanced or nontraditional nursing practice, be especially careful in selecting a policy because routine policies may not cover these activities.
- To ensure that your insurance coverage will be effective, adjust your coverage based on changes in areas of practice, rates, and scope of coverage. If you do adjust your coverage, make sure that your old and new policies overlap to avoid a gap in your coverage.
- No insurance policy will cover you for acts outside your scope of practice or licensure or for intentional wrongdoing.
- Be prepared to uphold all obligations specified in the policy; failure to do so may void the policy and cause personal liability for any damages.

Document the time, the date, the representative's name, and his instructions. Then hand-deliver the lawsuit papers to him and get a signed and dated receipt, or send the papers by certified mail with a return receipt requested.

Most policies require the health care facility or your private insurer to provide legal counsel, to pay all the expenses related to the lawsuit, and to pay damages in a settlement or as awarded in a judgment. The contract also spells out your and the insurer's rights and obligations and contains exclusionary clauses.

Attorney selection tips

If you're sued for malpractice, you may be faced with the added worry of hiring your own attorney. This can happen if you don't have malpractice insurance, if you're dissatisfied with the attorney your insurer provides, or if your insurer uses a policy defense and refuses to cover you.

Here are several suggestions for selecting an attorney to meet your needs:

- Ask family members for the name of a malpractice attorney.
- If you work in a health care facility with a legal services department, find out if your employer will provide you with an attorney or refer you to one.
- If you have a relative or friend who is an attorney or judge, ask him for a referral to a competent malpractice attorney.
- If you belong to a professional association, seek a referral to an attorney from the association.
- Contact the American Association of Nurse Attorneys.
- If none of these solutions applies to you, ask for a referral from your local bar association, lawyer referral service, or area law school (listed in the telephone directory). Try to find an attorney who's experienced in medical and nursing malpractice cases.
- Interview more than one attorney. Ask each candidate how long he thinks the lawsuit will take and what his fees are.
- Before you hire anyone to defend you, ask other health care professionals if they've heard of the attorney you're thinking of using. Find out about his reputation.
- Finally, try to choose an attorney who you feel understands your case and will work in your best interest.

When you notify your insurer that you've been named in a lawsuit, the company will first consider whether it must cover the alleged conduct. This is done by checking for any policy violations, such as giving late notice of the lawsuit, giving false information on your insurance application, or failing to pay a premium on time. If your insurer is certain you've committed such a violation, it can refuse to cover you.

If your insurer thinks you've committed a violation but isn't sure it has the evidence to support a policy defense, it may send you a certified letter saying that it might not have to defend you but will do so while reserving the right to deny coverage later, to withdraw from the case, or to take other actions. Meanwhile, the company will seek a declaration of its rights from the court.

If the court decides your insurer does not have to defend you, the company will withdraw from the case. Usually, an insurer takes this action only after careful consideration because refusing to defend you may give you grounds for suing the insurance company. In the rare event that your insurer does refuse to cover you, find your own attorney to defend you in the malpractice suit and advise you in your dealings with your insurer.

Finding an attorney

If you have your own malpractice coverage, your policy may allow you to select an attorney from a defined group, such as the American Association of Nurse Attorneys, or it may allow you to select an attorney of your choice. You need an attorney who specializes in defending nursing malpractice lawsuits. Names are available from your local state bar association. The attorney selected — called your *attorney of record* — is legally bound to do everything necessary to defend you. (See *Attorney selection tips.*)

If your policy doesn't allow you to select your own attorney and you're dissatisfied with the attorney selected, discuss this problem with a company representative. If you can't reach an agreement, hire your own attorney.

Working with your attorney

Once you have an attorney, he will obtain a copy of the plaintiff's medical record. Examine the complete record, including nurses' and consultation notes, X-ray and laboratory reports, flow sheets, and doctors' orders. The attorney will uncover every relevant detail about the case against you by using discovery devices—legal procedures for obtaining information.

Create your own legal file by asking your attorney to send you copies of all documents and correspondence pertaining to the case. Try to maintain a file that's as complete as your attorney's files. If you don't understand a document, ask your attorney to explain it. File documents in chronologic order in your own file system, such as folders or a loose-leaf notebook. Be sure to keep your files separate from your attorney's files; any notes you've written on them could be subpoenaed.

Protecting your assets

Some doctors and nurses deliberately remain uninsured—a policy known as "going bare"—because they believing it reduces their chances of being sued. This belief is a fallacy. A judgment can still be obtained against uninsured health care providers, whose homes, cars, and wages can be garnished. Filing bankruptcy is no defense either; it may buy some time, but judgments can last for years, during which time any earnings can be assigned. You wouldn't think of "going bare" to avoid paying a guest who fell on your porch steps, so why try to avoid accountability to your patient? Insurance is the best protection against loss of your assets and wages.

Your attorney's pretrial role

Your attorney will explain the legal process to you from complaint to appeal. (See *Understanding the legal process,* pages 354 and 355.) He'll file the appropriate legal documents in response to the subpoena you were served, and he'll ask for your help in preparing the response to the allegations made against you. In preparing your defense, he'll also ask you to review details and clarify specific points. Remember that all discussions between you and your attorney are privileged (confidential) communications that are protected by law. Your attorney can't disclose any information that you give him without your permission.

Because discussions with other people might result in information leaks that could compromise your case, your attorney will tell you not to discuss the lawsuit with anyone but him. He'll advise you not to mention the lawsuit to colleagues and, above all, not to contact the person suing you. All communication between you and the plaintiff should be through the attorneys who represent you.

Discovery devices include an interrogatory (written questions that require answers under oath) and a deposition (oral cross-examination under oath and before a court reporter). Your attorney will carefully prepare you to participate in these procedures and to testify

(Text continues on page 356.)

Understanding the legal process

Being named as a defendant in a malpractice lawsuit can be confusing as well as stressful. One of the best antidotes is knowing what to expect.

This chart summarizes the basic legal process from complaint to appeal. If you're ever involved in a lawsuit, your attorney will explain the specific procedures that your case requires.

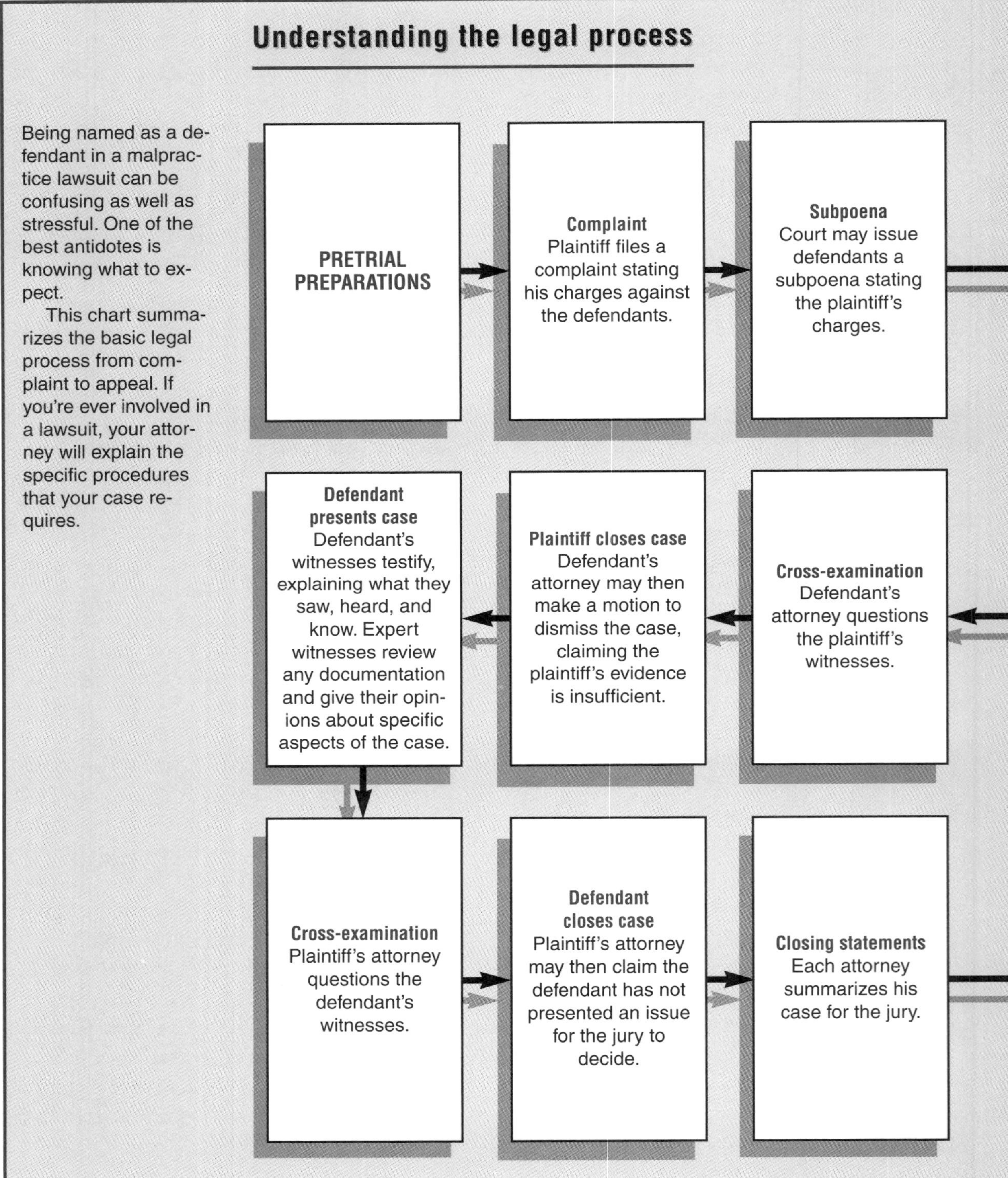

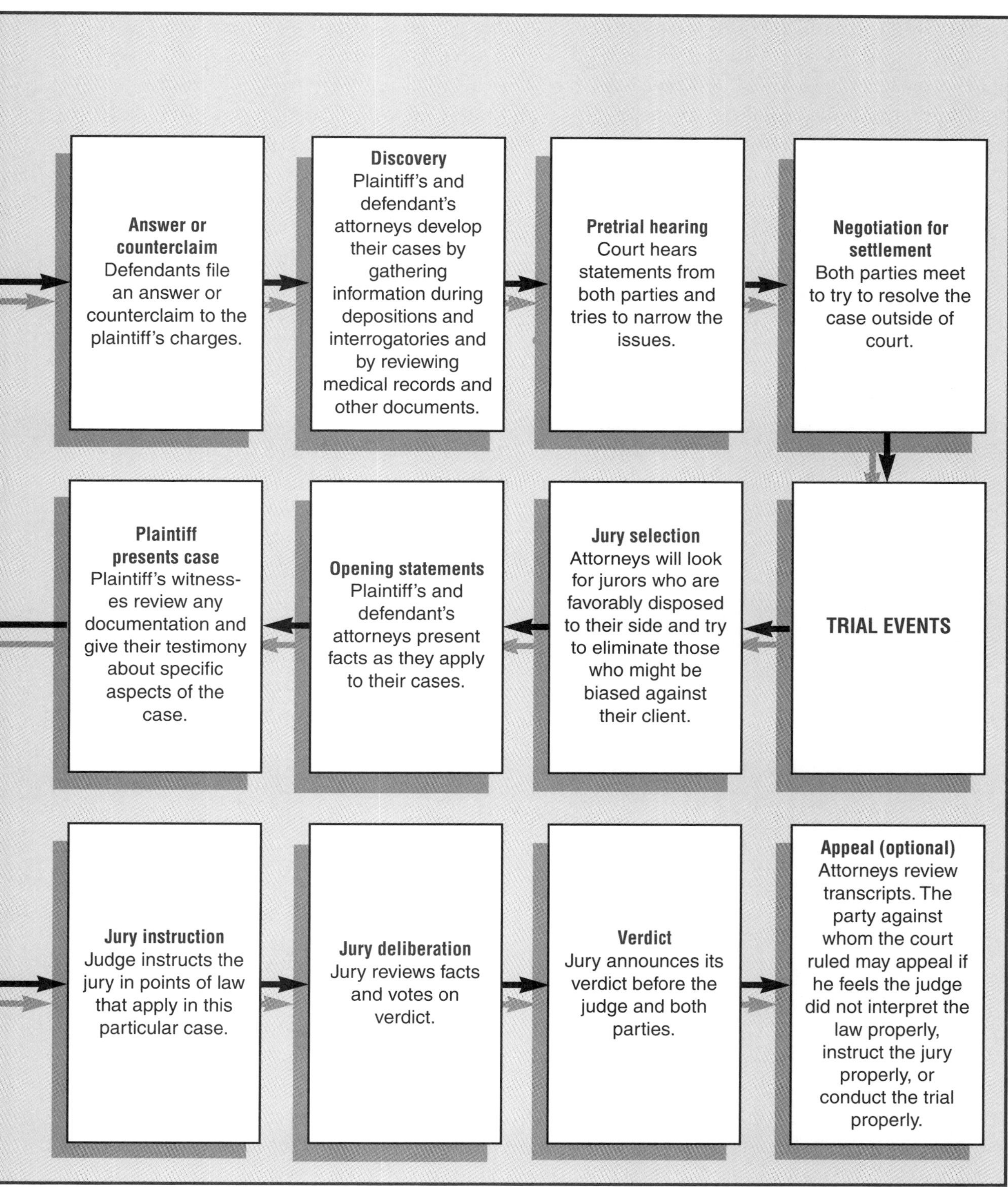
Answer or counterclaim
Defendants file an answer or counterclaim to the plaintiff's charges.
Discovery
Plaintiff's and defendant's attorneys develop their cases by gathering information during depositions and interrogatories and by reviewing medical records and other documents.
Pretrial hearing
Court hears statements from both parties and tries to narrow the issues.
Negotiation for settlement
Both parties meet to try to resolve the case outside of court.
TRIAL EVENTS
Jury selection
Attorneys will look for jurors who are favorably disposed to their side and try to eliminate those who might be biased against their client.
Opening statements
Plaintiff's and defendant's attorneys present facts as they apply to their cases.
Plaintiff presents case
Plaintiff's witnesses review any documentation and give their testimony about specific aspects of the case.
Jury instruction
Judge instructs the jury in points of law that apply in this particular case.
Jury deliberation
Jury reviews facts and votes on verdict.
Verdict
Jury announces its verdict before the judge and both parties.
Appeal (optional)
Attorneys review transcripts. The party against whom the court ruled may appeal if he feels the judge did not interpret the law properly, instruct the jury properly, or conduct the trial properly.

at the trial. He'll stress the importance of credibility by appearance, including dressing appropriately and presenting a professional demeanor. He'll rehearse with you the questions he'll ask at the trial and the questions he believes the plaintiff's attorney will ask you, and he'll probably discuss the best way to phrase your answers. Think carefully before you answer.

Remember, your attorney is your advocate, and he wants to win your case. He needs your cooperation to put forth a good defense. However, this doesn't mean that you must follow all your attorney's requests. If you think that he's asking you to do or say things that aren't in your best interest or that might damage your professional reputation, tell him. Resolve your differences *before* you go to court.

Surviving the deposition

During a deposition, the plaintiff's attorney questions you in the presence of your attorney and a court reporter. This process enables both parties to review each other's cases for strengths and weaknesses. The attorneys also observe the plaintiff and defendant during their separate depositions and gauge their credibility. The plaintiff may be present during your deposition, and you may be present during his.

Your attorney will explain the deposition procedure to you beforehand. He'll advise you to review all medical records in the case to help you recall important facts. During the actual deposition, the plaintiff's attorney has the right to inspect and copy any material you bring with you to aid your memory. Make sure that your attorney has a chance to inspect and approve this material first. Any materials you bring and make reference to may become part of the record as exhibits in the deposition.

At the start of the deposition, you'll be sworn in by the court reporter. As you answer questions under oath, the court reporter records everything so that a written transcript can be prepared later. This transcript may be used at trial to challenge your credibility on the stand, or the facts revealed in the deposition may cause the case to be settled before it goes to trial.

Your attorney will probably advise you to respond to all questions with simple answers and not to volunteer any additional information. If you have any doubts when responding to the other attorney's questions, avoid absolute answers. If you don't understand a question, ask the plaintiff's attorney for clarification. If you don't know the answer to a question, state that you don't know.

Memory fades with time, and even with the aid of medical records you won't be expected to recall the details of conversations that took place months or years earlier. If the case goes to court, however, you'll be held accountable for the answers you gave at the deposition.

Your attorney may object to some of the questions you're asked at the deposition; therefore, before answering anything, give him time to state his objection. If his objection is sustained (accepted), you won't have to answer the question. If he raises an objection but you still answer the question, the judge will rule on the objection at a later time. If that objection is sustained, your answer will be stricken from the record. Unless your attorney instructs you not to answer a question, you must give a response.

Defending yourself on the witness stand

While you're on the witness stand, the plaintiff's attorney may use several tactics to throw you off guard. Your attorney should discuss the following strategies with you.

Creating false security

The plaintiff's attorney knows that some jurors like and sympathize with nurses, so he won't want to antagonize the jury by being too hard on you. Instead, he'll try to make you "self-destruct" by creating a false sense of security, lulling you with politeness, respect, and even compliments. You may begin to let down your defenses and think "This attorney is really nice. He's only trying to be fair with me, so why was I so worried?" Then, in the same friendly way, he'll ask a question such as "Isn't it possible that you didn't document giving Mr. Smith his heart medication *because you didn't give it,* not because you forgot? Isn't it just possible?"

If you concede, you'll set the stage for one of two things. Either the attorney will carry his argument further, gently giving you enough rope to hang yourself, or he'll end his cross-examination abruptly, then pick up the point later, with a vengeance, in his summation to the jury. Always remember that the plaintiff's attorney is not your friend. Don't be lulled by his friendly demeanor or his winning personality. Stay on guard, and just answer his questions directly and briefly.

Asking leading questions

A leading question is one that suggests an answer, such as "Isn't it true that the medication was green?" In direct questioning (when your attorney questions you), leading questions aren't allowed. However, in cross-examination (when the plaintiff's attorney questions you), almost every question is a leading question. The attorney will never ask you a question such as "What happened when you examined the patient?" That offers you too much leeway to give an answer he doesn't want the jury to hear. Instead, he'll say something like "Isn't it true that the patient was sweating?" or "Isn't it a fact that Mrs. Smith complained about her arm?" Your answer should be a simple "yes" or "no." Of course, the attorney is hoping that you'll say more and give him the chance to charge ahead and upset you and disrupt your testimony.

Some nurses want to be helpful. Attorneys recognize this and try to use it to their advantage. You may want the jury to hear more than a simple yes or no. But wait until redirect questioning, when your own attorney questions you again after cross-examination. If he thinks you should expand on an answer, he'll ask the appropriate questions.

Before you answer a question from either attorney, take time to formulate your answer. As in the deposition, keep your answers to the absolute minimum — "yes" or "no" whenever possible. Don't stray from the main point; answer only the question that was asked.

Questioning your recollection

Because most cases don't come to trial until several years after the incident, one of the plaintiff's attorney's most effective techniques is to attack your recollection. The questioning might go like this:

ATTORNEY: Mrs. Brown, how many years ago did this happen?

NURSE: Five.

ATTORNEY: How many patients do you see a week?
NURSE: About 80.
ATTORNEY: Then that would be about 4,000 patients a year, would it not?
NURSE: Yes.
ATTORNEY: Which would come to 20,000 patients in 5 years, wouldn't it?
NURSE: Yes.

If you never charted the incident, the attorney might not attack your memory of it directly. Instead, he might just end the questioning abruptly and pick up the point again during his closing statement. If you *did* chart the incident, he might question you further, hoping that you'll contradict yourself.

Obviously, the wise approach is to chart everything that is relevant. But suppose you didn't record a particular incident that you remember well? Inform your attorney of this before the trial, and tell him why the incident is so vivid in your mind. Do you remember it because of certain people involved or because of where it occurred? This information will give your attorney the chance, either before or after cross-examination, to let you explain to the jury why you remember the incident even though you didn't document it.

The importance of charting everything is illustrated in this case: A patient died a few days after leaving the hospital against medical advice. His family filed suit against the hospital, alleging that the medical staff had failed to adequately warn him about the risks of leaving. A nurse testified that the patient had told her he was leaving no matter what the doctors said, but she hadn't noted this on the chart.

Instead of accusing the nurse of giving false testimony, the plaintiff's attorney questioned her about the importance of nurses' notes. He got her to concede that she wasn't likely to remember every patient she treated years ago. But under redirect questioning by the hospital's attorney, the nurse explained that even though she cared for hundreds of patients each year, she remembered those who left against medical advice.

Catching you in a contradiction

You'll need to carefully read the patient's chart and your signed pretrial deposition before the case comes to court. If you haven't read these documents, or you're not sure how to answer a question, always ask to see the chart to refresh your memory. If you don't know something, simply say that you don't; avoid trying to guess. In either case, the jury won't hold it against you.

If you read your deposition before the trial and disagree with something you said, tell your attorney. This allows him to defuse a potentially damaging situation. During his questioning, he'll let you explain why you've changed your mind. For example, you might say, "I've had a lot of time to recollect since the deposition. Then, I was a little confused and didn't understand the question." This perfectly logical explanation would look like a poor excuse if it came out for the first time under cross-examination.

Uncovering your bias

Another common technique is to weaken the nurse's testimony by trying to show that she's biased in favor of the facility or someone she works with who also is involved in the lawsuit. For example, the nurse may have a social relationship with her nurse-manager, a hospital administrator, or members of a doctor's family.

This tactic usually works very effectively on witnesses who haven't been adequately prepared by their attorneys. It may unnerve and embarrass them. In one case, a nurse testified that a patient arrived in the emergency department intoxicated and on diazepam but refused to be admitted to the hospital. The nurse said that she gave the patient the hospital's number to call if he needed help but that she never documented this. When the patient died 4 days later, the family alleged that he'd never been told he could be admitted and had never been given the hospital's number.

Here's how the questioning by the plaintiff's attorney went:

ATTORNEY: You know the hospital administrator pretty well, don't you? The fact is, you bought a house from him, didn't you?

NURSE: Yes.

ATTORNEY: And isn't it a fact that your children play with his children?

NURSE: Yes.

ATTORNEY: You wouldn't want to do anything to hurt his or the hospital's reputation, would you?

NURSE: No.

The nurse's answers were absolutely correct. But she hesitated, blushed, and was obviously ill at ease. Although the jury believed her and returned a verdict for the hospital, the nurse's credibility could have been seriously damaged.

Having social relationships with people you work with is normal, and jurors expect it. Don't be afraid to admit such relationships — just don't act evasive about it. If the plaintiff's attorney tries to give the impression that you're afraid of losing your job, simply say, "I took the oath, and I'm here to tell the truth as I know it."

Uncovering bias against the patient

The plaintiff's attorney may also try to undermine your testimony by showing that you disliked the patient. Don't deny the truth — if the patient was hard to like, admit it. Just be sure to explain why you felt this way and that your feelings didn't interfere with your giving him the best possible care. Jurors don't expect you to like everyone. They'll empathize with you for providing good nursing care under difficult conditions and may even respect you for it. If you have a difficult patient, document it in objective terms.

Making you defensive

If you give the plaintiff's attorney the opportunity, he may get tough with you. For example, in one case, an attorney asked a nurse why she hadn't immediately recorded a patient's vital signs when he was admitted to the emergency department. The nurse explained that the patient had needed immediate care, so she'd jotted his vital signs on the bed sheet, where everyone could see them.

Under cross-examination, the nurse said that she resented being accused of "incompetence." The attorney gave her a surprised look and replied, "Did you ever hear me use the word 'incompetence'? You're saying it, but I'm not thinking that." Although the facts won this case for the hospital, the nurse could have lost her credibility with the jurors by planting the word *incompetence* in their minds.

If a plaintiff's attorney is ever rude to you, don't be rude in return, and don't lose your temper. This may only make the jurors think, "If she's like this here, what's she like in the hospital?" And don't disagree with an attorney just to disagree. This will only create more problems for you and cause you to be on the stand longer.

A FINAL THOUGHT

As you expand your nursing expertise and take on more patient care responsibilities, you'll also be accepting greater legal risks. But you don't have to resign yourself to malpractice litigation. If you meet accepted standards of care and document that care meticulously, you'll be doing everything in your power to prevent or defend against a lawsuit.

Selected references

"Advice, p.r.n. Inappropriate Charting: Writing a Wrong," *Nursing97* 27(3):12, 14, March 1997.

Carroll, M.M. "Nursing Malpractice and Corporate Negligence: How Is the Standard of Care Determined?" *Journal of Nursing Law* 3(3):53-60, 1996.

"Defending Yourself on Many Fronts: Malpractice Isn't All You Should Worry About after a Patient Care Incident. Here's What You Need to Know..." reprinted with permission from *NSO Risk Advisor,* January 1997, *Missouri Nurse* 66(4):4, July-August 1997.

Nurse's Legal Handbook, 3rd ed. Springhouse, Pa.: Springhouse Corp., 1996.

Vernon, J. "Legal Lines: Could You Be Sued for Malpractice?" *Neonatal Network* 16(8):73-75, December 1997.

Wickens, R. *Professional Liability,* 3rd ed. Philadelphia: Coronet Books, 1996.

Wilkinson, A.P. "Nursing Malpractice: How to Avoid Your Day in Court," *Nursing 98* 28(6):34-40, June 1998.

Appendices
Glossary
Index

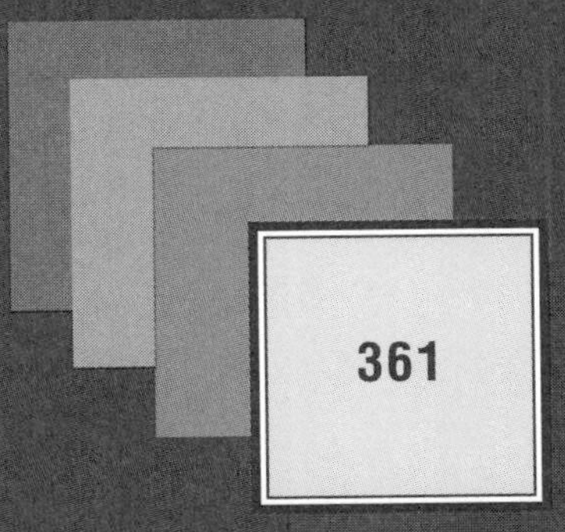

NANDA Taxonomy I, Revised

The North American Nursing Diagnosis Association (NANDA) endorsed its first nursing diagnosis taxonomic structure, NANDA Taxonomy I, in 1986. This taxonomy was revised in 1989, 1994 and, most recently, 1998. The taxonomy that appears here represents the currently accepted classification system for nursing diagnoses.

This classification system, which appears below, consists of nine human response patterns and their definitions: Exchanging: Mutual giving and receiving; Communicating: Sending messages; Relating: Establishing bonds; Valuing: Assigning worth; Choosing: Selection of alternatives; Moving: Activity; Perceiving: Reception of information; Knowing: Meaning associated with information; and Feeling: Subjective awareness of information.

Pattern 1: Exchanging

1.1.2.1	Altered nutrition: More than body requirements
1.1.2.2	Altered nutrition: Less than body requirements
1.1.2.3	Altered nutrition: Risk for more than body requirements
1.2.1.1	Risk for infection
1.2.2.1	Risk for altered body temperature
1.2.2.2	Hypothermia
1.2.2.3	Hyperthermia
1.2.2.4	Ineffective thermoregulation
1.2.3.1	Dysreflexia
1.2.3.2	Risk for autonomic dysreflexia
1.3.1.1	Constipation
1.3.1.1.1	Perceived constipation
1.3.1.1.2	Colonic constipation
1.3.1.2	Diarrhea
1.3.1.3	Bowel incontinence
1.3.1.4	Risk for constipation
1.3.2	Altered urinary elimination
1.3.2.1.1	Stress incontinence
1.3.2.1.2	Reflex urinary incontinence
1.3.2.1.3	Urge incontinence
1.3.2.1.4	Functional urinary incontinence
1.3.2.1.5	Total incontinence
1.3.2.1.6	Risk for urinary urge incontinence
1.3.2.2	Urinary retention
1.4.1.1	Altered (specify type) tissue perfusion (renal, cerebral, cardiopulmonary, gastrointestinal, peripheral)
1.4.1.2	Risk for fluid volume imbalance
1.4.1.2.1	Fluid volume excess
1.4.1.2.2.1	Fluid volume deficit
1.4.1.2.2.2	Risk for fluid volume deficit
1.4.2.1	Decreased cardiac output
1.5.1.1	Impaired gas exchange
1.5.1.2	Ineffective airway clearance
1.5.1.3	Ineffective breathing pattern

1.5.1.3.1	Inability to sustain spontaneous ventilation
1.5.1.3.2	Dysfunctional ventilatory weaning response
1.6.1	Risk for injury
1.6.1.1	Risk for suffocation
1.6.1.2	Risk for poisoning
1.6.1.3	Risk for trauma
1.6.1.4	Risk for aspiration
1.6.1.5	Risk for disuse syndrome
1.6.1.6	Latex allergy
1.6.1.7	Risk for latex allergy
1.6.2	Altered protection
1.6.2.1	Impaired tissue integrity
1.6.2.1.1	Altered oral mucous membrane
1.6.2.1.2.1	Impaired skin integrity
1.6.2.1.2.2	Risk for impaired skin integrity
1.6.2.1.3	Altered dentition
1.7.1	Decreased adaptive capacity: Intracranial
1.8	Energy field disturbance

Pattern 2: Communicating

2.1.1.1	Impaired verbal communication

Pattern 3: Relating

3.1.1	Impaired social interaction
3.1.2	Social isolation
3.1.3	Risk for loneliness
3.2.1	Altered role performance
3.2.1.1.1	Altered parenting
3.2.1.1.2	Risk for altered parenting
3.2.1.1.2.1	Risk for altered parent/infant/child attachment
3.2.1.2.1	Sexual dysfunction
3.2.2	Altered family processes
3.2.2.1	Caregiver role strain
3.2.2.2	Risk for caregiver role strain
3.2.2.3.1	Altered family process: Alcoholism
3.2.3.1	Parental role conflict
3.3	Altered sexuality patterns

Pattern 4: Valuing

4.1.1	Spiritual distress (distress of the human spirit)
4.1.2	Risk for spiritual distress
4.2	Potential for enhanced spiritual well being

Pattern 5: Choosing

5.1.1.1	Ineffective individual coping
5.1.1.1.1	Impaired adjustment
5.1.1.1.2	Defensive coping
5.1.1.1.3	Ineffective denial
5.1.2.1.1	Ineffective family coping: Disabling
5.1.2.1.2	Ineffective family coping: Compromised
5.1.2.2	Family coping: Potential for growth
5.1.3.1	Potential for enhanced community coping
5.1.3.2	Ineffective community coping
5.2.1	Ineffective management of therapeutic regimen (individual)
5.2.1.1	Noncompliance (specify)
5.2.2	Ineffective management of therapeutic regimen: Families
5.2.3	Ineffective management of therapeutic regimen: Community
5.2.4	Effective management of therapeutic regimen: Individual
5.3.1.1	Decisional conflict (specify)
5.4	Health-seeking behaviors (specify)

Pattern 6: Moving

6.1.1.1	Impaired physical mobility
6.1.1.1.	Risk for peripheral neurovascular dysfunction
6.1.1.1.2	Risk for perioperative positioning injury
6.1.1.1.3	Impaired walking

6.1.1.1.4	Impaired wheelchair mobility
6.1.1.1.5	Impaired wheelchair transfer ability
6.1.1.1.6	Impaired bed mobility
6.1.1.2	Activity intolerance
6.1.1.2.1	Fatigue
6.1.1.3	Risk for activity intolerance
6.2.1	Sleep pattern disturbance
6.2.1.1	Sleep deprivation
6.3.1.1	Diversional activity deficit
6.4.1.1	Impaired home maintenance management
6.4.2	Altered health maintenance
6.4.2.1	Delayed surgical recovery
6.4.2.2	Adult failure to thrive
6.5.1	Feeding self-care deficit
6.5.1.1	Impaired swallowing
6.5.1.2	Ineffective breast-feeding
6.5.1.2.1	Interrupted breast-feeding
6.5.1.3	Effective breast-feeding
6.5.1.4	Ineffective infant feeding pattern
6.5.2	Bathing or hygiene self-care deficit
6.5.3	Dressing or grooming self-care deficit
6.5.4	Toileting self-care deficit
6.6	Altered growth and development
6.6.1	Risk for altered development
6.6.2	Risk for altered growth
6.7	Relocation stress syndrome
6.8.1	Risk for disorganized infant behavior
6.8.2	Disorganized infant behavior
6.8.3	Potential for enhanced organized infant behavior

Pattern 7: Perceiving

7.1.1	Body image disturbance
7.1.2	Self-esteem disturbance
7.1.2.1	Chronic low self-esteem
7.1.2.2	Situational low self-esteem
7.1.3	Personal identity disturbance
7.2	Sensory-perceptual alterations (specify as visual, auditory, kinesthetic, gustatory, tactile, olfactory)
7.2.1.1	Unilateral neglect
7.3.1	Hopelessness
7.3.2	Powerlessness

Pattern 8: Knowing

8.1.1	Knowledge deficit (specify)
8.2.1	Impaired environmental interpretation syndrome
8.2.2	Acute confusion
8.2.3	Chronic confusion
8.3	Altered thought processes
8.3.1	Impaired memory

Pattern 9: Feeling

9.1.1	Pain
9.1.1.1	Chronic pain
9.1.2	Nausea
9.2.1.1	Dysfunctional grieving
9.2.1.2	Anticipatory grieving
9.2.1.3	Chronic sorrow
9.2.2	Risk for violence: Self-directed or directed at others
9.2.2.1	Risk for self-mutilation
9.2.3	Post-trauma syndrome
9.2.3.1	Rape-trauma syndrome
9.2.3.1.1	Rape-trauma syndrome: Compound reaction
9.2.3.1.2	Rape-trauma syndrome: Silent reaction
9.2.4	Risk for post-trauma syndrome
9.3.1	Anxiety
9.3.1.1	Death anxiety
9.3.2	Fear

Documentation Guidelines for Common Nursing Diagnoses

After you've explored your patient's chief complaint, performed an assessment, and analyzed the findings, you can formulate your nursing diagnoses (or problem list) and develop a plan of care. This plan will specify patient outcomes and the interventions to achieve them. Completing the process requires documenting your findings and activities. For your reference, this appendix provides documentation guidelines for the most commonly used nursing diagnoses.

Activity intolerance, risk for

related to immobility

Definition

Accentuated risk of extreme fatigue or other physical symptoms following simple activity

Documenting assessment findings

Chart assessment findings related to the following:

- history of present illness
- age
- past experience with immobility or prescribed bed rest
- cardiovascular status, including blood pressure, heart rate and rhythm at rest and with activity, complete blood count, skin temperature and color, edema, chest pain or discomfort
- respiratory status, including arterial blood gas (ABG) levels, breath sounds, pain or discomfort associated with respiration, and rate, rhythm, depth, and pattern of respirations at rest and with activity
- neurologic status, including level of consciousness (LOC), orientation, mental status, sensory status, motor status
- musculoskeletal status, including range of motion (ROM), muscle size, strength, tone, and functional mobility as follows:
  - 0 = completely independent
  - 1 = requires use of equipment or device
  - 2 = requires help, supervision, or teaching from another person
  - 3 = requires help from another person and equipment or device
  - 4 = dependent; doesn't take part in activity.

Documenting expected outcomes

Record appropriate patient outcomes on the plan of care. Possible outcomes include:

- Patient maintains muscle strength and ROM, as indicated by use of functional mobility scale.
- Patient carries out isometric exercise regimen.

- Patient communicates understanding of rationale for maintaining activity level.
- Patient avoids risk factors that may lead to activity intolerance.
- Patient performs self-care activities to tolerance level.
- Vital signs remain within prescribed range during periods of activity (specify).

Documenting interventions

Chart interventions related to:

- patient's expressed motivation to maintain maximum activity level within restrictions imposed by illness
- patient's physiologic response to increased activity (times and dates of vital signs: blood pressure, respirations, heart rate and rhythm)
- patient repositioning and turning (including times and assistive devices used)
- patient's functional level (use a functional mobility scale)
- prescribed ROM and other exercises (including times and assistive devices used, such as trapezes)
- patient teaching (including reason for treatment regimen and signs and symptoms of overexertion, such as dizziness, chest pain, and dyspnea) and patient's response
- patient's ability to perform activities of daily living (ADLs)
- evaluation of expected outcomes.

Airway clearance, ineffective

related to decreased energy or fatigue

Definition

Anatomic or physiologic obstruction of the airway that interferes with normal ventilation

Documenting assessment findings

Chart the defining characteristics as verbalized by the patient and your physical assessment findings, for example:

- defining characteristics: anxiety, apprehension, chest pain, choking or gasping, fever, inability to cough, ineffective cough, fatigue, decreased activity tolerance, dyspnea, tachypnea, nasal flaring, noisy respirations
- history of present illness
- patient's perception of ability to clear airway
- knowledge of physical condition
- neurologic status, including LOC, orientation, sensory status, and motor status
- respiratory status, including symmetry of chest expansion; use of accessory muscles; cough (productive or nonproductive); respiratory rate, depth, and pattern; breath sounds; sputum characteristics (color, consistency, amount, odor, and changes from patient's norm); palpation for fremitus; percussion of lung fields; ABG levels; hemoglobin and hematocrit; pulmonary function studies
- psychosocial status, including interest, motivation, and knowledge.

Documenting expected outcomes

Record appropriate patient outcomes on the plan of care. Possible outcomes include:

- Airway remains patent.
- Adventitious breath sounds are absent.
- Chest X-ray shows no abnormality.
- Oxygen level in normal range.
- Patient breathes deeply and coughs to remove secretions.
- Patient expectorates sputum.
- Patient demonstrates controlled coughing techniques.

- Ventilation is adequate.
- Patient shows no signs of pulmonary compromise.
- Patient demonstrates skill in conserving energy while attempting to clear airway.
- Patient states understanding of changes needed to diminish oxygen demands.

Documenting interventions

Chart interventions related to:

- patient's perception of ability to cough
- observed respiratory status and other physical findings
- patient positioning and repositioning (including times)
- airway and pulmonary clearance maneuvers (such as coughing and deep breathing, suctioning to stimulate cough and clear airways, aerosol treatments, postural drainage, percussion and vibration) and patient's response
- sputum characteristics (including amount, odor, consistency)
- prescribed medication administration (including expectorants, bronchodilators, and other drugs)
- amount of fluid intake to help liquefy secretions
- oxygen administration (including times, dates, equipment, and supplies)
- test results, including ABG levels and hemoglobin values, and reportable deviations from baseline levels
- endotracheal intubation
- patient teaching
- evaluation of expected outcomes.

Anxiety

related to situational crisis

Definition

Feeling of threat or danger to self arising from an unidentifiable source

Documenting assessment findings

Chart the defining characteristics as verbalized by the patient and your physical assessment findings, for example:

- defining characteristics: shortness of breath or smothering sensation; palpitations; sweating; cold, clammy hands; dry mouth; dizziness; light-headedness; nausea, diarrhea, or other abdominal distress; hot flashes or chills; frequent urination; difficulty swallowing; motor tension (including trembling, twitching, shakiness, muscle tension, aches, soreness, and restlessness); easy fatigability; keyed-up feeling; difficulty concentrating; insomnia; irritability
- reason for hospitalization, including patient's perception of problem, onset of problem, recent stressors, life changes, other precipitating events
- mental status, including orientation to time, place, or person; insight regarding current situation; judgment; abstract thinking; mood; affect; recent and remote memory; thought processes; thought content
- coping and problem-solving ability
- ability to perform ADLs
- sleep habits
- dietary and nutritional status
- available support systems, including family or significant other, friends, clergy, health care agencies.

Documenting expected outcomes

Record appropriate expected outcomes on the plan of care. Possible outcomes include:

- Patient identifies factors that elicit anxious behaviors.

- Patient discusses activities that tend to decrease anxious behaviors.
- Patient practices progressive relaxation techniques ____times a day.
- Patient copes with current medical situation (specify) without demonstrating severe signs of anxiety (specify for individual).

Documenting interventions

Chart interventions related to:

- patient's expressions of anxiety and feelings of relief
- observed signs of patient's anxiety
- time spent with patient, duration of anxious episodes, and emotional support given to patient and family
- comfort measures
- patient teaching (including clear, concise explanations of anything about to occur, relaxation techniques such as guided imagery, progressive muscle relaxation, and meditation)
- referrals to community or professional mental health services
- patient's involvement in making decisions related to care
- evaluation of expected outcomes.

Body image disturbance

Definition

Negative perception of self that makes healthful functioning more difficult

Documenting assessment findings

Chart the defining characteristics as verbalized by the patient and your physical assessment findings, for example:

- defining characteristics: actual change in structure or function, missing body part, inability to look at or touch body part, hiding or overly exposing body part, nonverbal or verbal response to actual or perceived change in structure or function, trauma to nonfunctioning part
- physiologic changes
- behavioral changes
- patient's and family's perception of the patient's present health problem
- patient's usual pattern of coping with stress
- patient's role in the family
- patient's past experiences with health problems
- sleep pattern
- appetite
- hobbies and interests
- occupational history
- ethnic background and cultural perceptions.

Documenting expected outcomes

Record appropriate expected outcomes on the plan of care. Possible outcomes include:

- Patient acknowledges change in body image.
- Patient communicates feelings about change in body image.
- Patient participates in decision making about his care (specify).
- Patient talks with someone who has experienced the same problem.
- Patient demonstrates ability to practice two new coping behaviors.
- Patient expresses positive feelings about self.

Documenting interventions

Chart interventions related to:

- patient's observed coping patterns and responses to change in structure or function

APPENDICES

of body part (such as touching or not touching)
- patient's participation in self-care
- patient's perception of self, prostheses, adaptive equipment, and limitations
- patient's focus on or denial of specific body parts
- patient's involvement in decision making related to care
- patient's response to nursing interventions
- patient teaching (including information on how bodily functions are improving or stabilizing and specific coping strategies)
- referrals to a mental health professional, a support group, or another person who has had a similar problem
- positive reinforcement of patient's efforts to adapt and use coping strategies
- evaluation of expected outcomes.

BREATHING PATTERN, INEFFECTIVE

related to decreased energy or fatigue

Definition

Change in rate, depth, or pattern of breathing that alters normal gas exchange

Documenting assessment findings

Chart the defining characteristics as verbalized by the patient and your physical assessment findings, for example:

- defining characteristics: dyspnea, especially on exertion; paradoxical breathing pattern; inspiration longer than expiration; decreased energy; fatigue
- history of respiratory disorder
- respiratory status, including rate and depth of respiration, breath sounds, symmetry of chest expansion, use of accessory muscles, presence of cough, anterior-posterior chest diameter, palpation for fremitus, percussion of lung fields, and pulmonary function studies
- neurologic and mental status, including LOC and emotional status
- knowledge, including current understanding of physical condition and physical, mental, and emotional readiness to learn.

Documenting expected outcomes

Record appropriate expected outcomes on the plan of care. Possible outcomes include:

- Patient's respiratory rate stays within ± 5 of baseline.
- ABG levels return to baseline.
- Patient reports feeling comfortable when breathing.
- Patient reports feeling rested each day.
- Patient demonstrates diaphragmatic pursed-lip breathing.
- Patient achieves maximum lung expansion with adequate ventilation.
- Patient demonstrates skill in conserving energy while carrying out ADLs.

Documenting interventions

Chart interventions related to:

- patient's expressions of comfort in breathing, emotional state, understanding of medical diagnosis, and readiness to learn
- physical condition related to pulmonary assessment (including respiratory rate and depth, auscultated breath sounds, and reportable changes)
- test results such as ABG levels
- prescribed medication and oxygen administration (including dates, times, dosages, routes, adverse effects, equipment, and supplies)
- comfort measures (including supporting upper extremities with pillows, providing

an over-bed table with a pillow to lean on, or elevating the head of the bed)
- airway suctioning to remove secretions
- patient teaching (including pursed-lip breathing, abdominal breathing, relaxation techniques, medications [dosage, frequency, reportable adverse effects], activity and rest, and diet)
- scheduling of activities to allow periods of rest
- evaluation of expected outcomes.

Cardiac output, decreased

related to reduced stroke volume as a result of mechanical or structural problems

Definition

Cardiovascular or respiratory symptoms resulting from insufficient blood being pumped by the heart

Documenting assessment findings

Chart the defining characteristics as verbalized by the patient and your physical assessment findings, for example:

- defining characteristics: oliguria or anuria, ascites, cyanosis, dyspnea, orthopnea, mental status change, pallor of skin and mucous membranes, cold and clammy skin, cough, frothy sputum, fatigue
- mental status, including orientation and LOC
- cardiovascular status, including history of valvular disorder, capillary heart disease, or myopathy; skin color, temperature, turgor, and capillary refill time; jugular vein distention; hepatojugular reflux; heart rate and rhythm; heart sounds; blood pressure; peripheral pulses; electrocardiogram (ECG); exercise ECG; echocardiogram; and phonocardiogram
- respiratory status, including respiratory rate and depth, breath sounds, chest X-ray, and ABG levels
- renal status, including weight, intake and output, and urine specific gravity.

Documenting expected outcomes

Record appropriate expected outcomes on the plan of care. Possible outcomes include:

- Patient maintains hemodynamic stability: pulse not less than ____ and not greater than ____ beats/minute; blood pressure not less than ____ and not greater than ____ mm Hg.
- Patient exhibits no arrhythmias.
- Skin remains warm and dry.
- Patient exhibits no pedal edema.
- Patient achieves activity within limits of prescribed heart rate.
- Patient expresses sense of physical comfort after activity.
- Heart's workload diminishes.
- Patient maintains adequate cardiac output.
- Patient performs stress-reduction techniques every 4 hours while awake.
- Patient states understanding of signs and symptoms, prescribed activity level, diet, and medications.

Documenting interventions

Chart interventions related to:

- patient's needs and perception of problem
- observed physical findings (including LOC, heart rate and rhythm, blood pressure, auscultated heart and breath sounds)
- reports of abnormal findings (including times, dates, and names)
- intake and output measurements, daily weight
- observation of pedal or sacral edema

- interventions for life-threatening arrhythmias, as ordered
- skin care measures to enhance skin perfusion and venous flow
- increasing patient's activity level within limits of prescribed heart rate
- observed pulse rate before and after activity
- patient's response to activity
- dietary restrictions as ordered
- patient teaching (including desired skills related to diet, prescribed activity, and stress reduction techniques; procedures and tests; chest pain and other reportable symptoms; medications [name, dosage, frequency, therapeutic and adverse effects]; simple methods for lifting and bending)
- administration of and response to oxygen therapy
- evaluation of expected outcomes.

Constipation

related to personal habits

Definition

Interruption of normal bowel elimination pattern characterized by infrequent or absent stools

Documenting assessment findings

Chart the defining characteristics as verbalized by the patient and your physical assessment findings, for example:

- defining characteristics: decreased appetite; fever; decreased bowel movement frequency; hard, formed stools; straining during defecation; reported decreased intake of fluid, food, or fiber
- history of bowel disorder or surgery
- GI status, including nausea and vomiting, usual bowel habits, change in bowel habits, stool characteristics (color, amount, size, consistency), pain, inspection of abdomen, auscultation for bowel sounds, palpation for masses and tenderness, percussion for tympany and dullness, laxative or enema use, medications (iron, narcotics)
- nutritional status, including dietary intake, appetite, current weight, and change from normal weight
- activity status, type and duration of exercise, and occupation (sedentary, having restricted access to bathroom)
- knowledge, including understanding of need for regular bowel habits, ability and motivation to change current patterns, and understanding of relationship between laxative and enema use, activity, and constipation.

Documenting expected outcomes

Record appropriate expected outcomes on the plan of care. Possible outcomes include:

- Elimination pattern returns to normal.
- Patient moves bowels every ____day(s) without laxative or enema.
- Patient states understanding of causative factors of constipation.
- Patient gets regular exercise.
- Patient describes changes in personal habits to maintain normal elimination pattern.
- Patient states plans to seek help resolving emotional or psychological problems.

Documenting interventions

Chart interventions related to:

- frequency of bowel movements and characteristics of stools
- administration of laxatives or enemas and their effectiveness
- patient's weight (weekly)

- referrals to or consultations with nutritional staff
- patient's expressions of concern about change in diet, activity level, use of laxatives or enemas, and bowel pattern
- establishment of daily schedule
- adherence to dietary recommendations
- observed diet, activity tolerance, and characteristics of stools
- patient teaching (about high-fiber diet, increased fluid intake, exercise, importance of responding to urge to defecate, and long-term effects of laxatives or enemas)
- evaluation of expected outcomes.

Coping, ineffective individual

related to situational crisis

Definition

Inability to use adaptive behaviors in response to difficult life situations, such as loss of health, a loved one, or job

Documenting assessment findings

Chart the defining characteristics as verbalized by the patient and your physical assessment findings, for example:

- defining characteristics: reported or observed change in usual communication patterns, chronic fatigue or worry, evidence of situational crisis, excessive drinking, inappropriate use of defense mechanisms, insomnia, irritability, irritable bowel, muscular tension, overeating or loss of appetite, verbal expression of inability to cope or seek help, verbal manipulation, inability to fulfill role expectations, meet basic needs, or solve problems
- coping behaviors
- problem-solving techniques usually employed to cope with life problems
- degree of physical and emotional impairment
- diversional activities
- financial resources
- occupation
- patient's perception of present health problem or crisis
- support systems, including family, companion, friends, and clergy.

Documenting expected outcomes

Record appropriate expected outcomes on the plan of care. Possible outcomes include:

- Patient communicates feelings about the present situation.
- Patient becomes involved in planning own care.
- Patient expresses feeling of having greater control over present situation.
- Patient uses available support systems, such as family and friends, to aid in coping.
- Patient identifies at least two coping behaviors.
- Patient demonstrates ability to use two healthful coping behaviors.

Documenting interventions

Chart interventions related to:

- patient's perception of current situation and what it means
- patient's efforts at self-care
- patient's coping behaviors and patient's evaluation of their effectiveness
- patient's verbal expression of feelings indicating comfort or discomfort
- observed patient behaviors
- nursing interventions to help patient cope and patient's responses
- patient teaching (about treatments and procedures)
- referrals to counselors and support groups

- patient's verbalization of factors that exacerbate the inability to cope
- evaluation of expected outcomes.

Denial

related to fear or anxiety

Definition

Conscious or unconscious attempt to disavow the knowledge or meaning of an event to reduce anxiety or fear to the detriment of health

Documenting assessment findings

Chart the defining characteristics as verbalized by the patient and your physical assessment findings, for example:

- defining characteristics: doesn't admit impact of disease on lifestyle, doesn't admit fear of death or invalidism, doesn't perceive personal relevance or danger of symptoms, minimizes symptoms, reports self-treatment to relieve symptoms
- perception of present health, including awareness of diagnosis, perception of personal relevance or impact on lifestyle, and description of symptoms
- degree of physical and emotional functional impairment
- mental status, including general appearance, affect, mood, memory, orientation, communication, thinking process, perception, abstract thinking, judgment, and insight
- coping behaviors
- problem-solving strategies
- support systems, including family or significant other, friends, and clergy
- financial resources
- belief system, including values, norms, and religion
- self-concept, including self-esteem and body image.

Documenting expected outcomes

Record appropriate expected outcomes on the plan of care. Possible outcomes include:

- Patient describes knowledge and perception of present health problem.
- Patient describes lifestyle and reports any recent changes.
- Patient expresses knowledge of stages of grief.
- Patient demonstrates behavior associated with grief process.
- Patient discusses present health problem with doctor, nurses, and family members.
- Patient indicates by conversation or behavior an increased awareness of reality.

Documenting interventions

Chart interventions related to:

- patient's perception of health problem, including its severity and potential impact on lifestyle
- patient's verbalization of feelings related to present problem
- mental status (baseline and ongoing)
- communications with doctor (to assess what patient has been told about illness)
- patient's knowledge of grief process
- patient's behavioral responses
- interventions implemented to assist patient
- patient's response to nursing interventions
- patient teaching and patient's response
- evaluation of expected outcomes.

Diarrhea

related to malabsorption, inflammation, or irritation of bowel

Definition

Interruption of normal elimination pattern characterized by frequent, loose stools

Documenting assessment findings

Chart the defining characteristics as verbalized by the patient and your physical assessment findings, for example:

- defining characteristics: abdominal pain and cramping, hyperactive bowel sounds, increased frequency or urgency of defecation, loose liquid stools, stool color changes and, possibly, bloody, mucoid, fatty, or bulky stool
- history of bowel disorder or surgery
- GI status, including nausea and vomiting, usual bowel habits, change in bowel habits, stool characteristics (color, amount, size, consistency), pain, inspection of abdomen, auscultation for bowel sounds, palpation for masses and tenderness, percussion for tympany and dullness, laxative and enema use, medications (especially antibiotics), stool culture, upper GI series, barium enema
- nutritional status, including dietary intake, change from normal diet, appetite, current weight, change from normal weight, and food irritants and contaminants
- fluid and electrolyte status, including intake and output, urine specific gravity, skin turgor, mucous membranes, serum potassium and sodium, and blood urea nitrogen
- psychosocial status, including personality, stressors (finances, job, marital discord, disease process), coping mechanisms, support systems, lifestyle, and recent travel.

Documenting expected outcomes

Record appropriate expected outcomes on the plan of care. Possible outcomes include:

- Patient controls diarrhea with medication.
- Elimination pattern returns to normal.
- Patient regains and maintains fluid and electrolyte balance.
- Skin remains intact.
- Patient discusses causative factors, preventive measures, and changed body image.
- Patient practices stress-reduction techniques daily.
- Patient seeks persons with similar condition or joins a support group.
- Patient demonstrates ability to use ostomy devices if diarrhea results from colorectal surgery.

Documenting interventions

Chart interventions related to:

- patient's expressions of concern about diarrhea, causative factors, and adaptation to changes in body image if diarrhea results from colorectal surgery.
- administration and observed effects of antidiarrheal medications
- intake and output measurements and daily weight
- observed stool characteristics and frequency of defecation
- skin condition (especially decreased skin turgor or excoriation)
- bowel sounds (auscultation findings)
- patient teaching (including causes, prevention, cleaning of perineal area and comfort, dietary restrictions, stress reduction, preoperative instruction about ileostomy or colostomy and abdominal surgery, and postoperative instructions about ostomy equipment)
- referrals to support groups (such as ostomy clubs) if appropriate
- evaluation of expected outcomes.

Fluid volume deficit

related to active loss

Definition

Excessive loss of body fluid and electrolytes

Documenting assessment findings

Chart the defining characteristics as verbalized by the patient and your physical assessment findings, for example:

- defining characteristics: dry mucous membranes; dry or cold, clammy skin; fever; rapid, shallow respirations; thirst; weakness; weight loss; oliguria; increased urine concentration; poor turgor of skin or tongue
- history of fluid loss, such as vomiting, nasogastric (NG) tube drainage, diarrhea, hemorrhage
- vital signs
- fluid and electrolyte status, including weight, intake and output, urine specific gravity, skin turgor, mucous membranes
- laboratory studies, including serum electrolytes, blood urea nitrogen, hemoglobin, hematocrit, and stool cultures.

Documenting expected outcomes

Record appropriate expected outcomes on the plan of care. Possible outcomes include:

- Vital signs remain stable.
- Skin color and temperature are normal.
- Electrolyte levels stay within normal range.
- Patient produces adequate urine volume.
- Patient has normal skin turgor and moist mucous membranes.
- Urine specific gravity remains between 1.005 and 1.010.
- Fluid and blood volume return to normal.
- Patient expresses understanding of factors that caused fluid volume deficit.

Documenting interventions

Chart interventions related to:

- vital signs
- patient's complaints of thirst, weakness, dizziness, and palpitations
- interventions to control fluid loss and patient's response
- observed skin and mucous membrane condition and other physical findings (including signs of fluid and electrolyte imbalances, such as tachycardia, dyspnea, or hypotension)
- intake and output and significant changes (including amount and characteristics of urine, stools, vomitus, wound drainage, NG drainage, chest tube drainage, and any other output)
- urine specific gravity (including times and dates)
- administration of any fluids, blood or blood products, or plasma expanders and patient's response
- patient's daily weight and abdominal girth
- patient teaching (about fluid loss and ways to monitor fluid volume at home, such as by measuring intake and output and body weight daily)
- evaluation of expected outcomes.

Gas exchange impairment

related to altered oxygen supply

Definition

Interference in cellular respiration resulting from inadequate exchange or transport of oxygen and carbon dioxide

Documenting assessment findings

Chart the defining characteristics as verbalized by the patient and your physical assessment findings, for example:

- defining characteristics: anxiety, confusion, dyspnea, inability to move secretions, irritability, decreased mental acuity, restlessness, somnolence, cyanosis
- neurologic status, including LOC, orientation, and mental status
- respiratory status, including respiratory rate and depth, symmetry of chest expansion, use of accessory muscles, cough, sputum, palpation for fremitus, percussion of lung fields, auscultation for breath sounds, ABG levels, pulmonary function studies
- cardiovascular status, including skin color and temperature, heart rate and rhythm, blood pressure, and complete blood count
- activity status, including such functional capabilities as ROM and muscle strength, ADLs, and occupation.

Documenting expected outcomes

Record appropriate expected outcomes on the plan of care. Possible outcomes include:

- Patient maintains respiratory rate within ± 5 of baseline.
- Patient expresses a feeling of comfort.
- Patient coughs effectively.
- Patient expectorates sputum.
- Patient maintains sufficient fluid intake to prevent dehydration: ____ml/24 hours.
- Patient performs ADLs to level of tolerance.
- Patient has normal breath sounds.
- Patient's ABG levels return to baseline: ____ pH; ____ Pao_2; ____ $Paco_2$.
- Patient performs relaxation techniques every 4 hours.
- Patient correctly uses breathing devices to improve gas exchange and increase oxygenation.

Documenting interventions

Chart interventions related to:

- patient's complaints of dyspnea, headache, or restlessness or expression of well-being
- observed physical findings (including vital signs, auscultation results, pulmonary status, cardiac rhythm)
- medication and oxygen administration (including times, dates, dosages, route, adverse effects, equipment and supplies) and patient's response
- patient positioning and repositioning and times; bronchial hygiene measures, such as coughing, percussion, postural drainage, suctioning
- intake and output measurements
- reportable signs of dehydration or fluid overload
- test results, including ABG levels
- endotracheal intubation and mechanical ventilation measures (including equipment and supplies used)
- patient teaching (including relaxation techniques and other measures to lower demand for oxygen)
- patient's ability to perform ADLs
- evaluation of expected outcomes

Hopelessness

related to failing or deteriorating physiologic condition

Definition

Subjective state in which an individual sees few or no available alternatives or personal choices and cannot mobilize energy on own behalf

Documenting assessment findings

Chart the defining characteristics as verbalized by the patient and your physical assessment findings, for example:

- defining characteristics: decreased appetite, initiative, and involvement in care (nonverbal cues include minimal eye contact, shrugging in response to questions, turning away from speaker; verbal cues include frequent sighing and negativity); increased sleep; decreased verbalization and affect
- nature of current medical diagnosis
- patient's and responsible caregiver's knowledge of diagnosis and prognosis
- actual or perceived self-care deficits (specify)
- mental status, including cognitive functioning, affect, and mood
- communication, including verbal (speech content, quality, quantity) and nonverbal (body positioning, eye contact, facial expression)
- available support systems, including clergy, family, and friends
- past experience with loss, including body part or function, death, residence, or employment
- history of depression, bipolar disease, or other psychiatric illness
- coping mechanisms and decision-making ability
- nutritional status, including alteration in appetite or body weight
- sleep pattern
- motivation level, including personal hygiene, therapies (physical and occupational therapy), and use of diversional activities
- developmental stage (Erikson's model), including age and role in family.

Documenting expected outcomes

Record appropriate expected outcomes on the plan of care. Possible outcomes include:

- Patient identifies feelings of hopelessness regarding current situation.
- Patient demonstrates more effective communication skills, including direct verbal responses to questions and increased eye contact.
- Patient resumes appropriate rest and activity pattern.
- Patient participates in self-care activities and in decisions regarding care planning.
- Patient participates in diversional activities (specify).
- Patient identifies social and community resources for continued assistance.

Documenting interventions

Chart interventions related to:

- patient's mental status
- patient's verbal and nonverbal communication
- patient's medical regimen
- increasing patient's feelings of hope and self-worth, and involvement in self-care and patient's response (including time spent communicating, talking, or sitting with patient)
- medication administration and comfort measures
- referrals to ancillary services, such as dietitian, social worker, clergy, mental health clinical nurse specialist, or support groups
- patient teaching (including diversional activities, self-care instruction, and discharge planning)
- patient's response to comfort measures
- evaluation of expected outcomes.

Incontinence, functional
related to sensory or mobility deficits

Definition
Involuntary and unpredictable passage of urine in socially unacceptable situations, in which patient usually does not recognize warning signs of bladder fullness

Documenting assessment findings
Chart the defining characteristics as verbalized by the patient and your physical assessment findings, for example:
- defining characteristics: nocturia, voiding that occurs before reaching an appropriate site or receptacle, failure to perceive bladder fullness
- history of mental retardation, trauma, alcohol abuse, and medication use
- age
- sex
- vital signs
- genitourinary status, including extent of clothing wetness from urine, frequency of incontinence, palpation of bladder, urine leakage when standing or sitting, voiding pattern
- fluid and electrolyte status, including intake and output, mucous membranes, skin turgor, urine specific gravity, and blood urea nitrogen, creatinine, and serum electrolyte levels
- neuromuscular status, including manual dexterity, mental status, mobility, motor ability to start and stop urine stream, rectal examination (muscle tone, prostate size, fecal impaction), and sensory ability to perceive bladder fullness
- psychosocial status, including behavior before and after voiding, coping skills, support from family or significant other, perception of health problem, self-concept, and stressors (finances, job, change in environment).

Documenting expected outcomes
Record appropriate expected outcomes on the plan of care. Possible outcomes include:
- Patient discusses impact of incontinence on self and others.
- Patient voids in appropriate situation using suitable receptacle.
- Patient voids at specific times.
- Patient has no wet episodes.
- Patient maintains fluid balance; intake equals output.
- Complications are avoided or minimized.
- Patient and family members demonstrate skill in managing incontinence.
- Patient and family members identify resources to assist with care following discharge.

Documenting interventions
Chart interventions related to:
- patient's expression of concern about incontinence and motivation to participate in self-care
- voiding pattern
- intake and output
- hydration status
- bladder elimination procedures (including bladder training, commode use times, toileting regimen, episodic wetness or dryness, use of external catheter, use of protective pads and garments)
- skin condition and care (including use of protective pads and garments)
- patient teaching (including toileting environment, time, and place; alcohol and fluid intake; techniques for stimulating void-

ing reflexes; techniques for reducing anxiety)
- patient's response to treatment regimen and patient teaching
- referrals to appropriate counselors and support groups
- family involvement in assisting patient with toileting
- evaluation of expected outcomes.

INFECTION, RISK FOR
related to external factors

Definition
Presence of internal or external hazards that threaten physical well-being

Documenting assessment findings
Chart assessment findings related to the following:
- health history, including accidents, allergies, falls, hyperthermia, hypothermia, poisoning, seizures, trauma, exposure to pollutants
- sensory or perceptual changes (auditory, gustatory, kinesthetic, olfactory, tactile, visual)
- circumstances of present situation that could lead to infection
- neurologic status, including LOC, mental status, and orientation
- laboratory studies, including clotting factors, hemoglobin and hematocrit, platelet count, serum albumin, white blood cell (WBC) count, and cultures of blood, body fluid, sputum, urine, and wounds.

Documenting expected outcomes
Record appropriate expected outcomes on the plan of care. Possible outcomes include:
- Temperature stays within normal range.
- WBC count and differential stay within normal range.
- No pathogens appear in cultures.
- Patient maintains good personal and oral hygiene.
- Respiratory secretions are clear and odorless.
- Urine remains clear yellow and odorless and exhibits no sediment.
- Patient shows no evidence of diarrhea.
- Wounds and incisions appear clean, pink, and free of purulent drainage.
- I.V. sites show no signs of inflammation.
- Patient shows no evidence of skin breakdown.
- Patient consumes ____ ml of fluid and ____ g of protein daily.
- Patient states infection risk factors.
- Patient identifies signs and symptoms of infection.
- Patient remains free of all signs and symptoms of infection.

Documenting interventions
Chart interventions related to:
- temperature readings (including dates and times and reporting of elevations)
- test procedures (including dates, times, and sites of obtained test specimens)
- test results (including WBC count and cultures of urine, blood, respiratory secretions, and wound drainage) and reporting of any abnormal results
- skin condition and wound care
- preventive measures (including personal hygiene, oral hygiene, airway suctioning, coughing, and deep-breathing measures)
- catheter management procedures (including dates and times of all catheter insertions, removals, and site care)

- equipment and supplies (including particulars of humidification or nebulization of oxygen)
- sanitary measures (for example, providing tissues and disposal bag for expectorated sputum)
- fluid intake
- nutritional intake
- isolation and other precautions
- patient teaching (including toileting and hygiene, hand-washing technique, factors that increase infection risk, and infection signs and symptoms)
- patient's response to nursing interventions
- episodes of loose stools or diarrhea
- evaluation of expected outcomes.

Injury, risk for

related to sensory or motor deficits

Definition

Accentuated risk of physical harm caused by sensory or motor deficits

Documenting assessment findings

Chart assessment findings related to the following:

- age
- nature of sensory or motor deficit
- health history, including cerebral function, mobility, sensory function, and use of adaptive devices
- psychological status, including substance abuse, familiarity with surroundings, mental status, coping skills, and self-concept
- medication use, including understanding of medications, compliance with prescribed regimen, use of over-the-counter medications, and interactions
- medication history
- knowledge, including understanding of safety precautions
- pain or fatigue
- laboratory studies, including complete blood count and differential, coagulation studies
- diagnostic tests, including chest and cranial X-rays
- sensory status, including hearing, vision, touch, and taste.

Documenting expected outcomes

Record appropriate expected outcomes on the plan of care. Possible outcomes include:

- Patient identifies factors that increase potential for injury.
- Patient assists in identifying and applying safety measures to prevent injury.
- Patient and family members develop strategy to maintain safety.
- Patient performs ADLs within sensorimotor limitations.

Documenting interventions

Chart interventions related to:

- observed factors that may cause or contribute to injury
- safety measures (side rails, positioning, use of call button and bed controls, orienting patient to environment, keeping bed in low position, and close night watch)
- statements by patient and family members about potential for injury due to sensory or motor deficits
- observed or reported unsafe practices
- interventions to decrease risk of injury to patient and patient's response
- patient teaching (including safe ways to improve visual discrimination, to decrease risk of burns from sensory loss, to use hearing aids and mobility assistive devices, and

to ensure household, automobile, and pedestrian safety)
- evaluation of expected outcomes.

Knowledge deficit
related to lack of exposure

Definition
Inadequate understanding of information or inability to perform skills needed to practice health-related behaviors

Documenting assessment findings
Chart the defining characteristics as verbalized by the patient and your physical assessment findings, for example:
- defining characteristics: needs information and lacks familiarity with information resources; inaccurate follow-through of instructions; inappropriate behaviors
- psychosocial status, including age, learning ability (affective, cognitive, and psychomotor domain), decision-making ability, developmental stage, financial resources, health beliefs and attitudes, interest in learning, knowledge and skill regarding current health problem, obstacles to learning, support systems (willingness and capability of others to help patient), usual coping pattern
- neurologic status, including LOC, memory, mental status, and orientation.

Documenting expected outcomes
Record appropriate expected outcomes on the plan of care. Possible outcomes include:
- Patient communicates a need to know.
- Patient states or demonstrates understanding of what has been taught.
- Patient demonstrates ability to perform new health-related behaviors as they are taught, and lists specific skills and realistic target dates for each.
- Patient sets realistic learning goals.
- Patient states intention to make needed changes in lifestyle, including seeking help from health care professionals when needed.

Documenting interventions
Chart interventions related to:
- patient's statements of known or unknown information and skills, expressions of need to know, and motivation to learn
- patient teaching (including learning objectives, teaching methods used, information imparted, skills demonstrated) and patient's responses
- referrals to resource people or organizations that can continue instructional activities after discharge
- evaluation of expected outcomes.

Mobility impairment
related to pain or discomfort

Definition
Limitation of physical movement

Documenting assessment findings
Chart the defining characteristics as verbalized by the patient and your physical assessment findings, for example:
- defining characteristics: pain related to movement; decreased muscle strength, control, mass, or endurance; impaired coordination; imposed restriction of movement, including mechanical and medical protocol; inability to move purposefully within the environment (including bed mobility, transfer, and ambulation); limited ROM; reluctance to attempt movement

- patient's verbal and nonverbal expressions of pain and discomfort
- characteristics of pain, including environmental and cultural influences, intensity, location, quality, and temporal factors
- history of recent surgery, injury, or disorder causing pain or discomfort
- medication history
- musculoskeletal status, including coordination, gait, muscle size and strength, muscle tone, ROM, and functional mobility as follows:
  - 0 = completely independent
  - 1 = requires use of equipment or device
  - 2 = requires help, supervision, or teaching from another person
  - 3 = requires help from another person and equipment or device
  - 4 = dependent; does not participate in activity
- psychosocial status, including coping mechanisms, lifestyle, personality, stressors (disease process, finances, job, marital discord), and support from family members.

Documenting expected outcomes

Record appropriate expected outcomes on the plan of care. Possible outcomes include:

- Patient states relief from pain.
- Patient displays increased mobility.
- Patient shows no evidence of complications, such as contractures, venous stasis, thrombus formation, or skin breakdown.
- Patient attains highest degree of mobility possible within confines of disease.
- Patient or family member demonstrates mobility regimen.
- Patient states feelings about limitations.

Documenting interventions

Chart interventions related to:

- patient's observed daily functional ability and changes (use functional mobility scale)
- patient's expressed feelings and concerns about immobility and its impact on his lifestyle, and his willingness to participate in care
- observed impairments and pain
- prescribed treatment regimen for underlying condition and patient's response to treatment and nursing interventions
- medication administration and other supportive measures (including padding extremities to prevent skin breakdown and ensuring correct height of crutches)
- prescribed ROM exercises
- patient repositioning (include times)
- progressive mobilization up to limits of patient's tolerance for pain (bed to chair to ambulation)
- patient and family teaching (including instructions for using crutches and walkers; practicing techniques to control pain, such as distraction and imaging; understanding need for mobility despite pain; performing ROM exercises, transfers, skin inspection, and mobility regimen) and patient's response
- referrals to counselor, support group, or social service agency
- evaluation of expected outcomes.

Noncompliance

related to patient's value system

Definition

Unwillingness to practice prescribed health-related behaviors

APPENDICES

Documenting assessment findings

Chart the defining characteristics as verbalized by the patient and your physical assessment findings, for example:

- defining characteristics: reported or observed challenge to beliefs and value systems, complications, exacerbation of symptoms, failure to keep appointments, failure to progress, inability to set or attain mutual goals, failure to adhere to the treatment regimen
- age
- health beliefs
- patient's perceptions of health problem, treatment regimen, and importance of complying with treatment regimen
- patient's ability to learn and perform prescribed treatments (activity, diet, medications)
- financial resources
- cultural and ethnic influences
- religious influences
- educational and language background.

Documenting expected outcomes

Record appropriate expected outcomes on the plan of care. Possible outcomes include:

- Patient identifies factors that influence noncompliance.
- Patient contracts with nurse to perform ____ (specify behavior and frequency).
- Patient uses support systems to modify noncompliant behavior.
- Patient demonstrates a level of compliance that does not interfere with physiologic safety.

Documenting interventions

Chart interventions related to:

- patient's stated reasons for noncompliance
- observed specific noncompliant behaviors
- promoting compliance (including negotiations and terms agreed upon with patient as well as positive reinforcements provided) and patient's response
- daily progress in complying with treatment regimen
- referrals to counselors or support groups
- evaluation of expected outcomes.

NUTRITION ALTERATION: LESS THAN BODY REQUIREMENTS

related to inability to digest or absorb nutrients because of biological factors

Definition

Change in normal eating pattern that results in changed body weight

Documenting assessment findings

Chart the defining characteristics as verbalized by the patient and your physical assessment findings, for example:

- defining characteristics: abdominal pain, diarrhea or steatorrhea, halitosis, coated tongue, hyperactive bowel sounds, reported weight loss despite adequate caloric intake or reported inadequate caloric intake, digestive problems, changes in bowel habits, pressure ulcers, pale conjunctivae or mucous membranes, weakness of muscles required for chewing or swallowing
- GI assessment, including antibiotic therapy, stool characteristics (color, amount, size, consistency), pain or discomfort, nausea and vomiting, usual bowel pattern, history of GI disorder or surgery, inspection and palpation of abdomen, auscultation for bowel sounds, palpation for masses and tenderness, and percussion for tympany and dullness

- nutritional status related to change in type of food tolerated, financial resources, height and weight, meal preparation, serum albumin level, sociocultural influences, usual dietary pattern, weight fluctuations over past 10 years
- intrapersonal or interpersonal factors, including internal or external cues that trigger desire to eat, rate of food consumption, and stated food preferences
- psychosocial status
- activity level
- coping behaviors
- body image as determined by perception of observer and self-perception.

Documenting expected outcomes

Record appropriate expected outcomes on the plan of care. Possible outcomes include:

- Patient tolerates oral, tube, or I.V. feedings without adverse effects.
- Patient takes in ____ calories daily.
- Patient gains ____ lb weekly.
- Patient shows no further evidence of weight loss.
- Patient and family or significant other communicate understanding of special dietary needs.
- Patient and family or significant other demonstrate ability to plan diet after discharge.

Documenting interventions

Chart interventions related to:

- daily weight
- daily fluid intake and output measurements (include volume and characteristics of any vomitus and stools—a clue to nutrient absorption)
- parenteral fluid administration
- daily food intake from prescribed diet
- electrolyte levels
- consultations with dietary department or nutritional support team
- any abnormal findings.

If the patient receives tube feedings, document interventions related to:

- concentration and delivery of regular feeding formula or one containing food-coloring additives (especially in patient with altered LOC or diminished gag reflex)
- use of supportive equipment, such as an infusion pump
- degree of elevation of head of bed during feeding
- feeding tube placement.

If the patient receives total parenteral nutrition, document interventions related to:

- monitored blood glucose levels and urine specific gravity (at least once each shift)
- monitored bowel sounds (once each shift)
- oral hygiene
- patient teaching (including the reasons for the current treatment regimen, principles of nutrition suited to the patient's specific condition, meal planning, and preoperative instructions if applicable)
- evaluation of expected outcomes.

Pain

related to physical, biological, or chemical agents

Definition

An unpleasant sensory and emotional experience arising from actual or potential tissue damage or described in terms of such damage

Documenting assessment findings

Chart the defining characteristics as verbalized by the patient and your physical assessment findings, for example:

- defining characteristics: changes in muscle tone (may range from listless to rigid), diaphoresis, increased or decreased respiratory rate, stated pain and description, preoccupation with discomfort (self-focusing)
- descriptive characteristics of pain, including location, quality, intensity on a scale of 1 to 10, temporal factors, and sources of relief
- physiologic variables, such as age and pain tolerance
- psychological variables, such as body image, personality, previous experience with pain, anxiety, and possible secondary gain
- sociocultural variables, including culture or ethnicity, attitude, values, cognitive style, sex, and birth order
- environmental variables, such as the setting and time.

Documenting expected outcomes

Record appropriate expected outcomes on the plan of care. Possible outcomes include:

- Patient identifies pain characteristics.
- Patient articulates factors that intensify pain and modifies behavior accordingly.
- Patient states and carries out appropriate interventions for pain relief.
- Patient expresses a feeling of comfort and relief from pain.

Documenting interventions

Chart interventions related to:

- patient's description of physical pain, pain relief, and feelings about pain
- observed physical, psychological, and sociocultural responses to pain
- prescribed medication administration (including times, dates, dosages, routes, adverse effects) and comfort measures (such as massage, relaxation techniques, heat and cold applications, repositioning, distraction, and bathing)
- patient's response to nursing interventions
- patient teaching (about pain and pain-relief strategies) and patient's response
- evaluation of expected outcomes.

SKIN INTEGRITY IMPAIRMENT, RISK FOR

Definition

Presence of risk factors for interruption or destruction of skin surface

Documenting assessment findings

Chart assessment findings related to the following:

- history of skin problems, trauma, chronic debilitating disease, or immobility
- age
- integumentary status, including color, elasticity, hygiene, lesions, moisture, sensation, quantity and distribution of hair, temperature and blood pressure, texture, and turgor
- musculoskeletal status, including anesthetic area, muscle strength and mass, joint mobility, paralysis, and ROM
- nutritional status, including appetite, dietary intake, hydration, present weight, and change from normal weight
- hemoglobin and hematocrit values
- serum albumin levels
- psychosocial status, including ADLs, mental status, occupation (involving sun exposure), and recreational activities.

Documenting expected outcomes

Record appropriate expected outcomes on the plan of care. Possible outcomes include:

- Patient maintains muscle strength and joint ROM.
- Patient sustains adequate food and fluid intake.
- Patient maintains adequate skin circulation.
- Patient communicates understanding of preventive skin care measures.
- Patient and family demonstrate preventive skin care measures.
- Patient and family correlate risk factors and preventive measures.
- Patient experiences no skin breakdown.

Documenting interventions

Chart interventions related to:

- skin condition and any changes
- repositioning patient as scheduled and ordered (including dates and times)
- ambulation or active ROM exercises to improve circulation and mobility (including dates and times)
- use of skin care devices and supplies (such as foam mattress, sheepskin, alternating pressure mattress, lotions and powders) and effectiveness of interventions
- nutritional intake
- hydration status
- weekly risk factor potential and score (use the Braden Scale)
- patient teaching (including the need to implement preventive measures to promote skin integrity, good personal hygiene habits, signs of skin breakdown, patient and responsible caregiver's demonstrated skill in carrying out preventive skin care measures) and patient's response
- evaluation of expected outcomes.

SLEEP PATTERN DISTURBANCE

related to internal factors, such as illness, psychological stress, drug therapy, or biorhythm disturbance

Definition

Inability to meet individual need for sleep or rest arising from internal or external factors

Documenting assessment findings

Chart the defining characteristics as verbalized by the patient and your physical assessment findings, for example:

- defining characteristics: waking up earlier or later than desired, difficulty falling asleep, interrupted sleep, not feeling well rested, disorientation, irritability, lethargy, listlessness, restlessness, dark circles under eyes, expressionless face, frequent yawning, fleeting nystagmus, ptosis of eyelids, hand tremor, speech problems
- age
- daytime activity and work patterns
- time the patient usually retires
- number of hours of sleep patient usually requires in order to feel rested
- problems associated with sleep, including early-morning awakening, falling asleep, staying asleep, nightmares, or sleepwalking
- quality of sleep
- sleeping environment
- activities associated with sleep, including bath, drink, food, or medication
- personal beliefs about sleep.

Documenting expected outcomes

Record appropriate expected outcomes on the plan of care. Possible outcomes include:

- Patient identifies factors that prevent or disrupt sleep.

- Patient performs relaxation exercises at bedtime.
- Patient sleeps ____ hours a night.
- Patient reports feeling well rested.
- Patient shows no physical signs of sleep deprivation.
- Patient exhibits no sleep-related behavioral symptoms, such as restlessness, irritability, lethargy, or disorientation.

Documenting interventions

Chart interventions related to:

- patient's complaints about sleep disturbances
- patient's report of improvement in sleep patterns
- observed physical and behavioral sleep-related disturbances
- interventions used to alleviate sleep disturbances (such as pillows, bath, food or drink, reading material, TV, soft music, quiet environment) and patient's response
- prescribed medication and patient's response
- patient teaching (including reason for treatment, relationship of regular exercise and sleep, and relaxation techniques, such as imagery, progressive muscle relaxation, and meditation)
- evaluation of expected outcomes.

Swallowing impairment

related to neuromuscular impairment

Definition

Inability to move food, fluid, or saliva from the mouth through the esophagus

Documenting assessment findings

Chart the defining characteristics as verbalized by the patient and your physical assessment findings, for example:

- defining characteristics: choking (aspiration) spells, difficulty in swallowing, coughing, stasis of food in oral cavity
- history of neuromuscular, cerebral, or respiratory disease
- age
- sex
- nutritional status, including appetite, dietary intake, hydration, current weight, and change from normal weight
- neurologic status, including cognition; gag reflex; LOC; memory; motor ability; orientation; symmetry of face, mouth, and neck; sensory function; and tongue movement
- diagnostic tests, including barium swallow, chest X-ray, and fluoroscopy.

Documenting expected outcomes

Record appropriate expected outcomes on the plan of care. Possible outcomes include:

- Patient shows no evidence of aspiration pneumonia.
- Patient achieves adequate nutritional intake.
- Patient maintains weight.
- Patient maintains oral hygiene.
- Patient and responsible caregiver demonstrate correct eating or feeding techniques to maximize swallowing.

Documenting interventions

Chart interventions related to:

- patient's expressed feelings about current condition
- observed and reported swallowing impairment, as evidenced by cyanosis, dyspnea, or choking

- nursing interventions and patient's response (include times of turning and repositioning and degree of elevation of head during mealtimes and for 30 minutes after)
- respiratory assessments and airway suctioning (including dates and times, instances of cyanosis, dyspnea, or choking)
- daily intake and output and weight measurements
- referrals to dietitian and other health services such as dysphagia rehabilitation team
- oral hygiene and comfort measures
- patient teaching (about positioning, dietary requirements, oral hygiene, and stimuli and feeding techniques to improve mastication, promote swallowing, and decrease aspiration)
- evaluation of expected outcomes.

Tissue perfusion alteration (cardiopulmonary)

related to decreased cellular exchange

Definition

Decrease in cellular nutrition and respiration due to decreased capillary blood flow

Documenting assessment findings

Chart the defining characteristics as verbalized by the patient and your physical assessment findings, for example:

- defining characteristics: chest pain with or without activity, cold and clammy skin, chest congestion, urination difficulties (decreased or absent), fatigue, palpitations, peripheral edema, shortness of breath, cyanosis, pallor of skin and mucous membranes
- health history, including presence of diabetes mellitus, high cholesterol, hypertension, obesity, smoking, stressful lifestyle, or family history of heart disease
- neurologic status, including LOC, mental status, and orientation
- cardiovascular status, including blood pressure; heart rate and rhythm; heart sounds; peripheral pulses; capillary refill; skin color, temperature, and turgor; hepatojugular reflux; jugular vein distention; and history of congenital heart disease or valvular disorder
- diagnostic tests, including chest X-ray, ECG, exercise ECG, echocardiogram, nuclear isotope studies, and cardiac angiography
- respiratory status, including respiratory rate and depth, ABG levels, and breath sounds
- renal status, including intake and output, urine specific gravity, and weight
- integumentary system, including cyanosis, pallor, and peripheral edema.

Documenting expected outcomes

Record appropriate expected outcomes on the plan of care. Possible outcomes include:

- Patient attains hemodynamic stability: pulse not less than ____ and not greater than ____ beats/minute; blood pressure not less than ____ and not greater than ____ mm Hg.
- Patient does not exhibit arrhythmias.
- Skin remains warm and dry.
- Patient's heart rate remains within prescribed limits while he carries out ADLs.
- Patient maintains adequate cardiac output.
- Patient modifies lifestyle to minimize risk of decreased tissue perfusion.

Documenting interventions

Chart interventions related to:

- patient's perception of health problems and health needs
- observed physical findings (including heart rate, blood pressure, central venous pressure, pulse rate, temperature, skin color, respiratory rate, and breath sounds)
- observed response to activity
- test procedures (including ECG to monitor heart rate and rhythm and results of creatine kinase, lactate dehydrogenase, and ABG analysis)
- prescribed medication administration and oxygen therapy (including dates, times, dosages, routes, adverse effects, equipment, and supplies)
- patient positioning and repositioning to enhance vital capacity and to avoid lung congestion and skin breakdown
- patient teaching (about need for low-fat, low-cholesterol diet; nitroglycerin or other medications, including possible adverse effects; activity level; stress management; risk factors for heart and lung disease; need to avoid straining with bowel movements; and benefits of quitting smoking)
- evaluation of expected outcomes.

URINARY ELIMINATION PATTERN ALTERATION

related to sensory or neuromuscular impairment

Definition

Alteration or impairment of urinary function

Documenting assessment findings

Chart the defining characteristics as verbalized by the patient and your physical assessment findings, for example:

- defining characteristics: reported dysuria, frequency, hesitancy, incontinence, nocturia, retention, or urgency
- history of urinary tract disease, trauma, surgery, or infection
- history of sensory or neuromuscular impairment
- vital signs
- genitourinary status, including characteristics of urine, cystometry, pain or discomfort, palpation of bladder, postcatheterization problems, presence and amount of residual urine, use of urinary assistive devices, urinalysis, and voiding pattern
- fluid and electrolyte status, including inspection of mucous membranes, intake and output, skin turgor, urine specific gravity, and blood urea nitrogen, creatinine, and serum electrolyte levels
- neuromuscular status, including degree of neuromuscular function present, motor ability to start and stop urinary stream, and sensory ability to perceive bladder fullness
- sexuality status, including capability, concerns, habits, and sexual partner
- psychosocial status, including coping skills, family or significant other, patient's perception of health problem, self-concept, and stressors (finances, job).

Documenting expected outcomes

Record appropriate expected outcomes on the plan of care. Possible outcomes include:

- Patient discusses impact of urologic disorder on self and others.
- Patient maintains fluid balance: Intake equals output.
- Patient voices increased comfort.
- Complications are avoided or minimized.

- Patient and family members demonstrate skill in managing urinary elimination problem.
- Patient and family members identify resources to assist with care after discharge.

Documenting interventions

Chart interventions related to:

- observed neuromuscular status
- observed voiding pattern
- patient's expression of concern about the urologic problem and its impact on body image and lifestyle
- patient's motivation to participate in self-care
- intake and output and fluid replacement therapy
- medication administration
- bladder training (including times and dates of commode use, Kegel exercises to strengthen sphincter)
- intermittent catheterization (record dates, times, volume eliminated spontaneously, volume eliminated via catheter, bladder balance)
- external catheterization of male patient (including time and date of condom catheter application and changes, supplies used, skin condition of penis, and hygiene)
- indwelling urinary catheterization (including time and date of catheter insertion and changes, condition and care of urinary meatus, type of drainage system used, and volume drained)
- suprapubic catheterization (including time and date of catheter insertion and changes, dressing changes, type of drainage system used, and supplies used)
- supportive care measures (including pain control and hydration, prompt response to call light, and bed in close proximity to bathroom), their effectiveness, and patient's response
- patient teaching (including signs and symptoms of full bladder, home catheterization techniques and management, signs and symptoms of autonomic dysreflexia, management of autonomic dysreflexia, and emergency measures)
- referrals of patient and family members to counselors and support groups
- evaluation of expected outcomes.

VERBAL COMMUNICATION IMPAIRMENT

related to decreased circulation to brain

Definition

Decreased ability to speak, understand, or use words appropriately

Documenting assessment findings

Chart the defining characteristics as verbalized by the patient and your physical assessment findings, for example:

- defining characteristics: reported or observed disorientation; dyspnea; impaired articulation; reported inability or lack of desire to speak, to identify objects, to modulate speech, to name words, or to speak in sentences; incessant verbalization, phonation difficulties, stuttering or slurring; perseveration, loss of association of ideas, flight of ideas
- neurologic status, including LOC, orientation, cognition, memory (recent and remote), insight, and judgment
- speech characteristics, including pattern (garbled, incomprehensible, difficulty forming words), language and vocabulary, level of comprehension and expression,

and ability to use other forms of communication (eye blinks, gestures, pictures, nods)
- motor ability
- circulatory status, including pulse rate, blood pressure, and a history of cardiac and circulatory problems
- respiratory status, including dyspnea and use of accessory muscles.

Documenting expected outcomes

Record appropriate expected outcomes on the plan of care. Possible outcomes include:
- Staff consistently meets patient's needs.
- Patient maintains orientation.
- Patient maintains effective level of communication.
- Patient answers direct questions correctly.

Documenting interventions

Chart interventions related to:
- patient's current level of communication, orientation, and satisfaction with communication efforts
- changes in speech pattern or level of orientation
- observed speech deficits, expressiveness and receptiveness, and ability to communicate
- diagnostic test results
- supplies or equipment used to promote orientation (TV, radio, calendars, reality orientation boards)
- promoting effective communication and patient's response
- evaluation of expected outcomes.

APPENDIX C

ANA Standards of Nursing Practice

In 1991, the American Nurses Association (ANA) developed standards of clinical nursing practice that provide guidelines for determining quality nursing care. In updating previous standards, the ANA addressed not only care but also performance standards and established measurement criteria for evaluating whether a nurse's activities meet those standards.

Standards of care

Nursing care standards are based on the steps of the nursing process — assessment, nursing diagnosis, outcome identification, planning, implementation, and evaluation.

Standard I: Assessment

The nurse collects health data about the client. Measurement criteria are as follows:

- The nurse bases data collection priorities on the client's immediate health condition and needs.
- The nurse uses appropriate assessment techniques in collecting data.
- Data collection involves the client, significant others, and health care providers when appropriate.
- The data collection process is systematic and ongoing.
- Relevant data are documented in a retrievable form.

Standard II: Nursing diagnosis

The nurse analyzes the assessment data in determining diagnoses. Measurement criteria are as follows:

- Diagnoses are derived from the assessment data.
- Diagnoses are validated with the client, significant others, and health care providers when possible.
- Diagnoses are documented in a manner that facilitates the determination of expected outcomes and plan of care.

Standard III: Outcome identification

The nurse identifies expected outcomes individualized to the client. Measurement criteria are as follows:

- Outcomes are derived from the diagnoses.
- Outcomes are documented as measurable goals.
- Outcomes are mutually formulated with the client and health care providers when possible.
- Outcomes are realistic and related to the client's present and potential capabilities.
- Outcomes are attainable in relation to resources available to the client.

- Outcomes include a time estimate for attainment.
- Outcomes provide direction for continuity of care.

Standard IV: Planning

The nurse develops a plan of care that prescribes interventions to attain expected outcomes. Measurement criteria are as follows:

- The plan of care is individualized to the client's condition or needs.
- The plan of care is developed with the client, significant others, and health care providers when appropriate.
- The plan of care reflects current nursing practice.
- The plan of care is documented.
- The plan of care provides for continuity of care.

Standard V: Implementation

The nurse implements the interventions identified in the plan of care. Measurement criteria are as follows:

- Interventions are consistent with the established plan of care.
- Interventions are implemented in a safe and appropriate manner.
- Interventions are documented.

Standard VI: Evaluation

The nurse evaluates the client's progress toward attainment of outcomes. Measurement criteria are as follows:

- Evaluation is systematic and ongoing.
- The client's responses to interventions are documented.
- The effectiveness of interventions is evaluated in relation to outcomes.
- Ongoing assessment data are used to revise diagnoses, outcomes, and the plan of care as needed.
- Revisions in diagnoses, outcomes, and the plan of care are documented.
- The client, significant others, and health care providers are involved in the evaluation process when appropriate.

Standards of Professional Performance

Nursing performance standards include guidelines for quality of care, performance appraisal, education, collegiality, ethics, collaboration, research, and resource utilization.

Standard I: Quality of care

The nurse systematically evaluates the quality and effectiveness of nursing practice. Measurement criteria are as follows:

- The nurse participates in quality-of-care activities, as appropriate to the individual's position, education, and practice environment. Such activities may include:
  - identification of aspects of care important for quality monitoring
  - identification of indicators used to monitor quality and effectiveness of nursing care
  - collection of data to monitor quality and effectiveness of nursing care
  - analysis of quality data to identify opportunities for improving care
  - formulation of recommendations to improve nursing practice or client outcomes
  - implementation of activities to enhance the quality of nursing practice

- participation on interdisciplinary teams that evaluate clinical practice or health services
- development of policies and procedures to improve quality of care.

■ The nurse uses the results of quality-of-care activities to initiate changes in practice.

■ The nurse uses the results of quality-of-care activities to initiate changes throughout the health care delivery system as appropriate.

Standard II: Performance appraisal

The nurse evaluates nursing practice in relation to professional practice standards and relevant statutes and regulations. Measurement criteria are as follows:

■ The nurse engages in performance appraisal on a regular basis, identifying areas of strength as well as areas for professional and practice development.

■ The nurse seeks constructive feedback regarding practice.

■ The nurse takes action to achieve goals identified during performance appraisal.

■ The nurse participates in peer review as appropriate.

Standard III: Education

The nurse acquires and maintains current knowledge in nursing practice. Measurement criteria are as follows:

■ The nurse participates in ongoing educational activities related to clinical knowledge and professional issues.

■ The nurse seeks experiences to maintain clinical skills.

■ The nurse seeks knowledge and skills appropriate to the practice setting.

Standard IV: Collegiality

The nurse contributes to the professional development of peers, colleagues, and others. Measurement criteria are as follows:

■ The nurse shares knowledge and skills with colleagues and others.

■ The nurse provides peers with constructive feedback regarding their practice.

■ The nurse contributes to an environment that is conducive to clinical education of nursing students as appropriate.

Standard V: Ethics

The nurse's decisions and actions on behalf of clients are determined in an ethical manner. Measurement criteria are as follows:

■ The nurse's practice is guided by the standard nurses' code.

■ The nurse maintains client confidentiality.

■ The nurse acts as a client advocate.

■ The nurse delivers care in a nonjudgmental and nondiscriminatory manner that is sensitive to client diversity and that preserves and protects the client's autonomy, dignity, and rights.

■ The nurse seeks available resources to help formulate ethical decisions.

Standard VI: Collaboration

The nurse collaborates with the client, significant others, and health care providers in providing client care. Measurement criteria are as follows:

■ The nurse communicates with the client, significant others, and health care providers regarding client care and nursing's role in the provision of care.

■ The nurse consults with health care providers for client care as needed.

■ The nurse makes referrals, including provisions for continuity of care, as needed.

Standard VII: Research

The nurse uses research findings in practice. Measurement criteria are as follows:

- The nurse uses interventions substantiated by research as appropriate to the individual's position, education, and practice environment.
- The nurse participates in research activities as appropriate to the individual's position, education, and practice environment. Such activities may include:
  - identification of clinical problems suitable for nursing research
  - participation in data collection
  - participation in a unit, organization, or community research committee or program
  - sharing of research activities with others
  - conducting research
  - critiquing research for application to practice
  - using research findings in the development of policies, procedures, and guidelines for client care.

Standard VIII: Resource utilization

The nurse considers factors related to safety, effectiveness, and cost in planning and delivering client care. Measurement criteria are as follows:

- The nurse evaluates factors related to safety, effectiveness, and cost when two or more practice options would result in the same expected client outcome.
- The nurse assigns tasks or delegates care based on the needs of the client and the knowledge and skill of the provider selected.
- The nurse assists the client and significant others in identifying and securing appropriate services available to address health-related needs.

APPENDIX D

JCAHO Nursing Care and Documentation Standards

The 1998 standards for accreditation of hospitals developed by the Joint Commission on Accreditation of Healthcare Organizations (JCAHO) include identification of goals, functions, and standards for provision of patient care. In contrast to previous years, the new guidelines place greater emphasis on integration of services from a variety of providers so that goals, functions, and standards reflect the combined responsibilities of those providing patient care. The standards are written to address patient needs, rather than identifying discrete responsibilities of separate providers.

In addition, the standards stress the value of continuous, rather than episodic, accreditation so that ongoing data collection, assessment, intervention, and evaluation can be performed. The Orion Project, an initiative to develop a continuous accreditation process on a regional level is being tested in Pennsylvania, Arizona, Tennessee, and Georgia. The outcome of this pilot program may provide additional options for how accreditation of health care organizations is conducted.

The selected standards that follow address assessment of patients, care of patients, leadership, management of human resources, and nursing.

Assessment of patients

The standards associated with this function clearly show the new focus on performance-improvement processes, and address the hospital's responsibility to collect data about each patient's physical and psychosocial status and health history, to analyze that data, and to make patient care decisions based on this information.

- Each patient's physical, psychological, and social status is assessed.
- Nutritional status is assessed when warranted by the patient's needs or condition.
- Functional status is assessed when warranted by the patient's needs or condition.
- Diagnostic testing necessary for determining the patient's health care needs is performed.
- The need for discharge planning assessment is determined.
- Each admitted patient's initial assessment is conducted within a time frame specified by hospital policy.
- Before surgery, the patient's physical examination and medical history, any indicated diagnostic tests, and a preoperative diagnosis are completed and recorded in the patient's medical record.
- Possible victims of abuse are identified using criteria developed by the hospital.

APPENDICES

- Pathology and clinical laboratory services and consultation are readily available to meet patients' needs.
- Each patient is reassessed at points designated in hospital policy.
- Staff members integrate the information from various assessments of the patient to identify and assign priorities to his care needs.
- The hospital has defined patient assessment activities in writing.
- A registered nurse assesses the patient's need for nursing care in all settings where nursing care is provided.
- The assessment process for an infant, child, or adolescent patient is individualized.
- The special needs of patients who are receiving treatment for emotional or behavioral disorders are addressed by the assessment process.
- The special needs of patients who are receiving treatment for alcoholism or other drug dependencies are addressed by the assessment process.

Care of patients

The selected standards that follow apply to all disciplines providing care to patients, and are to be applied collaboratively to ensure integration and continuity of care. The responsibilities of individual providers are determined by their professional credentials, licensure, and scope of practice; the type of care being provided; the experience level of the individual provider; and hospital policies and job descriptions.

- Care, treatment, and rehabilitation are planned to ensure that they are appropriate to the patient's needs and severity of disease, condition, impairment, or disability.
- Care is planned and provided in an interdisciplinary, collaborative manner by qualified individuals.
- Patient care procedures (such as bathing) are performed in a manner that respects privacy.
- Patients' progress is periodically evaluated against care goals and the plan of care and, when indicated, the plan or goals are revised.
- Medication use processes are organized and systematic throughout the hospital.
- Each patient's nutrition care is planned.

Leadership

The selected leadership standards that follow clearly show the new focus on patient care and the integration of services. JCAHO specifies that leadership should be inclusive, not exclusive; should encourage staff participation in shaping the hospital's vision and values; should develop leaders at every level who help to fulfill the hospital's mission, vision, and values; should accurately assess the needs of patients and other users of the hospital's services; and should develop an organizational culture that focuses on continuously improving performance to meet these needs.

- The leaders provide for hospital planning.
- Each hospital department has effective leadership.
- Patient care services are integrated throughout the hospital.
- The hospital's leaders set expectations, develop plans, and manage processes to measure, assess, and improve the quality of the hospital's governance, management, and clinical and support activities.

- All leaders participate in interdisciplinary, interdepartmental performance-improvement activities.
- The leaders allocate adequate resources for measuring, assessing, and improving the hospital's performance.

Management of Human Resources

The goal of the management of human resources function is to identify and provide the right number of competent staff members to meet the needs of patients; adequate staffing is the responsibility of all hospital leaders, not solely of the human resources department. Hospital leaders are responsible for considering the hospital's mission, the case mix of patients including degree and complexity of care, technology used in patient care, and the expectations of patients, hospital, and other customers in identifying how patient care will be delivered.

- The hospital's leaders define the qualifications and performance expectations for all staff positions.
- The hospital provides an adequate number of staff members whose qualifications are consistent with job responsibilities.
- The leaders ensure that the competence of all staff members is assessed, maintained, demonstrated, and improved continually.
- An orientation process provides initial job training and information and assesses the staff's ability to fulfill specified responsibilities.
- Ongoing in-service (and other) education and training maintain and improve staff competence.
- The hospital assesses each staff member's ability to meet the performance expectations stated in his job description.
- The hospital addresses a staff member's request not to participate in any aspect of patient care.

Nursing

Standards related to the nurse-executive position focus on responsibilities. Qualifications for the position are outlined in the intent statements and include education at the master's level or equivalent. The nurse-executive, registered nurses, and other designated nursing staff members write nursing policies and procedures, nursing standards of patient care, standards of nursing practice, and standards to measure, assess, and improve patient outcomes.

- Nursing services are directed by a nurse-executive who is a registered nurse qualified by advanced education and management experience.
- The nurse-executive has the authority and responsibility for establishing standards of nursing practice.
- Nursing policies and procedures, nursing standards of patient care, and standards of nursing practice are approved by the nurse-executive or a designee.
- The nurse-executive and other nursing leaders participate with leaders from the governing body, management, medical staff, and clinical areas in planning, promoting, and conducting organization-wide performance-improvement activities.

APPENDIX E

Nursing Organizations

Academy of Medical-Surgical Nurses
East Holly Avenue, Box 56
Pitman, NJ 08071-0056
(609) 256-2323
http://www.amsn.inurse.com

Alabama State Nurses Association
360 N. Hull Street
Montgomery, AL 36104-3658
(334) 262-8321

Alaska Nurses Association
237 E. 3rd Avenue #3
Anchorage, AK 99501
(907) 274-0827

American Association of Critical-Care Nurses*
101 Columbia
Aliso Viejo, CA 92656-1491
(800) 899-2226
http://www.aacn.org

American Association of Neuroscience Nurses*
224 N. Des Plaines
Chicago, IL 60661
(312) 993-0043
http://www.aann.org

American Association of Nurse Anesthetists*
222 S. Prospect Avenue
Park Ridge, IL 60068-4001
(708) 692-7050
http://www.aana.com

American Association of Occupational Health Nurses*
2920 Brandywine Road, Suite 100
Atlanta, GA 30341
(770) 455-7757

American Association of Spinal Cord Injury Nurses
7520 Astoria Boulevard
Jackson Heights, NY 11370-1177
(718) 803-3782

American College of Nurse-Midwives*
818 Connecticut Ave., NW, Suite 900
Washington, DC 20006
(202) 728-9860
http://www.midwife.org

American Nurses Association
600 Maryland Avenue, SW, Suite 100 West
Washington, DC 20024-2571
(202) 554-4444
http://www.nursingworld.org

**Certification program available*

American Radiological Nurses Association
2021 Spring Road, Suite 600
Oak Brook, IL 60523
(708) 571-9072

American Society of Post Anesthesia Nurses*
6900 Grove Road
Thorofare, NJ 08086
(609) 845-5557

Arizona Nurses Association
1850 E. Southern Avenue, Suite 1
Tempe, AZ 85282
(602) 831-0404

Arkansas Nurses Association
804 N. University
Little Rock, AR 72205-2920
(501) 664-5853

Association of Operating Room Nurses*
2170 S. Parker Road, Suite 300
Denver, CO 80231-5711
(303) 755-6300
http://www.aorn.org

Association of Women's Health, Obstetric, and Neonatal Nurses
2000 L Street, NW
Washington, DC 20005
(202) 261-2400

Colorado Nurses Association
5453 E. Evans Place
Denver, CO 80222
(303) 757-7483
http://www.nurses-co.drg/cna

Connecticut Nurses Association
377 Research Parkway, Suite 2D
Meriden, CT 06450
(203) 238-1207
http://www.nursingworld.org/snas/CT

Delaware Nurses Association
2644 Capitol Trail, Suite 330
Newark, DE 19711
(302) 368-2333

District of Columbia Nurses Association
5100 Wisconsin Avenue, NW, Suite 306
Washington, DC 20016
(202) 244-2705

Emergency Nurses Association
216 Higgins Road West
Park Ridge, IL 60068
(708) 698-9400

Florida Nurses Association
P.O. Box 536985
Orlando, FL 32853-6985
(407) 896-3261
http://www.floridanurse.org

Georgia Nurses Association
1362 W. Peachtree Street, NW
Atlanta, GA 30309
(404) 876-4624

Hawaii Nurses Association
677 Ala Moana Boulevard, Suite 301
Honolulu, HI 96813
(808) 531-1628
http://www.hawaiinurses.org

**Certification program available*

Idaho Nurses Association
200 N. 4th Street, Suite 20
Boise, ID 83702-6001
(208) 345-0500

Illinois Nurses Association
300 S. Wacker Drive, Suite 2200
Chicago, IL 60606
(312) 360-2300
http://www.nursingworld.org/snas/IL

Indiana State Nurses Association
2915 N. High School Road
Indianapolis, IN 46224
(317) 299-4575

Intravenous Nurses Society, Inc.*
Fresh Pond Square
10 Fawcett Street
Cambridge, MA 02138
(617) 441-3008

Iowa Nurses Association
1501 42nd Street, Suite 471
West Des Moines, IA 50266
(515) 225-0495
http://www.Iowanurses.org

Kansas State Nurses Association
700 S.W. Jackson, Suite 601
Topeka, KS 66603
(913) 233-8638
http://www.nursingworld.org/snas/KS

Kentucky Nurses Association
1400 S. 1st Street
P.O. Box 2616
Louisville, KY 40201
(502) 637-2546
http://www.Kentucky-nurses.org

Louisiana State Nurses Association
5700 Florida Boulevard, Suite 720
Baton Rouge, LA 70806-4820
(225) 201-0993
http://www.nursingworld.org/LA

Maine State Nurses Association
P.O. Box 2240
295 Water Street
Augusta, ME 04338-2240
(207) 622-1057

Maryland Nurses Association
849 International Drive, Suite 255
Linthicum Heights, MD 20910
(410) 859-3000

Massachusetts Nurses Association
340 Turnpike Street
Canton, MA 02021
(617) 821-4625

Michigan Nurses Association
2310 Jolly Oak Road
Okemos, MI 48864
(517) 349-5640

Minnesota Nurses Association
1295 Bandana Boulevard, North, Suite 140
St. Paul, MN 55108-5115
(612) 646-0927
http://www.mnnurses.org

Mississippi Nurses Association
31 Woodgreen Place
Madison, MS 39110
(601) 898-0670
http://www.geocities.com/Hotsprings/spa/8365

**Certification program available*

Missouri Nurses Association
1904 Bubba Lane
P.O. Box 105
Jefferson City, MO 65510
(573) 636-4623

Montana Nurses Association
104 Broadway, Suite G-2
P.O. Box 5718
Helena, MT 59604
(406) 442-6710

National Association of Orthopaedic Nurses, Inc.
East Holly Avenue, Box 56
Pitman, NJ 08071-0056
(609) 256-2310
http://www./naon.inurse.com

National Association of Pediatric Nurse Associates and Practitioners*
1101 Kings Highway, North, Number 206
Cherry Hill, NJ 08034
(609) 667-1773
http://www.napnap.org

National Association of School Nurses, Inc.*
P.O. Box 1300
Scarborough, ME 04070-1300
(207) 883-2117
http://www.Vrmedia.com/nurses

Nebraska Nurses Association
715 S. 14th Street
Lincoln, NE 68508
(402) 475-3859

Nevada Nurses Association
P.O. Box 2777
Reno, NV 89505
(702) 323-1661
http://www.nursingworld.org/snas/NV

New Hampshire Nurses Association
48 West Street
Concord, NH 03301
(603) 255-3783

New Jersey State Nurses Association
1479 Pennington Road
Trenton, NJ 08618
(609) 883-5335
http://www.njsna.org

New Mexico Nurses Association
6020 Constitution, N.E. #4
Albuquerque, NM 87110
(505) 268-7744
http://www.nursingworld.org/snas/NM

New York State Nurses Association
11 Cornell Road
Latham, NY 12110
(518) 782-9400
info@nysna.org

North Carolina Nurses Association
103 Enterprise Street
Raleigh, NC 27607
(919) 821-4250
http://www.nursingworld.org/snas/NC/index.htm

North Dakota Nurses Association
549 Airport Road
Bismarck, ND 58504-6107
(701) 223-1385

**Certification program available*

Ohio Nurses Association
4000 E. Main Street
Columbus, OH 43213-2983
(614) 237-5414
http://www.nursingworld.org/snas/OH

Oklahoma Nurses Association
6414 N. Santa Fe, Suite A
Oklahoma City, OK 73116
(405) 840-3476
http://www.nursingworld.org/snas/OK

Oncology Nursing Society*
501 Holiday Drive
Pittsburgh, PA 15220-2749
(412) 921-7373
http://www.ons.org

Oregon Nurses Association
9600 S.W. Oak Street, Suite 550
Portland, OR 97223
(503) 293-0011
http://www.nursingworld.org/snas/OR

Pennsylvania Nurses Association
P.O. Box 68525
Harrisburg, PA 17106-8525
(717) 657-1222
http://www.nursingworld.org/snas/PA

Rhode Island State Nurses Association
550 South Water Street
Providence, RI 02906
(401) 421-9703
risna@internet.mci.com

South Carolina Nurses Association
1821 Gadsden Street
Columbia, SC 29201
(803) 252-4781
http://www.nursingworld.org/snas/SC

South Dakota Nurses Association
1505 S. Minnesota Avenue, Suite 3
Sioux Falls, SD 57105
(605) 338-1401
Southdakota.nurses@internet.mci.com

Tennessee Nurses Association
545 Mainstream Drive, Suite 405
Nashville, TN 37228
(615) 254-0350
http://www.tennurse.org

Texas Nurses Association
7600 Burnet Road, Suite 440
Austin, TX 78757
(512) 452-0645
http://www.texasnurses.org

Utah Nurses Association
455 East 400, South
Salt Lake City, UT 84111
(801) 322-3439
http://www.xmission.com:80/~una

Vermont State Nurses Association
1 Main Street #26
Winooski, VT 05404-2230
(802) 655-7123

Virginia Nurses Association
7113 Three Chopt Road, Suite 204
Richmond, VA 23226
(804) 282-1808

Virgin Islands Nurses Association
P.O. Box 4247
St. Thomas, VI 00803
(340) 776-7397

**Certification program available*

Washington State Nurses Association
2505 2nd Avenue, Suite 500
Seattle, WA 98121
(206) 443-9762

West Virginia Nurses Association
P.O. Box 1946
Charleston, WV 25327
(304) 342-1169

Wisconsin Nurses Association
6117 Monona Drive
Madison, WI 53716
(608) 221-0383

Wyoming Nurses Association
Majestic Bldg.
1603 Capitol Avenue
Cheyenne, WY 82001
(307) 635-3955

APPENDIX F

Commonly Accepted Abbreviations

ABBREVIATION	MEANING
AAA	abdominal aortic aneurysm
ABC	airway, breathing, circulation
ABG	arterial blood gas
a.c.	before meals
AC	assist control
ACE	angiotensin-converting enzyme
ACh	acetylcholine
ACLS	advanced cardiac life support
A.D.	auris dextra (right ear)
ADA	American Diabetes Association
ADH	antidiuretic hormone
ADLs	activities of daily living
AFIB	atrial fibrillation
AFL	atrial flutter
AFP	alpha-fetoprotein
A-G	albumin-globulin (ratio)
AHF	antihemophilic factor (factor VIII)
AICD	automatic implantable cardioverter-defibrillator
AIDS	acquired immunodeficiency syndrome
ALL	acute lymphocytic leukemia
ALS	amyotrophic lateral sclerosis
ALT	alanine aminotransferase
a.m.	morning
AMA	against medical advice American Medical Association
AMI	acute myocardial infarction
AML	acute myelocytic leukemia
amt.	amount
ANA	American Nurses Association antinuclear antibody
AP	apical pulse
APTT	activated partial thromboplastin time
ara-A	adenine arabinoside (vidarabine)
ara-C	cytosine arabinoside (cytarabine)
ARDS	acute respiratory distress syndrome
ARF	acute renal failure acute respiratory failure
AS	aortic sounds
As	astigmatism
A.S.	auris sinistra (left ear)
ASA	acetylsalicylic acid (aspirin)
ASD	atrial septal defect
ASO	antistreptolysin-O
AST	aspartate aminotransferase
ATP	adenosine triphosphate

APPENDICES

ABBREVIATION	MEANING
A.U.	each ear
AV	arteriovenous atrioventricular
AVM	arteriovenous malformation
BBB	bundle-branch block
B.B.B.	blood-brain barrier
BBT	basal body temperature
BCG	bacille Calmette-Guérin
BE	barium enema
b.i.d.	twice daily
BLS	basic life support
BM	bowel movement
BMR	basal metabolic rate
BP	blood pressure
BPH	benign prostatic hyperplasia (or hypertrophy)
BPM	beats per minute
BRB	bright red blood
BRP	bathroom privileges
BSA	body surface area
BUN	blood urea nitrogen
C	Celsius centigrade
CA	chronological age
CABG	coronary artery bypass grafting
CAD	coronary artery disease
cAMP	cyclic adenosine monophosphate
CAPD	continuous ambulatory peritoneal dialysis
caps	capsules
CBC	complete blood count
CBF	cerebral blood flow
cc	cubic centimeter
C.C.	chief complaint

ABBREVIATION	MEANING
CCNU	lomustine
CCU	cardiac care unit
CDC	Centers for Disease Control and Prevention
CEA	carcinoembryonic antigen
CF	cystic fibrosis
CFS	chronic fatigue syndrome
CGL	chronic granulocytic leukemia
C.H.	crown-heel
CHB	complete heart block
CHD	childhood disease congenital heart disease congenital hip disease
CHF	congestive heart failure
CK	creatine kinase
CK-BB	creatine kinase, brain
CK-MB	creatine kinase, heart
CK-MM	creatine kinase, skeletal muscle
cm	centimeter
CML	chronic myelogenous leukemia
CMV	cytomegalovirus
CNS	central nervous system
CO	cardiac output
c/o	complains of
comp	compound
COPD	chronic obstructive pulmonary disease
CP	capillary pressure cerebral palsy cor pulmonale creatine phosphate
CPK	creatine phosphokinase
CPAP	continuous positive airway pressure
cpm	counts per minute cycles per minute

ABBREVIATION	MEANING
CPR	cardiopulmonary resuscitation
C.R.	crown-rump
CRIS	controlled-release infusion system
C & S	culture and sensitivity
CSF	cerebrospinal fluid
CT	chest tube clotting time computed tomography
CV	cardiovascular
	central venous
CVA	cerebrovascular accident
CVP	central venous pressure
CXR	chest X-ray
d	day
/d	per day
D	dextrose
dB	decibel
D/C	discharge discontinue
D & C	dilatation and curettage
DD	differential diagnosis discharge diagnosis dry dressing
D & E	dilatation and evacuation
DES	diethylstilbestrol
D & I	dry and intact
DIC	disseminated intravascular coagulation
dil	dilute
disp	dispense
DJD	degenerative joint disease
DKA	diabetic ketoacidosis
dl	deciliter
DM	diabetes mellitus

ABBREVIATION	MEANING
DNA	deoxyribonucleic acid
DNR	do not resuscitate
D_5½NSS	dextrose 5% in 0.45% normal saline solution
DOA	date of admission dead on arrival
DS	double-strength
DSA	digital subtraction angiography
DSM-IV	*Diagnostic and Statistical Manual of Mental Disorders,* 4th ed.
DTP	diphtheria and tetanus toxoids and pertussis vaccine
DTR	deep tendon reflexes
DVT	deep vein thrombosis
D_5W	dextrose 5% in water
EBV	Epstein-Barr virus
EC	enteric-coated
ECF	extracellular fluid
ECG	electrocardiogram
ECHO	echocardiography
ECMO	extracorporeal membrane oxygenator
ECT	electroconvulsive therapy
ED	emergency department
EDTA	ethylenediamine tetra-acetic acid
EEG	electroencephalogram
EENT	eyes, ears, nose, throat
EF	ejection fraction
ELISA	enzyme-linked immunosorbent assay
elix.	elixir
EMG	electromyography
EMIT	enzyme-multiplied immunoassay technique
ENG	electronystagmography

ABBREVIATION	MEANING
EOM	extraocular movement
ER	emergency room expiratory reserve
ERCP	endoscopic retrograde cholangiopancreatography
ERV	expiratory reserve volume
ESR	erythrocyte sedimentation rate
ESWL	extracorporeal shock-wave lithotripsy
et	and
ETT	endotracheal tube
ext.	extract
F	Fahrenheit
FDA	Food and Drug Administration
FEF	forced expiratory flow
FEV	forced expiratory volume
FFP	fresh frozen plasma
FHR	fetal heart rate
fl., fld.	fluid
Fr.	French
FRC	functional residual capacity
FSH	follicle-stimulating hormone
FSP	fibrinogen-split products
FT_3	free triiodothyronine
FT_4	free thyroxine
FTA	fluorescent treponemal antibody (test)
FTA-ABS	fluorescent treponemal antibody absorption (test)
FUO	fever of undetermined origin
FVC	forced vital capacity
G	gauge
g, gm, GM	gram
GFR	glomerular filtration rate

ABBREVIATION	MEANING
GI	gastrointestinal
G6PD	glucose-6-phosphate dehydrogenase
gr	grain (about 60 mg)
gt.	gutta (drop)
GU	genitourinary
GVHD	graft-versus-host disease
GYN	gynecologic
h., hr.	hour
H	hypodermic injection
HBD	alpha-hydroxybutyrate dehydrogenase
HBIG	hepatitis B immunoglobulin
HbsAg	hepatitis B surface antigen
hCG	human chorionic gonadotropin
Hct	hematocrit
HDL	high-density lipoprotein
HDN	hemolytic disease of the newborn
heme+	Hematest positive
heme–	Hematest negative
HF	heart failure
Hgb	hemoglobin
hGH	human growth hormone
HIV	human immunodeficiency virus
HLA	human leukocyte antigen
HMO	health maintenance organization
HNKS	hyperosmolar nonketotic syndrome
HOB	head of bed
hPL	human placental lactogen
h.s.	at bedtime
HS	half-strength hour of sleep house surgeon

ABBREVIATION	MEANING
HSV	herpes simplex virus
HVA	homovanillic acid
Hz	hertz
HZV	herpes zoster virus
IA	internal auditory intra-arterial intra-articular
IABP	intra-aortic balloon pump
IC	inspiratory capacity
ICF	intracellular fluid
ICHD	Inter-Society Commission for Heart Disease
ICP	intracranial pressure
ICU	intensive care unit
ID	identification initial dose
I & D	incision and drainage
IDDM	insulin-dependent diabetes mellitus
IgM	immunoglobulin
IM	infectious mononucleosis
I.M.	intramuscular
IMV	intermittent mandatory ventilation
in.	inch
IND	investigational new drug
I/O	intake and output
IPPB	intermittent positive-pressure breathing
IRV	inspiratory reserve volume
IU	International Unit
IUD	intrauterine device
I.V.	intravenous
IVGTT	intravenous glucose tolerance test
IVH	intravenous hyperalimentation (now called total parenteral nutrition [TPN])
IVP	intravenous pyelography
IVPB	intravenous piggyback
J	joule
JCAHO	Joint Commission on Accreditation of Healthcare Organizations
JP	Jackson-Pratt (drain)
JVD	jugular venous distention
JVP	jugular venous pressure
kg	kilogram
17-KGS	17-ketogenic steroids
17-KS	17-ketosteroids
KUB	kidney-ureter-bladder
KVO	keep vein open
L	liter, lumbar
LA	left atrium long-acting
LAP	left atrial pressure leucine aminopeptidase
lb	pound
LBBB	left bundle-branch block
LD	lactate dehydrogenase
LDL	low-density lipoprotein
LE	lupus erythematosus
LES	lower esophageal sphincter
LGL	Lown-Ganong-Levine variant syndrome
LH	luteinizing hormone
LLL	left lower leg left lower lobe
LLQ	left lower quadrant
L/min	liters per minute
LOC	level of consciousness

ABBREVIATION	MEANING
LR	lactated Ringer's solution
LSB	left scapular border left sternal border
LSC	left subclavian
LTC	long-term care
LUQ	left upper quadrant
LV	left ventricle
LVEDP	left ventricular end-diastolic pressure
LVET	left ventricular ejection time
LVF	left ventricular failure
m	meter
M	molar (solution)
m^2	square meter
MAO	monoamine oxidase inhibitor
MAR	medication administration record
MAST	medical antishock trousers (pneumatic antishock garment)
mcg	microgram
MCH	mean corpuscular hemoglobin
MCHC	mean corpuscular hemoglobin concentration
MCV	mean corpuscular volume
MD	medical doctor muscular dystrophy
mEq	milliequivalent
mg	milligram
mgtt	microdrip or minidrop
MI	mitral insufficiency myocardial infarction
ml	milliliter
μl	microliter
MLC	mixed lymphocyte culture
mm	millimeter

ABBREVIATION	MEANING
mm^3	cubic millimeter
MMEF	maximal midexpiratory flow
Mmol	millimole
MRI	magnetic resonance imaging
M.R.x1	may repeat once
MS	mitral stenosis morphine sulfate multiple sclerosis
MUGA	multiple-gated acquisition (scanning)
MVI	multivitamin infusion
MVP	mitral valve prolapse
MVV	maximal voluntary ventilation
NC	nasal cannula
ng	nanogram
NG	nasogastric
NICU	neonatal intensive care unit
NIDDM	non-insulin-dependent (type 2) diabetes mellitus
NKA	no known allergies
NMR	nuclear magnetic resonance
Noct.	night
NPN	nonprotein nitrogen
N.P.O.	nothing by mouth
NR	nonreactive
N/R	not remarkable
NS, NSS	normal saline solution (0.9% sodium chloride solution)
¼NS	¼ normal saline solution (0.225% sodium chloride solution)
½NS	½ normal saline solution (0.45% sodium chloride solution)
NSAID	nonsteroidal anti-inflammatory drug
NSR	normal sinus rhythm

ABBREVIATION	MEANING
N/V	nausea and vomiting
OB	obstetric
OD	Oculus Dexter (right eye) overdose
OGTT	oral glucose tolerance test
OOB	out of bed
OR	operating room
OS	oculus sinister (left eye)
OTC	over-the-counter
OU	oculus uterque (each eye)
oz	ounce
P	pulse
PA	posteroanterior pulmonary artery
PABA	para-aminobenzoic acid
PAC	premature atrial contraction
$Paco_2$	partial pressure of arterial carbon dioxide
PACU	postanesthesia care unit
Pao_2	partial pressure of arterial oxygen
Pap	Papanicolaou smear
PAP	pulmonary artery pressure
PAT	paroxysmal atrial tachycardia
PAWP	pulmonary artery wedge pressure
p.c.	after meals
PCA	patient-controlled analgesia
PC X-ray	portable chest X-ray
PDA	patent ductus arteriosus
PE	physical examination pulmonary embolism
PEARL	pupils equal and reactive to light
PEEP	positive end-expiratory pressure
PEFR	peak expiratory flow rate

ABBREVIATION	MEANING
PEP	preejection period
per	by or through
PET	positron-emission tomography
pg	picogram
PICC	peripherally inserted central catheter
PID	pelvic inflammatory disease
PKU	phenylketonuria
p.m.	afternoon
PMI	point of maximum impulse
PML	progressive multifocal leukoencephalopathy
PMS	premenstrual syndrome
PND	paroxysmal nocturnal dyspnea postnasal drip
P.O.	by mouth
PP	partial pressure peripheral pulses
PR	by rectum
PRBC	packed red blood cells
p.r.n.	as needed
PROM	passive range of motion premature rupture of the membranes
pt., Pt.	patient pint
PT	prothrombin time
PTCA	percutaneous transluminal coronary angioplasty
PTH	parathyroid hormone
PTT	partial thromboplastin time
PUD	peptic ulcer disease
PVC	polyvinyl chloride premature ventricular contraction
q	every
q a.m.	every morning

ABBREVIATION	MEANING
q.d.	every day
q.h.	every hour
q.i.d.	four times daily
q.n.	every night
q.o.d.	every other day
QS	quantity sufficient
qt.	quart
R	by rectum respiration
RA	rheumatoid arthritis right atrium
RAF	rheumatoid arthritis factor
RAP	right atrial pressure
RAST	radioallergosorbent test
RBBB	right bundle-branch block
RBC	red blood cell
RDA	recommended daily allowance
RE	rectal examination
REM	rapid eye movement
RES	reticuloendothelial system
Rh	rhesus blood factor
RHD	rheumatic heart disease
RIA	radioimmunoassay
RL	right lateral Ringer's lactate (lactated Ringer's solution)
RLQ	right lower quadrant
RNA	ribonucleic acid
R/O	rule out
ROM	range of motion rupture of membranes
RR	respiratory rate
RRR	regular rate and rhythm
RSC	right subclavian
RSV	respiratory syncytial virus right subclavian vein Rous sarcoma virus
R/T	related to
RUQ	right upper quadrant
RV	residual volume right ventricle
RVEDP	right ventricular end-diastolic pressure
RVEDV	right ventricular end-diastolic volume
RVP	right ventricular pressure
Rx	prescription
SA	sinoatrial
Sao_2	arterial oxygen saturation
sat.	saturated
SC	subclavian
S.C., SQ	subcutaneous
SCID	severe combined immunodeficiency syndrome
sec	second
SGOT	serum glutamic oxaloacetic transaminase (now called aspartate aminotransferase [AST])
SGPT	serum glutamic pyruvic transaminase (now called alanine aminotransferase [ALT])
SHBG	sex hormone-binding globulin
SI	Système International d'Unités (International System of Units)
SIADH	syndrome of inappropriate antidiuretic hormone
SIDS	sudden infant death syndrome
Sig	write on label
SIMV	synchronized intermittent mandatory ventilation
SLE	systemic lupus erythematosus

ABBREVIATION	MEANING
SOB	shortness of breath
sol., soln.	solution
SR	sustained release
SRS-A	slow-reacting substance of anaphylaxis
stat	immediately
STD	sexually transmitted disease
supp	suppository
susp	suspension
SV	stroke volume
$S\bar{v}O_2$	mixed venous oxygen saturation
syr.	syrup
T	temperature
T, Tbs, tbsp	tablespoon
t, tsp	teaspoon
tab	tablet
TBG	thyroxine-binding globulin
TCA	tricyclic antidepressant
TENS	transcutaneous electrical nerve stimulation
TIA	transient ischemic attack
t.i.d.	three times daily
TIL	tumor-infiltrating lymphocyte
tinct., tr.	tincture
TLC	total lung capacity triple lumen catheter
TM	temporomandibular tympanic membrane
TMJ	temporomandibular joint
TNF	tumor necrosis factor
TO	telephone order
tol.	tolerate tolerates tolerated
tPA	tissue plasminogen activator

ABBREVIATION	MEANING
TPN	total parenteral nutrition
TRH	thyrotropin-releasing hormone
TSH	thyroid-stimulating hormone
UA	urinalysis
UCE	urea cycle enzymopathy
USP	United States Pharmacopeia
UTI	urinary tract infection
UV	ultraviolet
V, vag.	vaginal
VAD	vascular access device ventricular assist device
VAP	vascular access port
VDRL	Venereal Disease Research Laboratory (test)
VLDL	very low density lipoprotein
VMA	vanillylmandelic acid
VO	verbal order
$\dot{V}/\dot{Q}$	ventilation-perfusion ratio
VS	vital signs
VSD	ventricular septal defect
VSS	vital signs stable
V_T, Vt	tidal volume
WBC	white blood cell
WNL	within normal limits
w/o	without
WPW	Wolff-Parkinson-White syndrome
Z/G, ZIG	zoster immune globulin

APPENDIX G

Commonly Accepted Symbols

SYMBOL	MEANING
Pulses	
0	absent; not palpable
+1	weak or thready; hard to feel; easily obliterated by slight finger pressure
+2	normal; easily palpable; obliterated only by strong finger pressure
+3	bounding; readily palpable; forceful; not easily obliterated
Reflexes	
++++	very brisk; hyperactive
+++	increased, but not necessarily abnormal
++	average; normal
+	present, but diminished
0	absent
Heart murmurs	
1/6 or I/VI	faint; barely audible even to the trained ear; may not be heard in all positions
2/6 or II/VI	soft and low; easily audible to the trained ear
3/6 or III/VI	moderately loud; approximately equal to the intensity of normal heart sounds
4/6 or IV/VI	very loud, with a palpable thrill at the murmur site
5/6 or IV/VI	very loud, with a palpable thrill; audible with stethoscope in partial contact with chest
6/6 or VI/VI	extremely loud, with a palpable thrill; audible with stethoscope over but not in contact with chest
Apothecary symbols	
♏	minim (about 0.06 ml)
℞	Prescription
ʒ	dram
℥	ounce
Other symbols	
ā	before
āā	each
@	at
c̄	with
Ca	calcium
Cl	chloride
CO	cardiac output, carbon monoxide
CO_2	carbon dioxide
Hg	mercury

SYMBOL	MEANING
K	potassium
Ⓛ	left
(LA)	left arm
(LL)	left leg
Na	sodium
NaCl	sodium chloride
O_2	oxygen
Ⓡ	right
(RA)	right arm
(RL)	right leg
♀	female
♂	male
″	inches
#	number, pound
+	excess, plus, positive
–	deficiency, minus, negative
>	greater than
≥	greater than or equal to
<	less than
≤	less than or equal to
∧	diastolic blood pressure (commonly used on graphic forms)
∨	systolic blood pressure
≅	approximately equal to
≈	approximately
↑	increase
↓	decrease
?	questionable
ø, ȯ	none, no
1°	primary, first degree
2°	secondary, second degree
3°	tertiary, third degree

SYMBOL	MEANING
1:1	one-to-one
p̄	after
s̄	without
ss, s̄s̄, ṡṡ	one-half
×	times
ī̇	one
ī̇ī̇	two, etc.

Glossary

Accreditation Official recognition from a professional or government organization that a health care facility meets relevant standards

Advance directive Document used as a guideline for life-sustaining medical care of a patient with an advanced disease or disability, who is no longer able to indicate his own wishes; includes living wills and durable powers of attorney for health care

Barthel index and scale Functional assessment tool used to evaluate an older patient's overall well-being and self-care abilities; evaluates the ability to perform 10 self-care activities

Case management Model for management of health care facilities in which one professional — usually a nurse or a social worker — assumes responsibility for coordinating care so that patients move through the health care system in the shortest time and at the lowest cost possible

Charting by exception (CBE) Charting system that departs from traditional systems by requiring documentation of only significant or abnormal findings

Core charting Charting system that focuses on the nursing process; components include a database, plan of care, flow sheets, progress notes, and discharge summary

Clinical pathway Documentation tool used in managed care and case management in which a time line is defined for the patient's condition and for the achievement of expected outcomes; used by caregivers to determine on any given day where the patient should be in his progress toward optimal health; also known as a critical pathway

Damages The amount of money a court orders a defendant to pay the plaintiff, when the case is decided in favor of the plaintiff

Database Subjective and objective patient information collected during the nurse's initial assessment of the patient; includes information obtained by taking the patient's health history, performing a physical examination, and analyzing laboratory test results

Diagnosis-related group (DRG) System of classifying or grouping patients according to medical diagnosis for purposes of reimbursement of hospitalization costs under Medicare (For example, according to the DRG system, all patients admitted to the hospital for a coronary bypass receive the same reimbursement from Medicare regardless of actual cost to the hospital. If the patient's hospital bill totals less than the amount paid by Medicare, the hospital is allowed to keep the difference.)

Durable power of attorney for health care Legal document whereby a patient authorizes another person to make medical decisions for him should he become incompetent to do so

Focus charting Charting system that uses assessment data, first to evaluate patient-centered topics (or foci of concern) and then to document precisely and concisely

Health history Summary of a patient's health status that includes physiologic, psychological, cultural, and psychosocial data

Health maintenance organization (HMO) Organization that provides an agreed-upon health service to voluntary enrollees who prepay a fixed, periodic fee that is set without regard to the amount or kind of services received (People who belong to an HMO are cared for by member doctors with limited referrals to outside specialists.)

Incident report Formal report, written by doctors, nurses, or other staff members, that informs hospital administrators (and the hospital's insurance company) about an incident and that serves as a contemporary factual statement in the event of a lawsuit; also called an occurrence report

Incremental record Record kept according to time and occurrences

Independent practice association (IPA) model HMO Health maintenance organization that contracts with an association of doctors to provide doctor services to its members while the doctors maintain their independent practices

Informed consent Permission obtained from a patient to perform a specific test or procedure after the patient has been fully informed about the test or procedure

Interventions Nursing actions taken to meet a patient's health care needs; should reflect nurse's agreement with the patient on how to meet defined goals or expected outcomes

Joint Commission on Accreditation of Healthcare Organizations (JCAHO) Private, nongovernmental agency that establishes guidelines for the operation of hospitals and other health care facilities, conducts accreditation programs and surveys, and encourages the attainment of high standards of institutional medical care; members include representatives from the American Medical Association, American College of Physicians, and American College of Surgeons

Katz index Assessment tool used to evaluate a patient's ability to perform the basic functions of bathing, dressing, toileting, transfer, continence, and feeding

Learning outcomes Outcomes developed as part of a patient-teaching plan that identify what a patient needs to learn, how the nurse will teach him, and how she'll evaluate what he has learned

Living will Witnessed document indicating a patient's desire to be allowed to die a natural death, rather than be kept alive by life-sustaining measures; applies to decisions that will be made after a terminally ill patient is incompetent and has no reasonable possibility of recovery

Minimum data set (MDS) Standardized assessment tool that must be filled out for every patient admitted to a long-term care facility as mandated by the federal government

National Committee for Quality Assurance (NCQA) National accrediting body for managed care plans that annually evaluates the quality of managed care plans based on data collected from those plans that choose to submit information (The NCQA then sells its evaluations to employers, health consultants, and the media.)

Negligence Failure to exercise the care that a prudent person would exercise

North American Nursing Diagnosis Association (NANDA) Organization responsible for developing and categorizing nursing diagnoses and examining applications of nursing diagnoses in clinical practice, education, and research

Nursing diagnosis Clinical judgment made by a nurse about a patient's responses to actual or potential health problems or life processes; describes a patient problem that the nurse can legally solve; may apply to families and communities as well as individual patients

Nursing process Systematic approach to identifying a patient's problems and then taking nursing actions to address them; steps include assessing the patient's problems, forming a diagnostic statement, identifying expected outcomes, creating a plan to achieve expected outcomes and solve the patient's problems, implementing the plan or assigning others to implement it, and evaluating the plan's effectiveness

Occurrence screening Identification of adverse events through a review of medical records

Outcome criteria Standards by which measurable goals (outcomes) are objectively evaluated

Outcome documentation Charting that focuses on patient behaviors and responses to nursing care; documents the patient's condition in relation to predetermined outcomes included in the plan of care

Peer review organization (PRO) Basic component of a quality improvement program in which the results of health care given to a specific patient population are evaluated according to outcome criteria established by peers of the professionals delivering the care; promoted by professional organizations as a means of maintaining standards of care

Practice guidelines Sequential instructions for treating patients with specific health problems

Preadmission screening annual resident review (PASARR) Form used to assess the mental status of a patient before admission to a long-term care facility; required for Medicare or Medicaid reimbursement

Problem-intervention-evaluation (PIE) charting Charting system that organizes patient information according to the patient's problems; integrates the patient's plan of care into the progress notes in order to simplify the documentation process

Problem-oriented medical record (POMR) Method of organizing the medical record that consists of baseline data, a problem list, and a plan of care for each problem

Quality improvement Commitment on the part of a health care facility or several health disciplines to work together to achieve an optimal degree of excellence in the services rendered to every patient (State regulatory and accrediting agencies may require health care facilities to regularly monitor, evaluate, and seek ways to improve the quality of care.)

Resident assessment protocol (RAP) Form required by federal mandate for use in long-term care facilities that identifies the patient's primary problems and care needs and documents the existence of a plan of care

Risk management Identification, analysis, evaluation, and elimination or reduction of risks to patients, visitors, or employees; involves loss prevention and control and the handling of all incidents, claims, and other insurance- and litigation-related tasks

Slander To defame or speak falsely about a person; to damage a person's reputation

SOAP charting Structured method of recording progress notes in which data is organized into the following categories: Subjective, Objective, Assessment, and Planning

SOAPIE charting Structured method of recording progress notes in which data is organized into the following categories: Subjective, Objective, Assessment, Planning, Implementation, and Evaluation

SOAPIER charting Structured method of recording progress notes in which data is organized into the following categories: Subjective, Objective, Assessment, Planning, Implementation, Evaluation, and Revision

Tort A wrongful act other than a breach of contract; relief may be obtained in the form of damages or an injunction

Utilization review Program initiated by reimbursing agents to maintain control over health care providers; may focus on length of stay, treatment regimen, validation of tests and procedures, and verification of the use of medical supplies and equipment

Index

i refers to an illustration; t refers to a table.

B

INDEX

i refers to an illustration; t refers to a table.

INDEX

C

D

i refers to an illustration; t refers to a table.

i refers to an illustration; t refers to a table.

i refers to an illustration; t refers to a table.

G

H

i refers to an illustration; t refers to a table.

I

i refers to an illustration; t refers to a table.

J

K

i refers to an illustration; t refers to a table.

L

M

i refers to an illustration; t refers to a table.

N

i refers to an illustration; t refers to a table.

O

i refers to an illustration; t refers to a table.

i refers to an illustration; t refers to a table.

Q

R

i refers to an illustration; t refers to a table.

i refers to an illustration; t refers to a table.

U

V

WXYZ

i refers to an illustration; t refers to a table.